The Fork in the Road

The Divergence and Potential Rejoining of Traditional and Allopathic Medicine

Robert Elphin Smith, Ph.D.
with Maryse Bader Smith

Copyright © 2020 by Robert Elphin Smith

All rights reserved. This book or any portion thereof may not be reproduced or used in any manner whatsoever without the express written permission of the publisher except for the use of brief quotations in a book review.

Printed in the United States of America

First Printing, 2020

ISBN 9781708454203

Contents

Introduction _____ 4
Chapter 1: On the Nature of Healing _____ 8
Chapter 2: The Origins of Traditional Indigenous Medicine _____ 30
Chapter 3: Shamanism _____ 61
Chapter 4: Mystery Schools—Ancient and Modern _____ 92
Chapter 5: The Material and the Invisible,
or Is What We See All There Is? _____ 111
Chapter 6: The Development of Medicine in the West _____ 136
Chapter 7: The Spread of Greek Medicine _____ 161
Chapter 8: Paracelsus, the Middle Ages, and the Renaissance ___ 174
Chapter 9: Descartes, the Cartesian Dichotomy, Newton,
and Mathematical Models _____ 199
Chapter 10: Methodism: Hahnemann & Homeopathic Medicine ___ 218
Chapter 11: European Medicine in the 19th and 20th Centuries ___ 235
20th century _____ 248
Chapter 12: American Medicine in the 19th and 20th Centuries ___ 250
Chapter 13: The Impact of Western Science on Medicine:
Methods and Assumptions of Western Science _____ 268
Chapter 14: The Impact of Western Science on Medicine: Methods
and Assumptions of Western Medical Science, Continued ____ 288
Chapter 15: Modern Physics and Medicine The Modern Conflict in
Western Science—The Paradigm Is Shifting _____ 301
Conclusion: What We Have Learned About the Nature of Healing ___ 329
APPENDIX A: Prehistory Timeline _____ 341
APPENDIX B: Assumptions of Western (Materialistic) Science ___ 344
About the Author _____ 345

Introduction

Traditional medicine, practiced by indigenous cultures and in many parts of the world such as China and India, is new to many, but its ability to provide a superior first line of defense against most illness indicates the need for its better understanding by practitioners, patients and potential patients. Careful examination shows that such traditional forms of medicine have far closer ties to Western medicine than most realize. It began 5,000 years ago with the insights of sages, expanded upon during thousands of years of observation and study. Those insights and observations led to concepts and therapeutic procedures that paralleled developments in Greek medicine, the foundation of Western medicine.

Both traditional forms of medicine and Greek medicine developed similar concepts of the fundamental influences on an individual's health—for example, the four humors in Greek medicine and the five elements in Oriental medicine—and these early forms all recognized that harmony and balance between these elements were the key to a healthy life.

Hippocrates, the father of Western medicine and the ultimate Greek physician, has been described as the founder of holistic medicine, for his medicine was a medicine of mind, body and spirit. In China, physicians similarly understood the relationship among emotions, spiritual energy, and the health of the body. Both systems recognized the impact of diet and the environment on health.

Several traditional forms of medicine and Greek medicine all developed similar diagnostic procedures. For example, newcomers to Oriental medicine are amazed at the diagnostic information its practitioners obtain by palpating a patient's pulses. Few are aware that Greek physicians were using and describing the same pulses and their use two thousand years ago.

Western medicine turned away from Hippocrates in the second century AD, primarily due to the influence of the Roman physician, Galen, who sought to identify diseases and their treatment rather than focusing on the patient in his or her entirety. That separation widened when 17th Century mathematician-philosopher René Descartes declared body to be separate from mind and spirit. From that time on, Western medical science has studied the body as a machine. Medical research has greatly expanded our knowledge of biological mechanisms, and a wealth of medical technology has been developed. The result is a Western scientific medicine that is laboratory-based and disease-oriented. It excels in technology, diagnosis and the management of often life-threatening symptoms of acute illness, but it is limited to alleviating the patient's symptoms in many chronic conditions. How and when this "Fork in the Road" took place is, in part, what this book takes up.

In contrast, traditional forms of medicine continued to focus on observation and the perfection of methods to restore the patient's balance and harmony in all aspects of his or her physical, emotional and spiritual well-being. This approach is patient-oriented rather than disease-oriented. It detects and treats the imbalances that lead to an illness rather than focusing on the management of a patient's physical symptoms. It is particularly effective in treating chronic illness, often caused by a combination of the environmental, emotional, and dietary influences that these traditional medical forms have long studied. The goal is to help restore balance within the patient's body and life with a variety of treatments; again, using Oriental medicine as an example, through a combination of such therapies as acupuncture, herbs, diet, energy-balancing exercises such as Qi Gong, and bodywork.

With its ability to provide health care at a cost well below that of high-tech Western medicine, these traditional forms of medicine are both long-proven systems of holistic medicine and a major community asset.

Technically-advanced Western medicine and holistic forms of medicine are complementary medical systems, sharing similar heritages but each focusing on different aspects of medical care. There are emergency situations where there is no substitute for Western medical procedures. But for most medical problems, however, traditional forms provide an effective first line of defense against illness. By detecting internal imbalances, then restoring a patient's balance while symptoms are still minor, they can address causes and prevent the development of serious illness. The treatment of choice for many chronic illnesses, they are often a low-cost way of treating acute illness as well.

This book is divided into three parts. The first discusses the record of the art of healing in prehistory up to the time of Hippocrates and Plato. It addresses what has been learned in recent years of prehistory, then goes on to discuss shamanism, the origin of spiritual insights and of religious beliefs, and the origin of the art of healing and the principle of service to one's community. Shamanism, together with the insights of mystics, led to mystery schools, both ancient and modern, with healing being a major function of those mystery schools. It then addresses the question, "What is the source of the knowledge obtained by the shamans, the mystics, the prophets and by the dowsers of antiquity as well as the present?" Part One closes with the story of Aesculapius, the Greek god of healing and the predecessor of Hippocrates, and with healing by incubation in the temples of Aesculapius.

The second part focuses on the development of Western medicine after the time of Hippocrates to the present, including the influence of Cartesian and Newtonian science on the development of Western scientific medicine. Hippocrates was fully aware of the causal influence of mental, emotional and spiritual factors on illness, and he viewed the symptoms of an illness as expressions of the body's self-healing process—pain to alert the patient to a problem, fever and an increase in the number of white blood cells to assist the immune system in its healing task, edema at the site of a wound to facilitate the immune system's operation, and so on. Plato's student Aristotle modified his mentor's teaching, focusing not on the cause of illness but on the concept of disease as an entity. This part reviews Galen's influence, the concept of the separation of body from mind and spirit that was initially embraced in the 17th century writings of French philosopher René Descartes, the foundation of the American Medical Association (AMA), and the Flexner report.

The third part addresses the rejoining of the ancient art of healing with the science, including the medical science, of the twentieth century—a rejoining of the paths separated when the road forked following Hippocrates. Here, we begin at the turn of the twentieth century with Max Planck's discovery of quantum physics. Planck's discovery, augmented by those of Einstein, Bohr, Heisenberg, Schrödinger and later many others, proved to be the key to rejoining ancient traditions with modern science, rejoining the paths separated by the two-thousand-year-old fork in the road. Physicists have shown that there really is interconnectedness and instantaneous communication between all material particles.

New discoveries lead to new understanding, and this description of the fork—and rejoining—in the road is not intended to denigrate either modern science or Western scientific (allopathic) medicine. Symptom control can be lifesaving, for symptoms can kill, but allopathic medicine and symptom control do not address the cause of illness, focusing instead on antidotes for symptoms. As a result, our current health care system is both inordinately expensive and has led to dismal health statistics. Change is needed, a paradigm shift, and learning from Hippocrates and Plato as well as indigenous medical traditions, to look beyond the material, to recognize that the invisible, the mental, emotional and spiritual factors are too often the cause of illness as well as the key to its reversal and a healthier society as a whole.

Chapter 1
On the Nature of Healing

1.1 Healing vs. Curing

The first and very relevant question to be considered is "What is Healing?" Plato answered this question as follows: "The part can never be well unless the whole is well."[1] To heal is to make whole—mind, body and soul.

In order to define healing completely, we must first consider illness: We must recognize we have to examine not just physical symptoms, but the events in the patient's life that led to those symptoms. For example, if a divorce produced an emotional response that in turn led to a depressed immune system, and the depressed immune system resulted in breast cancer, we must recognize that the *key event* was the emotional response to the divorce. And the sequel: To heal we must counter that emotional response. Forgiveness often is involved in this process. Colin Tipping's *Radical Forgiveness*[2] provides a different perspective on forgiveness—that the perceived injury might lead to an upward step in the patient's spiritual growth and that therefore there is nothing to forgive. This concept is reinforced by Sherri Cortland's reference to "relationship villains" in her book *Windows of Opportunity*.[3] Reference should also be made to Dr. Lissa Rankin's *Mind Over Medicine*[4] and T. Edward Ross's *The Healing Mind*[5], both highly recommended.

In other cases a long-held belief system may be the culprit. In Chapter Three (Shamanism) I present cases where a belief system led to life-threatening illnesses. Once the belief system had been recognized and released, the patient was healed.

Cause often precedes symptoms by months or years (cancers, multiple sclerosis, etc), though the response can sometimes be immediate (for example, fainting in response to a sudden emotional shock). We note that an emotional cause can be involved in acute as well as chronic illness; for example, an immune system depressed by an emotional shock can be susceptible to a bacterium or virus that the body would otherwise shrug off. An example of the importance of a healthy immune system (not subject to emotional stress) is the story of the cholera germs imbibed by Claude Bernard described in Chapter Eleven. More familiar examples of this phenomenon are the student who catches a cold the day before an examination. We also note that the maximum incidence of heart attacks is at 9 am on Monday mornings. (cause?)

The mind and soul act to protect a person. The development of disease symptoms is a benevolent act, a way of calling attention to a serious problem. If the problem is threatening to the mind, then so will symptoms be threatening to the body. As an example, if the subconscious mind is faced with a serious problem, that problem may be expressed as a serious disease. Consider the patient with painful hemorrhoids described by Upledger and cited later in this chapter.

How is cause detected? There are many methods, with *careful history taking* by the health practitioner being foremost. Physician Dr. Lissa Rankin has found countering the stress of life to be more important than diet, exercise and other life-supporting habits. In her book, *Mind Over Medicine*[6], Dr. Rankin describes steps she takes to augment the usual medical intake interview, to include in her medical intake interview questions regarding her patient's feeling fulfilled by life, whether her patient's life makes her happy, by her relationships, by whether she feels that she is meeting her goals in life, and most importantly, *"What do you think might be at the root of your illness?"* and *"What does your body need in order to heal?"*[7]

Dr. Rankin also describes a case of self-healing after a patient took control of her life and met the needs she needed in order to heal. Stress frequently causes illness. Harvard physician and physiologist Walter B. Cannon described how the body responds to the stress of danger in his book, *The Wisdom of the Body*[8] in 1932, and Cannon's observations were expanded by Canadian physician and physiologist Hans Selye in his *The Stress of Life*[9] in 1956. Cannon's colleague, Dr. Edmund Jacobson, focused on the stresses of daily life and suggested methods of relaxing to counter those stresses in his book *You Must Relax*[10], published in 1934. More recently, Harvard physician and physiologist Herbert Benson has written of how to counter these stresses in *The Relaxation Response.*[11] Dr. Rankin has expanded upon Benson's work by combining his procedure with issues she has found important to address in order that self-healing can take place. Relaxation sets the stage for self-healing, and Dr. Rankin has made good use of this fact.

Energy bodies (the "auras" seen by clairvoyants) can be detected by a variety of methods. Hands may be used, as is the case with many shamans. Pulses are studied in a meditative state by Tibetan, Chinese, Japanese, ancient Greeks, *Unani Tibb* healers, and many others. Vision, both normal and subtle, can be used. The Canadian healer Adam (*Dream Healer: A True Story of Miracle Healing*)[12] sees a holographic image of the body; others see diagnostic information in the energy bodies (auras, surrounding the physical body). Shamanic insight can be important, and on occasion a shaman will take the patient on a shamanic journey to identify the cause of an illness. Dreams can be useful. The Hawaiian *kahuna* Papa Henry Auwae found dreams valuable both in diagnosis and even specifying treatment, as did ancient Greek and also Chinese medicine.

This brings us to the question, "How is the cause healed?" If symptoms are life threatening, they must be managed, and allopathic Western Scientific Medicine (WSM) is then often valuable, though WSM is not the only way—many herbal practitioners, including contemporary shamans, are also capable of addressing acute symptoms. Part of the training of a complementary health practitioner is to recognize life-threatening symptoms and to refer patients to Western medicine when appropriate.

If symptoms are not life threatening, the health practitioner must assist the body's wisdom to deal with the problem. This could require balancing energies with acupuncture, acupressure, or energy medicine, by counseling regarding lifestyle and diet, as well as the use of herbal remedies—the aim being to detoxify the body, improve immune function, improve circulation, and to improve energy flow (Qi Gong, yoga, or Tai Chi may be useful here), possibly body work. All are often required in chronic disease.

Addressing emotional issues that are the underlying cause of the illness may be required in order to address the source of the patient's problem. *Counseling regarding an emotional cause* may be very important, and referral to a psychiatrist may be appropriate. For a Chinese medical perspective, Lonnie Jarrett's *Nourishing Destiny*[13] may be useful.

To address physical symptoms, consider the following: If an organ system needs support, provide that support with appropriate diet, with acupuncture, or with herbs. If an energy imbalance exists, correct it with diet, energy work, acupuncture, herbs, or bodywork.

Addressing the question, "What is healed?" requires recognition that the ultimate *cause* is almost always a function of mind or emotions (for example, a belief system or an emotional issue), and the healer needs to ascertain the cause and to heal mind. Then the body can heal.

Evidence from ancient and modern times show the importance of a holistic approach.

The physician-scientist Alexis Carrol commented in *Man the Unknown*, "Envy, hate, and fear, when these sentiments are habitual, are capable of starting organic changes and genuine disease."[14]

Tibetan Medicine, perhaps the most sophisticated medical system on the globe today, recognizes the importance of the spiritual in health and healing. Tibetan physician Dr. Pema Dorjee has written in his book, *Heal Your Spirit, Heal Yourself:*

"Tibetan medicine is a spiritual medical system based on the fundamental laws of the universe. As such it essentially reflects the workings of nature which apply to everything and everyone across the planet. At its very heart is the essential need for balance, harmony and a natural process of exchange, of giving and receiving. This Buddhist system and pure science which stresses the indivisible interdependence of mind, body and vitality has been transmitted to numerous inspired Tibetan physicians by various means."[15]

Tibetan medicine recognizes three mental poisons. The Buddha found these to be the causes of suffering. These are the root causes of most disease in Tibetan medicine:

1. Acquisitiveness, greed → To heal, go to → Generosity
2. Anger, hate → To heal, go to → Forgiveness, Compassion
3. Self-delusion (ignorance) → To heal, go to → Wisdom

Shamans, as we will discuss in Chapter Three, recognized that deep psychological problems often manifested themselves as illness, and the shamans recognized spiritual as well as psychological causes for illness. For example, Peruvian (Inca) healers recognize the role of unhealthy emotions as the cause of illness. To eliminate illness, first understand one's self, then go on to minimize the ego. That self-understanding, particularly when it leads to minimizing the ego, will eliminate the cause of illness. To minimize the ego, the Incas address *Supaycu* (known in the West as the "seven deadly sins")[16]:

1. Anger
2. Pride
3. Envy
4. Gluttony
5. Laziness
6. Greed
7. Lust

As far back as the Egyptian medicine of Thoth (Hermes Trismegistus) and Imhotep, it was recognized that one of the primary causes of disease was unhealthy, abnormal mental attitudes: depression, morbid emotions, hate, resentment, condemnation of one's self, criticism of others, jealousy, and possessiveness (note the similarity to Tibetan and Inca Medicines). The Egyptians felt that such unhealthy thinking resulted in ulcers, tumors, cancers, fevers, tuberculosis, paralysis, and all types of nervous conditions. Furthermore, the ancients considered germs as a creation of man's evil thoughts and actions. They considered germs to be a result, not a cause of disease. The European physician-scientists Béchamps and Enderlein have come to a similar conclusion, to be discussed in Chapter Eleven. It should be noted that symptoms can take time (or not) to disappear after cause is gone.

The many cases of Near Death Experiences (NDEs) provide useful information. Particularly relevant and valuable is the case of Anita Moorjani, described in her book, *Dying To Be Me: My Journey from Cancer, to Near Death, to True Healing*[17]. Anita was dying of cancer, in a coma and given only a few hours to live by her physician. In her NDE Moorjani was shown the cause of her cancer and, with the cause recognized and released, she was able to heal herself. She healed in days, to the astonishment of her physicians. Anita reports, "I was shown how diseases start on an energetic level before they become physical. If I chose to go on into life, the cancer would be gone from my energy, and my physical body would catch up very quickly. I then understood that when people have medical treatments for illnesses, it rids the illness only from their body but not from their energy, so the illness returns. I realized that if I went back, it would be with very healthy energy. Then the physical body would catch up to the energetic conditions very quickly and permanently." And so it did—Anita returned to life, and her cancer was healed within days. (Quotation from Anita Moorjani in Wayne Dyer, *Wishes Fulfilled*).[18]

I am reminded of the teaching of clairvoyant healer Rosalyn Bruyere, who taught the same concept of energy fields reported by Anita. Rosalyn provided overnight healing to a woman who had had an NDE so beautiful that her body had developed a serious food allergy, apparently a part of her body's effort to return her to the other side that had been so beautiful and loving. Once the cause of her food allergy was revealed and released, her body healed itself.

Rosalyn's teaching regarding the energy body's relationship to health has provided healing to many patients. Her observations have been verified by UCLA's Professor Valerie Hunt in experiments in which Professor Hunt measured surface potentials of patients in a shielded chamber with Rosalyn inside the chamber and reporting what she observed in the patient's auras. As Professor Hunt remarked to me, "Anyone can see auras if they have a million-dollar computer!"[19]

Always remember that *all healing is ultimately self-healing*. As a friend and professor of (allopathic) internal medicine described it, "We keep the patient happy while nature cures her."[20] As might be expected, curing is not an adequate response to chronic illness. The task of the healer is to help the patient heal her/himself. A recurrent theme in indigenous medicines is that key elements in healing are often *compassion, forgiveness* and *gratitude*.

In the case that cause is truly external, then symptoms represent the way the body fights back. Well known examples are fever and local immune responses at an infected wound. Thus, it may be best *not* to suppress a symptom. This may look like a "curing," but is not "healing."

Curing, the goal of Western scientific medicine (WSM), provides a marked contrast to healing. Healing not only restores the body to physical balance and encourages the patient's self-healing to restore the patient to full health, but healing also addresses the cause of the imbalance. Curing, unfortunately, focuses only on eliminating or relieving (managing) the physical symptoms of the illness. WSM has concentrated on developing methods of managing symptoms, thus on curing acute illnesses. "We keep the patient happy while nature cures her" is an apt description of the cures of WSM.

A shaman's perspective has been expressed by Alberto Villoldo in *Shaman, Healer, Sage*[21], "Curing is remedial and involves fixing whatever outer problem arises, such as patching a tire if you have a flat... It does not help you avoid the nails on the road... Healing is broader, more global, and complete. Healing transforms one's life, and often, though not always, produces a physical cure. I have seen many medical cures in which healing did not occur. I have also seen instances in which there was great healing but the patient passed away. ... While healing, we measure success by increased well-being, by a sense of newfound peace, empowerment, and a feeling of communion with all life."

Many problems are associated with curing (eliminating symptoms). Best known are the unfortunate "side effects" of drugs, radiation or surgery. It should be noted that side effects can be found with herbal treatments, even with acupuncture. This can be serious. Side effects are an important reason why a study in 2000 at Johns Hopkins found the medical profession to be the third leading cause of hospital deaths. (This is discussed in Chapter Eleven.)

It must also be recognized that symptoms play an important role in communicating the body's needs. There is real risk in the elimination of symptoms, disguising the underlying problem. The lethal effect of eliminating symptoms has been well illustrated by Upledger in his essay in *Healers on Healing*:

> The reason we need to clarify the difference between healing and curing is quite simple: Effective therapy—whatever its outer form—initiates, facilitates, and supports the patient's self-healing efforts, whereas the 'curing' process is one that provides a more temporary and perhaps only palliative effect. Although 'curing' may remove the symptoms of a disease from the outside, so to speak, it usually leaves the underlying causes of the symptoms untouched.
>
> For example, a physician might "cure" hemorrhoids by surgically removing them. If, however, the hemorrhoids are secondary to a congested liver that is due to chronic drinking, the problem will not be 'healed' until the patient resolves the underlying reason for the alcohol abuse. In this case, it might be better for the surgeon to leave the hemorrhoids intact, as a reminder and perhaps motivating force that will help focus the patient's attention on the alcohol abuse. In this way the real cause of the problem may one day be eradicated.
>
> A friend and general surgeon with more than thirty years' experience once confided to me that, in retrospect, he felt the majority of surgical procedures he had performed might be classified as excisions of the "vocal apparatuses" of the inner selves of his patients. He

meant that by removing certain organs or tissues, he was eliminating the bodily voices that were attempting to communicate the presence of deeper emotional or spiritual problems in need of attention.

Thus, to refer again to our previous example of an alcohol-abusing hemorrhoid patient, we must consider that although removal of the hemorrhoids might temporarily alleviate some of the symptoms, it also removes one avenue by which the inner self is attempting to focus attention on the alcohol problem. If the hemorrhoids are removed and the alcohol abuse continues, the inner self has no choice but to select another organ to use as an attention-getter.

The next "target" organ might be the gallbladder. And the surgeon removes the gallbladder, which may be full of gallstones. Certainly the surgeon feels justified in performing both surgeries, yet no attempt has been made to determine whether the patient's inner self is trying to relay some underlying message to the conscious mind. So now we have a heavily drinking patient without hemorrhoids or gallbladder who still has little or no idea why he or she is abusing alcohol. Perhaps the drinking is a means of escape from guilt feelings instilled during childhood by a parent. If so, the issue is left unexplored and the abuse continues until, eventually, the function of the liver begins to falter.

As the deterioration proceeds, the "inner voice" of the body's wisdom will feel an increasingly urgent need to contact the patient's conscious mind. It is likely that varicose veins will develop in the esophagus. The situation is now serious and life-threatening, requiring co-management by internal medicine specialists as well as surgeons. Once these veins are surgically dealt with, there is little remaining that can be removed, except the liver itself in the rare cases when a transplant may be undertaken. Usually, however, the internist must support the abused and failing liver until death intervenes.

Let's backtrack a little. Somewhere along the line, a psychiatrist may have been called in to deal with the compulsive alcohol abuse, or because the patient may have been recognized as suicidal. In either case, most of the drugs prescribed by the psychiatrist will probably have both mind-altering and hepatotoxic (liver-poisoning) qualities. Therefore, the "inner voice" will have even less chance of communicating with the drug-compromised conscious mind about the reason for the alcohol abuse (i.e., unresolved guilt), and the liver function will be further impaired by the toxic nature of the drugs. Finally, premature death occurs.

The cause of death will probably be recorded as "liver failure due to alcohol abuse." From our perspective, however, it might be as accurate to say that the cause of death was the hemorrhoidectomy performed without search for an underlying message or cause; or the second excision of the "inner voice", which was attempting to speak through the gallbladder.

Becoming aware of this inner voice is what I mean by the kind of self-discovery that leads to self-healing. In the case just discussed, treatment not only failed to make the patient aware of the inner voice, it ultimately suppressed it. This treatment led to a self-perpetuating cycle of deterioration. Short of a miracle, the process was probably not reversible once the varicose veins developed in the esophagus and the brain was numbed by mind-altering drugs. After all, what chance does the inner voice have against modern surgical technology and psychopharmacology?[22]

Returning to the issue of healing versus curing: clearly the healer's task is not merely to subdue symptoms. If the healer is to serve the patient well, he or she must find and heal the *cause* of the illness. Perhaps a belief system must be altered, or an emotional distress's perpetrator forgiven; in many cases the answer is recognition of gratitude for all one's blessings—in any case, setting the stage for self-healing to occur (see Chapter Three for examples of cases of apparently miraculous recoveries once cause was identified and healed). Eliciting the Relaxation Response may be useful in setting the stage for self-healing, as Dr. Rankin has found.

In Chinese medicine, reading pulses and the examination of the tongue are each valuable tools for getting at the issue of energy balance, but we must recognize that the symptom is often not the real problem. Bernard Lown, in *The Lost Art of Healing: Practicing in Medicine*[23], describes patients where the <u>Chief Complaint</u> was not the issue. *Careful listening* (listening to what *isn't* said, often more important than what *is* said) on the healer's part in taking the history of the patient is often the key to getting at cause and so to true healing. This takes time! Dr. Lown writes, "A physician committed to healing could not and should not focus on a <u>Chief Complaint</u> or even a diseased organ. If one were to help those who are sick, the stressful aspects of life had to be exposed. I have frequently heard a patient complain of a disabling discomfort, but after a thoroughgoing history identify a difficult social or family problem and dismiss the chief complaint. The most critical problems are invariably troubled family relations." The instruction to health practitioners is clear: **Listen** to the patient! Use Dr. Rankin's augmented medical intake form. ***Focus* on your patient!**

1.2 Cosmology

The context within which healing occurs is provided by the patient's cosmology, his or her view of reality. Our cosmologies, our belief systems, have an often unrecognized impact on our lives, and certainly they have a major impact on issues of curing vs. healing illness. Our cosmology provides answers to the question, "Who are we?"

Western (Cartesian and Newtonian) science has us as separate physical bodies (this perspective is called "material realism" by scientists—see the discussion of material realism in

Chapter Five). Western medicine addresses issues on how to restore those bodies to physical health (that is, to be symptom-free, and thus, "cured"). Therefore, WSM focuses on studying the machinery of the body and its pathology.

Indigenous medicines in contrast, do not separate the mental and spiritual from the physical, generally seeing us as "spiritual beings having a human experience." Thus, indigenous medicines make no separation between body, mind and soul. For example, Inca Jorge Luis Delgado, in *Andean Awakening,* comments, "In the Inca mind, there is no separation of the physical and the spiritual life of the people."[24] Similarly, Lewis Mehl-Madrona, M.D., observes, in *Coyote Healing,* "Most indigenous cultures, including Native American, believe that all physical and emotional healing is first spiritual healing."[25] Tibetan medicine provides another example of this perspective.

The implications of this contrast are enormous. Western Scientific Medicine sees humans from a material realism perspective, as separate parts of a clockwork universe, subject only to the concepts of Descartes, whose writings were unquestionably impacted by the 17th century Roman Inquisition, and, subsequently, the laws of Newtonian physics describing the interactions of separate bodies. This materialist perspective was in turn augmented by the chemical concepts of Robert Boyle, that flowed logically from Newtonian physics, together with Darwin's views of the "survival of the fittest" that followed in the 19th century.

In contrast, the indigenous healer sees us as part of a spiritual universe that is better described by quantum physics than Cartesian-Newtonian physics. In the quantum physics universe emotions and thoughts have important impacts on our lives and health that are missed when we focus only on the material level.

One additional and important contrast between Newtonian WSM and indigenous medicines is that WSM views us as individuals, as separate beings, whereas both indigenous medicines and modern physics recognize us as *all being interconnected*. This is again a profound difference, with major implications that will be discussed in depth in later chapters.

Closely related to the issue of cosmologies is the very personal question, *"What is the nature and purpose of being?"* WSM does not address this question, leaving the issue to philosophers and theologians. In contrast, indigenous medicines generally describe the purpose of being in physical bodies within their spiritual context, that purpose being an opportunity to learn and grow. The Inca as well as Eastern philosophies' view, for example, is that the purpose of life is self-realization, a spiritual pursuit. Note that this purpose is often reflected in our health, for if we incorporate only a material view of our lives, we may be subject to the three mental poisons of Tibetan medicine (anger, greed, ignorance).

We can summarize the difference in cosmologies and philosophies between Western and indigenous/holistic medicines as follows:

Western Medicine	**Indigenous-Holistic Medicine**
Materialist; body is a bio-chemical machine	Holistic; emotions affect mind and body
Disease-oriented	Patient-oriented
Cure: manage symptoms	**Heal:** Bring a patient to wholeness (Healing is only 20% medicine, 80% is spiritual, per *kahuna la'au lapa'au* Papa Henry Auwae)
We are separate beings	We are all interconnected, with each other and with all beings in nature.

Indigenous medicines' concept of healing is to bring about the restoration of balance, harmony, so that the body can heal itself. This philosophy is expressed in different ways:

In Hawaii this balance is expressed as *lokahi,* harmony both physical and emotional, within the individual, between the individual and his/her relationships, with the environment and with *akua* (God).

In the Greece of Hippocrates it was expressed as *eucrasia,* again, harmony and balance. In Chinese and Tibetan medicines it is expressed as the balance of yin and yang, of the elements, of humors.

In shamanic traditions, similar to that found in Hawaii, this approach has been described by Kalweit in *Shamans, Healers, and Medicine Men,* as follows, "The attainment of inner balance, or inner purification from imbalance, from conflicting forces, brings about the restoration of health and *joie de vivre.*"[26] And later Kalweit comments, "For the Navajo, healing is a harmonization of the psyche. For patients, the cosmological sand paintings bring about a balanced relationship of themselves with the universal forces. Religion, art, and psychotherapy come together, and at the apex of the unified vision of nature, earth, heaven, and humanity arises health and wholesomeness."[26]

Hawaiian medicine provides an example of this approach with *Ho'oponopono,* a—spiritual reconciliation process in which conflicts are resolved. *Kahuna* Nana Veary, in *Change We Must,* gives us the example of the child who caught a cold after a quarrel with a friend. When the friendship was repaired, the cold was healed, for the body had healed itself. In short, resolve the emotional issues as a predecessor to healing.[27]

Kahunas recognize guilt as a cause of disease. This is a form of self-punishment by the subconscious mind (*unihipili*). To repeat Papa Auwae's constant reminder—healing is 80% spiritual, only 20% medicine.

Native American medicine men and women recognized healing as involving multiple elements: "To heal requires spending time with patients, providing them with complete and undivided attention... There is healing power in relationships, and the intent of all persons involved to transform illness. Healing incorporates the power of the mind to transform the physical body, encompassing the self-healing response and the power of the inner healer who lives within us all."

Kalweit comments, "Healing a major illness requires profound life change—a transformation of one's relationships to all aspects of life.

"To heal requires recognition of the healing power of spirit and the spiritual dimension in our lives, including the role of ritual and ceremony in catalyzing change, in connecting us to nonphysical energies, in giving us a view of ourselves as capable of more than we had previously thought, and by enfolding us in the comfort of the Divine.

"The role of family and community is important in healing physical conditions and in serving as the unit for healing, instead of the isolated individual, as Western medicine believes. (Note: The Hallmark movie, *November Christmas,* provides an excellent example of the power of family and community in healing.)

"Healing incorporates the shamanic concepts of taking ourselves apart and reassembling the pieces, coupled with a story-based approach; life is a story that we weave, and healing requires an understanding of the story, the plot, and the characters and how to change them."[28]

Lewis Mehl-Madrona, M.D., comments in *Coyote Healing,* "Fundamentally, I believe that *all healing is spiritual healing.* Whatever else we do—including herbs, diet, radiation, surgery, or bodywork—we need to humbly ask for help from the spiritual realm. People who participate in a spiritual practice do better with any illness than those lacking religious beliefs. We must touch the earth and the ancestors, experience grace, and otherwise make ourselves available to the Divine for healing. Spirit is the spark in the chain that creates healing and miracles. Spirit cannot be ignored, whether it is to give our pain back to the earth or to accept healing from the earth, the angels, or God."[29]

This approach in found among indigenous cultures the world over. The Australian aboriginal healers use five principles with which they heal and create:

(1) **Willingness** to change

(2) **Acceptance** of the challenge required to heal (often releasing old belief systems)

(3) **Awareness** of what you are creating (*Love, Forgiveness, Gratitude* top the list of emotions that bring about healing)

(4) **Empowerment**—move beyond limitations (Mind + "Big Guy" can create *anything!*)

(5) **Focus**—the importance of intention.[30]

(See Gary and Robbie Holz, *Journey to the Heart: Secrets of Aboriginal Healing* for additional details.)[31]

1.3 The Power of Prayer and Meditation in Healing

Prayer and meditation are often powerful tools for establishing the cause of illness and assisting the healing process. Scientific studies (double-blind) have confirmed the power of prayer and meditation, but perhaps more dramatic examples are provided by personal experiences known to the author. David Rodman, a personal friend who lives in Hawaii and is an adopted member of a Lakota family, has given his permission to include the story of his recovery from serious atrial fibrillation. Here are David's words about his experience:

> On a Saturday morning in late August 1992, I was playing racquetball preparing for an annual tournament on Kauai, the Pineapple Open. I used to be able to play for hours at a time but on this day I couldn't last more than a few minutes. I was sweating profusely, light headed, and weak. When I got off the court I checked my pulse – and couldn't find one! After I cooled down a bit I was able to feel a pulse. It was extremely irregular.
>
> I went to my local HMO and was informed that I was suffering from AFib – atrial fibrillation. The cause and cure were not yet known. I needed to see a cardiologist. After a delay of a couple of weeks, I spent an hour with a cardiologist who told me that I seemed to have a condition called IHSS, that he needed to perform some additional tests to be sure, and we would discuss the options after that.

Within a few minutes of leaving the cardiologist's office I would be terrified to discover that IHSS (Ideopathic [cause unknown] Hypertrophic Subaortic Stenosis) is a condition from which otherwise healthy people suddenly drop dead with no warning. In other words, for no apparent reason the aorta closes up and the person dies. I made a will, got my affairs in order, and began to consider the actual possibility of not living forever.

I flew to Maui to get the echocardiogram done, and then met again with the cardiologist. He told me my heart is enlarged, that there is cardiomyopathy (unhealthy heart growth), and I had these options: (1) just live with the AFib; (2) cardioversion – that's a roadside procedure where they slap a truck starter across your chest, electrocute you, and hope your heart starts up again, in normal sinus rhythm this time; (3) ablation –crack open your chest and slice a matrix of little grooves on your heart, to break up the bad electric currents that cause the fibrillation. I went with (2) and that left me with a delay of several more weeks.

So during this forced hiatus, I had time to consider the flow, the pattern, the larger influences that were showing up so unsettlingly in my heart. The one really helpful bit of input from the world of medicine came from the Lown Clinic, a Boston group dedicated to arrhythmia. The doc who read my echocardiogram said no, you don't have IHSS, your heart is uniformly enlarged, not cardiomyopathic; and what's going on in your life such that you're so stressed out? "We treat patients," he explained, "not diseases." A marvelous point of view. And so I began to consider my own participation in my heart's rhythm.

My wife Judy provided immense support and really partnered with me on this journey. At her suggestion we began each day with a recitation of what we were grateful for. I was surprised one day to find myself saying I was grateful for being placed into this high-stakes exploration of my own role in my state of health. As my sister Linda put it, I got all the benefits of a heart attack without the heart attack.

Well, we did the cardioversion finally and after a couple of tries it worked and I came out of the general anesthesia feeling strong and fabulous.

During that year I had been paying a lot more attention to the aspects of my life that I don't control, I became serious about pursuing a spiritual path. Through a series of remarkable concordances I received an accelerated introduction to the Lakota inipi ceremony ("sweat lodge"). Although I considered myself an atheist, I found that the act of praying not only improved my sense of wellbeing, it was often followed by what I could only characterize as prayers answered.

As it happened, a friend who knew of my practice asked me to help build a sweatlodge while I was in AFib and waiting for the cardioversion to be done. I thought "Hm. What if I do this, and pray for relief? I wonder – I know my heart speeds up when I'm in there, maybe it will speed up to the point where it kind of over-rides the arrhythmia, and then it'll just slow down and stay in normal rhythm. Why not?" And that is exactly how it went. I did check in with the cardiologist beforehand, and he said he really could not recommend this, it would put a strain on my heart. Like electrocution doesn't, right?

Since then I've had the same experience about 6 times in 22 years. Every time, when I go into the inipi ceremony and pray, my heart settles back into normal rhythm. One time I realized I was in AFib and I just said "Hey, no problem, I'll jump in the lodge and it'll be fine." I did that, and it wasn't fine. I came out frightened and bummed – and Judy said "Did you pray?" Oops! She made me build up the fire and heat up the stones again and get back in there, and she came in and ran the ceremony and told me to just shut up and pray. And it worked. And it always has. Sometimes it does take longer than others, just as with cardioversion.

So what's going on here? Well I have some theories. First of all, you may be wondering exactly how does an atheist pray, anyway? I don't dwell on the question "to whom are you praying." What I am doing when I'm praying is placing myself into an attitude of supplication, respect, and focus on a desired outcome. An outcome that I can honestly characterize as "good" without reservation or evasion. I am acknowledging that I do not control everything, that there are powerful forces, influences, currents that shape our lives and that we do not cause, direct, or possess.

I believe that the honesty and integrity of the "good outcome" focus is important because it invites the unencumbered presence of those forces for which I may act as an antenna. It seems clear that our attitudes can influence our bodies and vice-versa, and that these influences are rarely conscious as they are occurring. Likewise, factors outside of our bodies obviously affect both our consciousness and our physical being. So part of my goal in prayer is to invite all of those influences to align in whatever way works for them, without getting bogged down in a quest for understanding of the mechanisms involved.

That idea of maintaining integrity in prayer also helps prevent me from just relinquishing all participation in my own healing. I can't pray without evasion for a healthy heart while I'm consuming foods that increase blood pressure or heart rate, getting no exercise, or otherwise choosing actions that work against the outcome I'm praying for. Using the religious language: pray, leave it all in God's hands, and remember that you and God are one. So – understand without blame how I have been choosing to suffer from this malady and how forces not under my control have been supporting or supported by that choice, choose differently, and align more consciously with forces that support a good outcome.

I do not propose a boycott of modern medicine. While symptoms and injuries are effectively modified and often resolved by the allopathic methodology, only a practice whose depth matches the depth of the contributory factors has a prayer of altering a pattern of pathology.[32]

The power of the invisible prayer made the difference.

My Hawaiian teacher, *Po'okela La'au Lapa'au* Papa Henry Auwae, was highly regarded by the Hawaiian medical profession, and he was provided with an office at Queen's Hospital in Honolulu whenever he visited Oahu. There he had worked with a Native Hawaiian hospital administrator and had come to know her well. At one point she was diagnosed with stomach cancer and was given six months to live by her oncologist. She went to Papa in despair; she was in her twenties and wanted to live. Papa put her on a restricted diet, gave her some herbs and—most importantly—sent her to the seashore to meditate. At the end of the day, he asked her about her insights from her meditation. Papa had her repeat this process for days. Result: I knew her as Papa's assistant fourteen years later.[33]

Psychiatrist Carlos Warter makes a comment in his book, *Who Do You Think You Are?* That provides a fitting close to this discussion of healing and curing: "The secret of the entire process is to learn to lead with our hearts instead of our heads."[34] If we can facilitate our patients' doing that, we will be true healers.

1.4 Summary

This chapter reviewed the difference between healing and curing. We have noted that symptoms can provide clues to cause, especially in chronic disease. Symptoms may also represent the body's healing response to the cause, whether that cause is internal or external, acute or chronic. We have emphasized that the task of the healer is to optimize the body's ability to heal itself, and that self-healing may well require addressing issues that caused the illness. We have also reviewed the importance of cosmologies, belief systems, and philosophies in determining a medical system's practices. Finally, we have noted the value of prayer and meditation, of leading from the heart instead of from the head, as aids to the body's self-healing.

Notes

1 Plato, *The Republic*.
2 Tipping, Colin *Radical Forgiveness: Making Room for the Miracle*, Marietta, GA, 2002.
3 Cortland, Sherri *Windows of Opportunity*, Ozark Mountain Publishing, 2009.
4 Rankin, M.D., Lissa *Mind Over Medicine: Scientific Proof That You Can Heal Yourself*, Carlsbad, CA, Hay House, 2013.
5 Ross II, T. Edward *The Healing Mind: The Way of the Dowser*, Danville, VT, American Society of Dowsers, 2013.
6 Rankin, M.D., Lissa *Mind Over Medicine: Scientific Proof That You Can Heal Yourself*, Carlsbad, CA, Hay House, 2013.
7 Ibid.
8 Cannon, M.D., Walter B. *The Wisdom of the Body*, W.W. Norton & Company, Inc., 1932.
9 Selye, M.D., Hans *The Stress of Life*, McGraw-Hill (2nd edition), 1978.
10 Jacobson, Edmund *You Must Relax: Practical Methods For Reducing the Tensions of Modern Living*, New York, McGraw-Hill, 1934.
11 Benson, M.D., Herbert *The Relaxation Response*, William Morrow Paperbacks (expanded edition), 2000.
12 Adam, *Dream Healer: A True Story of Miracle Healings*, 2006.
13 Jarrett, Lonnie *Nourishing Destiny*, Spirit Path Press (2nd edition), 1999.
14 Carrol, Alexis *Man the Unknown*, Harper & Bros., 1935.
15 Dorjee, Pema Janet Jones, and Terence Moore, *Heal Your Spirit, Heal Yourself: The Spiritual Medicine of Tibet*, Watkins Publishing LTD, 2005.
16 Huata, Willarupersonal communication.
17 Moorjani, Anita *Dying To Be Me: My Journey from Cancer, to Near Death, to True Healing*, Hay House, 2012.
18 Dyer, Wayne *Wishes Fulfilled: Mastering the Art of Manifesting*, Hay House, 2012.
19 Hunt, PhD, Valerie personal communication.
20 Cohn, MD, Jerry personal communication.
21 Villoldo, Alberto *Shaman, Healer, Sage*, Harmony, 2000.
22 Upledger, John E., Self-Discovery and Self-Healing, in *Healers on Healing*, Richard Carlson and Benjamin Shield, eds., 1989.
23 Lown, Bernard *The Lost Art of Healing*, Ballantine Books, 1999.
24 Delgado, Jorge Luis, *Andean Awakening*, Council Oak Books, 2006.
25 Mehl-Madrona, M.D., Lewis *Coyote Healing: Miracles in Native Medicine*, Bear & Company, 2003.
26 Kalweit, Holger *Shamans, Healers, and Medicine Men*, Shambhala, 1992.
27 Veary, Nana *Change We Must*, Institute of Zen Studies, 2001.
28 Kalweit, Holger *Shamans, Healers, and Medicine Men*, Shambala, 1992.
29 Mehl-Madrona, M.D., Lewis *Coyote Healing: Miracles in Native Medicine*,

Bear & Company, 2003.
30 Holz, Robbie personal communication.
31 Holz, Gary and Robbie, *Journey to the Heart: Secrets of Aboriginal Healing*, iUniverse, 2012.
32 Holz, David Rodman, personal communication.
33 Auwae, Papa Henry personal communication.
34 Warter, M.D., Ph.D., Carlos *Who Do You Think You Are?: The Healing Power of Your Sacred Self,* New York, Bantum Books, 1998.

Chapter 2
The Origins of Traditional Indigenous Medicine

2.1 Academia and Belief Systems

One of the problems faced by academia is its conformity to accepted dogma, to its Belief Systems. We award Nobel Prizes to those who make major advances in science, yet most academicians restrict themselves to accepted scientific dogma. This phenomenon has been well documented by Thomas Kuhn in his book, *The Structure of Scientific Revolutions*[35], in which he demonstrates that an older generation with an investment in a particular point of view has to die out before a younger generation can bring forth new ideas. This was emphasized to the author when he was discussing geology with the chairman of the university's Geology Department. The chairman commented that fifty years earlier no respectable academic geologist would admit to believing in Wegener's Continental Drift hypothesis, but that today every academic geologist believed in Plate Tectonics, (another name for what Wegener had postulated).

This phenomenon is not restricted to science—it pervades our culture. Every schoolchild knows that Columbus discovered America in 1492, and we celebrate Columbus Day every October. Yet, there is ample proof that Columbus was *not* the first European to discover America, with documentation from many sources that Columbus was preceded not only by Vikings, but also by Irish, Welsh, Scots, Italians, and Portuguese and as far back as Phoenicians, to say nothing of immigrants from Atlantis and Lemuria (for details see Harvard professor Barry Fells' *America B.C.*[36] and Charles Boland's *They All Discovered America*[37])

Similarly, it is accepted dogma that the original Native Americans were primitives who crossed the ice from Siberia and from there moved south. This dogma ignores the possibility—for which there is ample documentation—that those Americans may have been joined by more sophisticated immigrants who arrived by sea. An illustration of this phenomenon is provided by the recent discovery of the remains of a long buried but very modern city found underneath the Alaskan tundra. It was *not* a structure one would attribute to a group of primitive hunter-gatherers.

In recent years our understanding of history and prehistory has greatly advanced. Old paradigm geology and archeology subscribes to the assumptions and doctrines of gradualism and social Darwinism. We are now in the midst of a paradigm shift, as both theories are being challenged. There are now convincing data that contradict the old paradigm. Science made important discoveries in the twentieth century that provide information crucial to our ability to trace events that happened long ago. The first was carbon dating of ancient artifacts. This was followed by the development of DNA testing that made possible the establishment of genetic links between peoples often separated by large distances.

Thus, the record of prehistory is now being reevaluated. With that reevaluation we need to revisit the context of the prehistory of traditional/indigenous medicines. We shall now review that context, and with that comes a negation of the belief in Social Darwinism and the view that the "primitive" ancients had a science, including medical science, that was far inferior to ours.

2.2 The Geological Record

For the past 200 years the accepted geological record has been based on the dogma of Uniformism, the view that geological changes occur only very gradually. Per this view, sedimentary rocks are laid down over millennia, and igneous rocks are formed when magma surfaces, via volcanic action, again gradually, in geologic time. In contrast to this gradualism, it has been recognized that astronomical events—the effects of comets or asteroids impacting or approaching the earth—were the cause of fires (e.g., Siberia, 1908), earthquakes or floods resulting in the extinction of local flora and fauna (as much as over 90% of the earth's flora and fauna in the very ancient past).[38] In keeping with this perspective, the extinction of the dinosaurs was believed to have occurred at the end of the Cretaceous Period, circa 65,000,000 BCE. The cause of this extinction is believed to have been the impact of a meteor colliding with the earth in the region of the Gulf of Mexico, and the loss of solar radiation that followed.

Glacial cycles were believed to have occurred at about 20,000-year intervals for the last 700,000 years. The onset of the latest of four Pleistocene ice ages was dated at around 72,000 BCE, with its maximum around 16,000, BCE and ending between 8,000 and 10,000 BCE. The climate in non-glaciated areas during an ice age was believed to have been cold and dry. Sea levels were significantly lower than at present, and undersea ruins have been discovered of cities flooded when the sea level rose at the end of the last ice age.

There were several major floods between 95,000 and 48,000 BCE, and there was a major cataclysm and consequent deluge around 11,000 BCE. This date is corroborated by Mayan records, and we note that Plato's date for the destruction of Atlantis, which is based on Egyptian records, is around 9,600 BCE (could be as late as 8,600 BCE, depending on the source chosen).

2.3 Anthropological Record

The accepted anthropological record, per traditional academic anthropology, is as follows: The remains designated "Lucy" are dated at 3,500,000 BCE, and Homo Habilis ("Handy Man") is dated around 2,000,000 BCE, in the Early Pleistocene Ice Age. Homo Erectus ("Upright Man") is dated around 1,000,000 BCE, in the Old Stone Age (conventionally dated around 800,000 BCE, with tool making found around 700,000 BCE or earlier). Homo Sapiens ("Thinking Man") is dated around 270,000 BCE, when man's brain tripled in size from that of Homo Erectus. Neanderthal Man is dated at 70,000 to 30,000 BCE. Cro-Magnon Man appeared around 35,000 BCE in Europe, but probably existed in Asia as early as at least 80,000 BCE. The New Stone Age (Neolithic Age) is dated at 8,000 BCE.

The climate became warmer, but was still cold and wet at the end of the Ice Age, around 10,000 BCE. The temperature then rose, becoming warm and wet around 4,000 BCE. Per conventional anthropology, agriculture arose in the Fertile Crescent (Mesopotamia to Egypt) and was well established by 5,500 BCE, although we note (see below) that agriculture was established earlier in Mesoamerica.

The Bronze Age was established in Mesopotamia by 6,500 BCE. It was probably established earlier in America, but we have no records to prove this. We do know that ships were in use in the Near East around 6,000 BCE.

Malta was built between 10,000 and 8,000 BCE and was destroyed around 3,000 BCE, apparently due to a major tidal wave. It is interesting to note that the Mayan calendar began a new age at 3,113 BCE, and that Sumerian, Egyptian, and Chinese civilizations arose at this time. This was also the time period when Stonehenge was erected. Per these records, Sumer was established around 10,000 BCE, with the first cities dated at 5,500 BCE and an increase of cities established around 4,000 BCE. There is also evidence of Sumerian hospitals in Ur of Chaldea prior to 4,000 BCE.

There was a Mesopotamian Flood, dated by a Sumerian myth at around 4,000 BCE, probably the flood recorded in the Old Testament as "Noah's Flood." This flood was recorded at Ur of Chaldea at around the same time. In Ur of Chaldea there are royal graves around 3,500 BCE. The sacking of Ur, and migration of Abraham's family from Ur, occurred in 1,960 BCE.

Per the established record, Moses led the Hebrews out of Egypt in 1,334 BCE, and the first books of the Old Testament were written using Babylonian records during the Babylonian captivity of the Hebrews (586 BCE). This date would suggest that the record of Moses' leading the Hebrews out of Egypt was written 748 years after the Exodus.

Egypt's first pharaonic dynasty, per most academic Egyptologists, was established in 3,050 BCE, though the temple at Karnak is dated at 3,200 BCE. This raises an important point regarding chronology: in older Egyptian temples, there is evidence of a more sophisticated astronomy, as if the builders were well-versed in astronomy and imbedded that knowledge in their architecture. This knowledge was gradually lost. The Great Pyramids were far more sophisticated than were the later pyramids. The Great Pyramids appear to have been astronomical observatories or mystery school training sites, not tombs (as were the later and less- sophisticated pyramids). The inference is that Egypt was settled by sophisticated immigrants from Atlantis, who intermarried with the indigenous occupants of the region. As time passed, the knowledge of the Atlantean immigrants was lost and only retained in mythological records.

Similarly, recent discoveries in southwestern Egypt (Sahara) at Nabra Playa suggest a sophisticated knowledge of astronomy thousands of years before Egypt's pharaonic age[39].

A similar phenomenon occurred in Turkey's Göbeckli Tepe[40]. Dated at 8,600 BCE, Göbeckli Tepe is the oldest settlement known to archeology, and the site shares with Egypt the characteristic that the earliest ruins are more sophisticated than are later ruins.

2.4 New Evidence

Discoveries in the 20th century, by non-academic as well as academic historians, changed all this. In 1960, Charles Hapgood published studies (*Maps of the Ancient Sea Kings*[41]) of the Turkish admiral Piri Reis' Map, which showed accurate longitudes and depicted Antarctica with a shoreline that was ice-free. The Piri Reis Map was apparently drawn from earlier charts of ancient navigators, and those sources had to be drawn before 4,000 BCE. The most likely date for the source charts is between 10,000 and 13,000 BCE. Professor Hapgood also describes the Bauche Map, which shows Antarctica completely ice-free, suggesting a source date before 13,000 BCE.[42] The accuracy of these maps was verified by the seismic surveys conducted during the International Geophysical Year expeditions of 1949 and 1958. Antarctica was only rediscovered by Western navigators in 1848.

It should be noted that the accuracy and sophistication of the map-making of these ancient navigators implies a knowledge of both astronomy and of a highly sophisticated mathematics, including spherical trigonometry. It is important to note that with regard to medicine: *religion, science and healing* were closely related in the days of the ancients. Thus, we find the same teachers teaching the arts and sciences of civilization, including medicine, religion, mathematics, astronomy and astrology, and navigation. This is true of Thoth in Egypt, Quetzalcoatl in Mexico, Kukulkan in Central America (Maya), and Viracocha in the Andes. Those teachers were probably Atlanteans or Lemurians. Per the Troano Document found by archeologists and now in the British Museum (translated by Augustus Le Plongeon)[43], the Maya are descendants of the outer priesthood of Atlantis. The inner priesthood, known as Nakkals, is reported to have emigrated to Tibet prior to the destruction of Atlantis. This account conforms with the history of the Maya as they themselves describe it. Descendants of this outer priesthood of Atlantis remain among the Maya today and represent an unbroken line to Atlantis.[44]

We now have solid evidence of a major cataclysm around 9,500 BCE, and the geological record is being rewritten. The Pleistocene Ice Age is now recognized as much shorter than was previously thought (See Appendix A), and the cataclysm apparently originated with a supernova in the Vela star system. Fragments from that supernova reached the earth around 9,500 BCE, with consequences that will be described below.

Contradicting a belief in Social Darwinism, there is now strong evidence that pre-Deluge maritime civilizations were far more advanced scientifically, as was medical science, than was previously recognized. The Piri Reis and Bauche Maps provide strong evidence of advanced navigational, mathematical, and astronomical abilities, and the Ica Stones (discussed below) equally provide evidence of a sophisticated medical system.

The land bridge between Asia and Australia appears to have subsided much more recently than was previously thought, probably around 8,000 BCE. Nevertheless, ancient navigation to Australia still appears to have occurred, but from Antarctica and/or Lemuria.

2.5 Atlantis

Atlantis has been a fabled land ever since its mention by Plato[45] & [46], his description based on ancient Egyptian records.[47] Historian Andrew Collins, in his book, *Gateway To Atlantis*[48], has presented a scholarly and meticulous review of Plato's work, together with a review of all pertinent evidence, and has concluded that Atlantis *did* exist, and was most likely located in modern day Cuba and the Bahamas.[49] The location of this continent has been much disputed, with a possible location in Antarctica, or a more likely location in the western Atlantic Ocean. Remnants of the Atlantean language appear to be found in the Aymara language found in the Lake Titicaca region of Peru and Bolivia, and also in the Basque language in the Pyrenees (ancient Euskara, forerunner of modern Basque). Assuming a location for Atlantis in Antarctica, navigation from Antarctica to Australia would have been straightforward, an hypothesis advanced by Rand and Rose Flem-Ath in their book, *When the Sky Fell*[50]. Others, most prominently Plato, Collins, and Edgar Cayce[51], place Atlantis in the western Atlantic Ocean and believe it to have been destroyed in a cataclysm. Survivors of the cataclysm apparently went to the Americas as well as to Europe, Africa and Asia. Thoth, a spiritual leader in Atlantis, foresaw the cataclysm and left with his followers, founding Egyptian religion, medicine, writing, agriculture, and all the civilized arts.[52]

Survivors from Atlantis appear in widely different locations. There is a long-standing tradition that the Basques in the Pyrenees are descendants of survivors from Atlantis, with DNA evidence suggesting that these traditions are accurate. Survivors who went to Central America (Maya) have been mentioned above, and in 1402 Spanish sailors found inhabitants in the Canary Islands, Gauchos, who not only told of their ancestors' surviving the destruction of Atlantis, but had ruins of sophisticated structures dated at 30,000 BCE attributed to those ancestors. The sailors also found pottery, some dating to 20,000 BCE, and cave paintings almost identical to those found in caves in southern France. Blood analysis showed a connection between

The Origins of Traditional Indigenous Medicine 39

the mummies of the Canary Islands, survivors of Atlantis, and both the Basques and the Berbers of North Africa.[53]

Although written prior to the discovery of carbon dating, Robert Stacy-Judd's *Atlantis: Mother of Empires*[54] presents a scholarly work comparing cultures east and west that derived from Atlantis. Lewis Spence's *The History of Atlantis*[55] is similarly recommended.

Atlantis appears to have had different phases of existence, each ending due to major cataclysms. British hypnotherapist and past life regressionist Joanna Prentice and Stuart Wilson, in their book, *Atlantis and the New Consciousness* describe five phases of the continent's existence, as follows:

First Phase: 250,000 BCE – 150,000 BCE (Destroyed by volcanic activity)

Second Phase: 150,000 BCE – 100,000 BCE (Destroyed by the impact of a giant comet)

Third Phase: 100,000 BCE – 52,000 BCE (Destroyed when the use of anti-matter got out of control)

Fourth Phase: 28,000 BCE – 18,000 BCE (Destroyed by the violent shifting of the Earth's magnetic pole, which led to an Ice Age)

Fifth Phase: 16,000 BCE – 10,000 BCE (This includes the Golden Age from about 14,000 BCE to about 12,500 BCE.)[56]

(Destroyed by the shifting of the tectonic plates, which caused major earthquakes and tidal waves presumably as an aftermath of an object hitting earth as described by Allan and Delair in *Cataclysm!: Compelling Evidence of a Cosmic Catastrophe in 9500 B.C.*[57])

There was apparent contention in Atlantis between the materialists (associated with the Sons of Belial) and those who followed a spiritual path, the Children of the Law of One, who were led by their grand master, Thoth[58]. Foreseeing the destruction of Atlantis, Thoth led his followers to Egypt, and established the advanced civilization found in ancient Egypt. After many years in Egypt, many of Thoth's followers went to Tibet and established a monastery there. Others,—probably the same group led by Thoth, known among the Essenes as the

Kaloo, and who referred to Atlantis as the Old Land in the West—proceeded from Egypt to establish communities in other regions, including both the Essenes and the Druids. The Kaloo thus established a close relationship between the Essenes and the Druids and continued to guide them in the years that followed.[59]

Medicine in Atlantis was, according to Wilson and Prentis, primarily what we would today term spiritual healing and energy medicine.[60] Healing was described as "fundamentally a process of moving into resolution—that is, resolution in the way a musician understands this term: the release of drama and tension experienced when passing through discord and the restoration of concord. This can also be described as the transition from conflict into harmony."[61] Patients were encouraged to shed the drama of their "stories" (the *cause* of their illness), as the resolution of their discordant states would permit change, healing, and spiritual growth. Energy healing took place in healing temples and used crystals, light, color therapy, and odors (aromatherapy), that were used per the patient's needs—very much a holistic approach to healing.[62]

2.6 Lemuria

Lemuria (Mu) was apparently founded earlier than was Atlantis. Lemuria had a highly spiritual culture and may have been the site of the Garden of Eden. Survivors of the cataclysm that destroyed this land are found in northern Japan (Ainu), in New Zealand (the Waitaha, a sub-tribe of the Maori with a tribal memory of their land's submergence in 60,000 BCE)[63], and in Tibet (Bön), where they were joined by the inner Nakkal at the time of the destruction of Atlantis[64]. Memories of Lemuria, genetic traces and artifacts abound in North and South America. In North America, remnants of this heritage are found in Alaska and in the West Coast[65] and Southwest cultures, including Navajo, Piute and Hopi. In Central and South America are found the Maya and Olmecs in Mexico and Guatemala, as well as the pre-Inca culture in Peru and Bolivia. Off-shore discoveries of man-made structures have provided additional evidence of this long-lost but highly advanced civilization. [66]

Medical science in Lemuria was highly sophisticated. Healers made use of crystals, telepathic communication with the patient (getting at and healing the underlying *cause,* which would have enabled bodies to heal themselves), sound, and color, and they were highly trained as medical intuitives. Healers would visualize the patient as healed, whole, and perfect. They would use the blueprint of the etheric body and intend that the vision of the perfect body be attained, using sound or their visualization to attain the balance and harmony required to set the stage for the patient's self-healing. There is evidence that Lemurians were well aware of the value of stem cells for healing.[67]

2.7 Cataclysm

The Cataclysm that brought about the destruction of Atlantis seems to have been characterized by a pole shift, as well as multiple impacts of celestial objects in many locations. This Cataclysm apparently occurred between 15,000 and 9,000 BCE. As described in British scientists D. S. Allen and J. B. Delair's Cataclysm!: Compelling Evidence of a Cosmic Catastrophe in 9500 BC.[68] The pole shift produced a separation of the geographic and magnetic poles, the shift of 23 ½° being reflected in Egyptian and other paintings. The shift generated the Precession of the Equinoxes as well as changing seasons and the advent of agriculture. The cataclysmic changes were not only highly destructive but were followed by further global "adjustments" over the following 8,000 years. A major flood, (probably Noah's Flood,) occurred in the Black Sea around 5,600 BCE.[69] Thira (Santorini) erupted around 1,630 BCE, destroying the Minoan civilization on Crete.

2.8 Prehistoric Medicine

Several hours' drive south of Lima, and not far from Peru's Nazca Plain, lies the city of Ica. Ica contains the Cabrera Museum, established by the physician and biology professor, Dr. Javier Cabrera Darquea. One of Dr. Cabrera's patients gave him an engraved stone purchased from a local grave robber. Robbing graves is a local industry, to obtain artifacts that can be sold to tourists. Dr. Cabrera recognized the engraving as that of a species extinct for 4,000 years, and he immediately became intrigued. He put out the word that he was in the market for more of the engraved stones, and in time he amassed a collection of thousands of such stones. This established the Cabrera museum.[70]

The Cabrera Museum constitutes a library depicting a sophisticated culture long vanished. It is a library of astronomy, geography, and medicine. It depicts the lifestyle of a culture co-existing with dinosaurs (suggesting a date far earlier than provided by accepted history). The Ica stones have been examined by a geological laboratory but, in the absence of carboniferous material that could be carbon dated, the laboratory could only adjudge the stones as being "very old."

The science of the ancient Ica culture appears to have been very advanced. One of the Ica Stones includes a depiction of astronomers using telescopes to view an incoming celestial object in the night sky, suggesting that they saw a Cataclysm coming. They built caves as refuges, but they did not survive the Cataclysm. Per a very knowledgeable Inca shaman, this occurred in the final phase of the Lemurian civilization.[71] It is perhaps relevant to note that in coastal Peru a fossilized human skull has been found buried in Eocene rock, thus dating the fossil to 20,000,000 BCE. In marked contrast, there are depictions of dinosaurs on Mocha pottery, made by a Peruvian culture dated 0-800 CE.

Most relevant to this review of the history of medicine are Ica engravings depicting a very sophisticated and advanced medical knowledge. The engravings show that this culture understood the physiology of reproductive cycles. They show Caesarian surgery, using acupuncture as an adjunct to that surgery. Indicating an advanced medical skill, engravings depict details of a heart transplant procedure, and they even show brain transplants. Visiting the Cabrera Museum, the author, a medical school faculty member, was impressed by the sophistication of the Ica culture's medical techniques.

Details of the Ica library, together with photographs of several of the engraved stones, can be found in Barbara Hand

Clow's *Catastrophobia: The Truth Behind Earth Changes in the Coming Age of Light*.[72] (See also *The Message of the Engraved Stones of Ica*, by Javier Cabrera Darquea,[73] and *Secrets of the Ica Stones and Nazca Lines*, by Dennis Swift[74]). Clow also discusses details of events that occurred between the Cataclysm and the historic period, including the missing millennia in Egyptian records. She provides a description of an advanced urban farming culture around 7,000 BCE, probably as far back as 9,000 BCE, and an astronomical temple dated around 6,700 BCE.

2.9 Lost Knowledge

This brings us to the issue of lost knowledge, which is only now being recovered, but still only in part. The first cause of lost knowledge is egocentricity. The libraries of Alexandria and the Americas were destroyed due to religious beliefs. The initial destruction of Alexandria's library of ancient records and teachings was caused by fanatical Christians, with final destruction of the library caused by equally bigoted Muslims. The libraries of the Americas (Mayan and Aztec) were also destroyed by Christian priests, though a few records found their way to Europe and were thus preserved (e.g., the Dresden Codex and the Troano Document, mentioned earlier). Another motivation, that of wanting to destroy records of predecessors, similarly resulted in the destruction of libraries and documents in Carthage and China.

The forces of nature also resulted in barring knowledge of times past from those who would learn of our history. Submergence destroyed the libraries of Lemuria and Atlantis. Iron rusts, so we have more relics of the Bronze Age than we do of the Iron Age. Wood rots, so only in dry climates are organic materials preserved. It is in the dry climates of post-geological uplift—Peru, Chile, and Bolivia—that materials have been preserved that were lost in moister climates.

As a result of these challenges, we must rely on stone records, on mythology, and, most recently, the development of hypnotherapy procedures that have enabled us to reconstruct lost history. Engraved Ica Stones have been mentioned above.

The classic case of the use of apparent mythology also led to an important archeological discovery was that of the German investigator Heinrich Schliemann, who studied Homer's account of the Trojan Wars and, as a result, was able to unearth the site of Troy. The Minoan culture of Crete was unearthed in a similar fashion.

Careful study and analysis of remaining structures found in the Pacific Ocean, apparently the remnants of Lemurian civilization, reveal a highly sophisticate culture. Present-day meteorological and tectonic plate analysis suggests that massive structures at Nan Madol and at Easter Island were located at spots that would provide both meteorological and geologic protection for the civilizations[75].

2.10 Navigation

Reference has been made above to the Piri Reis and Bauche Maps, indicating that navigation was a very ancient art and indicated a high level of scientific sophistication at the time the original maps were drawn. However, navigation appears to have been far more ancient than even these documents suggest. Navigation from Asia to Australia by Homo Sapiens appears to have occurred between 80,000 and 58,000 BCE, and possibly as early as 120,000 BCE. Pacific islanders were navigating the Pacific around 33,000 BCE and, if Lemurian tales are correct, probably far earlier.

Navigation was not limited to the Pacific, however. A Babylonian priest wrote of Oannes of Nineveh in 13,000 BCE, describing him as a great teacher and a navigator who arrived in Sumer by sea around 15,600 BCE. The founding gods of India and Egypt have been similarly described. It is interesting to note that the cross is found on ancient statuary, including statues of Oannes, as a symbol of navigation.

Quetzalcoatl, Kukulcan, Viracocha, Thoth, as well as Oannes, were navigators. A navigator god of Mexico lived around 15,600 BCE. Viracocha, Oannes, and probably Quetzalcoatl and Kukulcan lived *prior* to the Deluge. There is some evidence that Oannes originated in Peru, and Peruvian navigation dates to around 10,000 BCE.

There is also evidence of trade across the Atlantic Ocean. Trade to Africa from Mexico appears to have occurred at least 4,500 BCE, in the pre-Mayan and pre-Toltec era of the negroid Olmecs. It is also likely that this trade included that with the Pacific continent of Lemuria.

2.11 Golden Age

There appears to have been a true Golden Age between 31,000 and 10,000 BCE, and it was in 10,000 BCE that mammoths, the American horse, and the saber-tooth tiger vanished. This was the time of Lemuria (although, according to the Waitaha of New Zealand, Lemuria was submerged around 60,000 BCE) and Atlantis, although the time of their founding was undoubtedly much earlier.[76] The Golden Age was a time of great intellectual accomplishment, of civilization, medicine, the arts, spiritual development, trade and peace—there were no walls on cities during this era, but there were seaports and extensive maritime as well as land-based trade.

An Egyptian civilization existed from 36,000 to 23,000 BCE, which would have been during the Cro-Magnon period and would have been prior to the Cataclysm. The Piri Reis map, with its source dated between 10,000 and 13,000 BCE, appears cartographically to be projected from Alexandria. This is presumably pre-deluge but could have been made by survivors of the Cataclysm.

It should be noted that pre-dynastic Egypt, 3,500 BCE, did not have any form of writing. Hieroglyphics suddenly appeared in complete and perfect form, and Thoth is credited with bringing writing from Atlantis to Egypt. Thoth, a spiritual leader and teacher from Atlantis, arrived in Egypt around 9,900 BCE, possibly via Nicaragua. The sphinx, according to geological studies and astroarcheology, was built around 10,400 BCE (per the latest information from geologist Robert Schoch, the Sphinx could possibly be dated as long ago as 34,000 BCE). The Great Pyramids, in contrast, appear most likely to have been built around 2,500 BCE, which would have followed the Malta flood. *The Egyptian Book of the Dead* was written around 3,000 BCE. This would have followed the Malta/Sumerian flood, possibly that of Noah. It appears that there was a highly developed pre-cataclysm civilization in Egypt, then a restored post-cataclysm and pre-Malta flood Egypt, which was then followed by the classical ancient Egypt of the Egyptologists.

According to Mayan records, there was a cataclysmic flood that occurred in 11,202 BCE, which would have been at the end of the last Ice Age. The great megaliths of the world, including those at Göbeckli Tepe, appear to have been built near to, or prior to, 9,500 BCE, the time of the great Cataclysm.[77]

2.12 Art

Cave art contributes to our understanding of cultures contemporary with that art. Probably the best-known example of this cave art is that of Chauvet in France, dated at 30,000 BCE. Equally as old is the cave art at Pedro Furada in Brazil, also dated around 30,000 BCE, art that depicts animals extinct around 10,000 BCE. The cave art at Lascaux in France is usually considered the work of Cro-Magnon man, but may have been painted by survivors from Atlantis, and is dated at 22,000 BCE. It too depicts animals extinct around 10,000 BCE.[78]

African cave art has been found, dated at 24,000 BCE. Both European and Siberian carvings have been found: those in Germany have been dated at 32,000 BCE, those in France at 22,000 and 20,000 BCE, and those in Siberia dated at 15,000 BCE.[79]

2.13 Culture

There were Caucasians in Northwest America in 7,300 BCE. According to Hopi tradition, their ancestors originated in Lemuria and Atlantis.[80]

The Americas hold the record of established cultures in antiquity. Artifacts of a Brazilian culture have been found as ancient as 50,000 BCE, and a maritime culture existed at Monte Verde in Chile around 30,000 BCE. Monte Alegre, also in Chile, is also dated at 30,000 BCE. Tiahuanaco, in Bolivia, was built probably in 10,150 BCE. The major Mayan site, Caracol, in Belize, was established prior to 7,500 BCE.[81]

Agriculture was established in the Americas well before it was developed in either Sumer or Egypt. The earliest evidence of agriculture was found in Brazil, dated around 32,000 BCE, with indications of agriculture before 8,000 BCE in the region of Oaxaca, Mexico, and in Belize around 9,000 BCE.[82]

Mummies found in the Americas date at least 3,000 years before they appeared in Egypt. In the marine culture at Chinchorro, in Chile, mummies have been discovered that date to 10,000 BCE, and others in Chile dated at 9,000 BCE. In Brazil mummies have been found that have been dated at 8,000 BCE. Mummies, presumably those of Lemurian émigrés, have been found in the Gobi Desert of China that are of red haired-Caucasians.[83]

There is evidence of a major copper and tin trade during the Bronze Age by the Phoenicians, presumably between the Americas and the Middle East. The Lake Titicaca region in Peru and Bolivia was a source of tin, and copper mining is known to have occurred in the Lake Superior region in the United States. After being attacked by Hittites, the Phoenicians moved from the Middle East to Carthage, where they were destroyed by the Romans in 146 BCE. There is a great amount of evidence of Phoenician presence in America, including at Olmec sites.[84]

2.14 Intellectual Achievements in Prehistory

Intellectually, the prehistoric cultures were clearly far advanced. The medicine depicted by the Ica Stones has been discussed above, as were astronomers studying the night sky. Astronomers were also knowledgeable about the Precession of the Equinoxes, which suggests a very long period of precise astronomical observation. It takes 26,000 years to measure one cycle of the precession, which implies measurements to at least 37,000 BCE, and probably earlier, if the astronomers measured one complete precession cycle. Or alternately, the astronomers may have tuned into another source (the Library of All

Knowledge, also known as the Zero Point Field, which will be discussed in a later chapter).

The Olmec/Mayan calendar, which, according to some records, came with the spiritual leaders from Atlantis, was the most accurate calendar ever developed until the recent development of the atomic clock. The Julian calendar defined a year as being 365.2500 days in length. The Gregorian calendar, which is still in use, defines the year as 365.2425 days, and the Mayan calendar as 365.2420 days per year. The atomic clock defines the year as 365.2422 days.[85]

That the ancient astronomers used telescopes, as shown in the Ica engravings, is confirmed by the ancient knowledge of the existence of the moons of Mars. Both the Mayans and the Sumerians knew of the existence of Uranus and Neptune, planets only discovered by Western science in 1781 and 1846, respectively.[86]

In mathematics, the ancients had a knowledge of zero long before western mathematicians recognized zero and its importance. As described earlier, spherical trigonometry was understood and used thousands of years before it was developed in the West. Similarly, the measurement of longitude was understood by the ancients, but not duplicated in the West until late in the 18th century.[87]

2.15 Ancient Religions

The religious beliefs of times past were benevolent: Quetzalcoatl (Toltec, "Feathered Serpent"), Kukulcan (Mayan, "Plumed Serpent"), and Viracocha (pre-Inca, Peru) all taught a humanitarian religion very similar to that taught by Jesus and Shakyamuni Buddha. All three were depicted as Caucasians who arrived by sea. (Lemurians were primarily Caucasian, with the red-haired mummies mentioned above; some Lemurians were apparently brown-skinned or Negroid.)

In medicine, the Paleolithic shamans (circa 77,000 BCE) were, per anthropological records, the first priest-healers. A subsequent chapter will be devoted to shamanic healing.

2.16 Religion and Healing

In Tibet, Bön healers are traditionally dated from the arrival of the Buddha Tonpa Shenrab, founder of Bön Buddhism at 16,000 BCE, perhaps from Lemuria. Religion and healing were closely related (Shakyamuni Buddha wrote medical texts, as did St. Hildegard von Bingen in the 11th century CE). Previous to Tonpa Shenrab, religion and healing in Tibet was that of North Asian shamanism.[88]

Sumer had hospitals and apparently a sophisticated medicine, together with their mathematics, astronomy and other sciences, dated around 3,000 BCE.

Quetzalcoatl, Kukulcan, and Viracocha all taught medicine as well as other arts of civilization prior to the deluge. They were spiritual leaders and healers as well. Nicaraguan statues show divergent characteristics, described as Sumerian, East Indian, Egyptian and Mayan. One statue shows a long beard and a chakra dot on the forehead.

There is evidence of a medical school at Monte Alban (Oaxaca, Mexico) in an undated, apparently pre-deluge time, with Negroid figures, a marine culture, and structures suggesting dates similar to Machu Picchu, ca. 2,500 BCE).[89] As mentioned earlier, the pre-Inca Ica Stones depict sophisticated surgery and acupuncture pre-Cataclysm, and probably represent Lemurian science and medicine. It is not surprising that the Spanish Conquistadors found Inca healers far superior to Spanish medicine when they conquered Peru.[90]

2.17 What Happened?

How was this superior knowledge of medicine and healing lost? There apparently was a Golden Age, with great teachers, high intellectual development, including medicine, science, trade between America, Sumer, Egypt, Africa and probably India, that began at least 31,000 BCE – 40,000 BCE and ended with the end of the Ice Age and cataclysms beginning around 11,000 BCE. Evidence suggests the sophisticated civilizations on Atlantis and Lemuria were destroyed in the same cataclysms, though the destruction apparently came in stages. The end of the Ice Age submerged portions of both, with subsequent approaches to the earth by Comet Enke causing further destruction (see Prehistory Timeline [Appendix A] for dates).

Plato used the destruction of Atlantis to illustrate an important point: *Human societies begin to self-destruct when their citizens no longer hold in regard organic relationships between the spiritual and the material spheres of existence.* [Emphasis added by author.] Imbalance in one, he suggests, sets up a similarly deteriorating resonance in the other. Note that surviving legends among the cultures of survivors suggest the accuracy of Plato's thesis.[91]

Atlantean survivors and their descendants developed Sumerian, Egyptian, Tibetan, East Indian, and American civilizations. American and Indian seaports, as well as Lemurian islands, were submerged as sea levels rose ca. 400-450 feet, though some Chilean, Peruvian and Bolivian coastal cities were preserved by a geologic uplift.

The Cataclysm not only destroyed cities but most of the intellectuals and the intellectual centers that had brought and taught a sophisticated knowledge of mathematics, astronomy, other sciences, including medicine and healing. However, those who survived left their mark on the new civilizations they founded.

As navigational knowledge was lost (navigational centers and universities were at seaports and were submerged and destroyed), and most trade was lost with it, though navigation did continue in Pacific islands up to the present and across the Atlantic by Phoenicians until the end of the Bronze Age.

2.18 Iron Age

The final blow to the Golden Age of civilization was the development of the Iron Age around 1,000 BCE. That ended the Bronze Age, so no longer was tin required from Bolivia or copper from Lake Superior, where copper mining severely decreased after 1,000 BCE. With superior iron weapons now available, which were harder than bronze weapons, military might became the rule of the day. Phoenician culture was demolished when

Rome destroyed Carthage in 146 BCE. Walled cities began to appear in Europe at the same time that navigation died out.

2.19 Traditional/Indigenous Medicines

Traditional medicines were characterized by the notable fact that, across millennia and across oceans, despite great cultural differences, they all teach very much the same thing: First, there is the concept that the basis of health is harmony and balance. In Greece, this was known as eucrasia, and in China, as the balance of yin and yang and of the five elements. In Hawaii this balance was known as lokahi, harmony within oneself, within relationships, with the environment, and with Akua (God).

Shamans strived to achieve harmony not only within their selves but with others and with the environment. (See more in Chapter Three) and note Holger Kalweit's comments in Shamans, Healers, and Medicine Men, which reflect traditional/indigenous medicines' insights:

> Basic health and well-being mean the panoramic perception of all levels of being.
>
> Healing means healing culture first, then people, and finally sickness.
>
> Holiness means feeling many—all—spheres of existence within oneself.
>
> We have lost this triad with its qualities of wisdom, happiness, and magic.
>
> Medicine people do not heal patients first. First they heal themselves, then all else.
>
> This is the "vision of knowledge," the vision of a new kind of medical practitioner. Primeval medicine and primal healing methods travel the inner way, in a quest for wholeness and health beyond the ego. The medicine of the shaman knows no pills and shots, does not seek to eliminate symptoms—*that would go against nature* [emphasis added]. Rather, it revives life and heals our relation with the world—for is illness not the clogging of our spiritual pores, a blockage of a global perception of the world, and "illness" only in our limited sense?

Shamanic healing means the healing of an entire life rather than just healing failing functions and disruptive pains. For shamans, healing involves philosophy, a view of life.[92]

This same spiritual view is reflected in Tibetan (see Chapter One and below), Australian, Native American ("all healing is first spiritual healing" [93]), Hawaiian ("healing is 80% spiritual, 20% medicine"[94]), and other traditional/indigenous healing systems.

2.20 Where Does This Knowledge Come From?

The origins of the knowledge from which the traditional/indigenous medical systems are derived is often from dreams, visions, prayer, meditation Also, in medieval Europe St. Hildegard von Bingen had "a vision from God" from which she wrote a medical textbook. Even though St. Hildegard had no medical training or experience, her herbal medicine is so effective that it is still in use today.

In Hawaiian medicine, (per Hawaiian genealogy chants), there is a connection to Egyptian, Greek, and Indian medicine. Both *kahunas* and patients are often taught in meditation or dreams. The dream may contain diagnostic or even treatment information. A notable example of such teaching occurred when cancer became a problem in Hawaii in the 20th century. *Kahunas*, through dreams and meditation, received the information that enabled them to very successfully treat this new disease, cancer.

Tibetans attribute their medicine to the Medicine Buddha. Tibetan sages, using visions, dreams, and meditations, developed perhaps the most sophisticated system of medicine in use today. This medicine will be discussed below.

In China, the Taoist sages were the source of a highly sophisticated medical system. These sages provided the spiritual basis of Chinese medicine, together with their insights into energy meridians.

Native American healers used prayers to *Wakan Tanka* (The Great Mystery), and to *Tunkashala* (Grandfather [Lakota]) in healing their patients. They would commune with spirits in sweat lodges, vision quests, other ceremonies, and dreams.

Dreams have been used in the diagnosis of illness by shamans in Zambia, as well.

Shamanic medicines throughout history have always included a major spiritual component. Sometimes this has involved asking spirits for help. "The souls of the dead are queried concerning impending fortune and misfortune, and their healing capacities are implored."—Kalweit.[95] Shamanic healing will be discussed further in Chapter Three.

Egyptian medicine was highly sophisticated, and it included recognizing a major spiritual aspect in health. Given the origins of the Hawaiians (per genealogy chants), it is not therefore surprising that Hawaiian medicine includes a major spiritual component.

Today we have a modern counterpart to the spiritual focus of these traditional/indigenous medicines. Anthroposophic medicine is a modern example of a Western medicine that incorporates the spiritual background of illness.

Just as there are similar philosophies in traditional/indigenous medicines, so there are similar diagnostic methods. Tibetan physicians obtain diagnostic information from their patients by sensing pulses while in a meditative state. The information so obtained may equal or surpass information about the patient's medical history and condition obtained with our finest Western technology. This was illustrated when a senior Tibetan physician, Yeshe Dhonden, was visiting Yale School of Medicine. As their guest, Dhonden was invited to examine the patient scheduled for exhibition at the day's Grand Rounds. Dhonden requested a urine sample from the patient, which he examined. He then assumed a meditative state and sensed her pulse for about 30 minutes. At the conclusion of his examination he described the patient as having a congenital heart defect many years earlier (she was then in her 60s), and described the sequelae that had followed. When the patient was presented at Grand Rounds, it was found that Dhonden's diagnosis had been absolutely accurate.[96]

Pema Dorjee, et al, in *Heal Your Spirit, Heal Yourself*, comments, "The physicians in Tibet built a whole philosophy upon the understanding of the close relationship between the process of thought and problems manifesting in the body, so naturally the life of the physician is attuned to this fundamental truth. There is accordingly a profound acceptance that it is our negative emotions that hinder our progress on the crucial road to health, and that the mind must be tamed and mastered. Conflict arises when we become the slave of the raw energy of emotion. When we use the mind as a route to relating positively to this energy, we begin to defuse the conflict and dilute the power of the emotion."[97]

The author is acquainted with a case similar to the Yale example cited above, but in Hawaiian medicine. A patient sensed that there was a problem with his heart. He went to a hospital for tests, and the laboratory tests could reveal no problems with his heart or his cardiovascular system. At his wife's urging, he then consulted Kahuna and native healer Papa Auwae. Papa, in a prayerful meditative state, used his hands to sense the patient's energy fields. Papa also measured his circulation time with a wristwatch, then diagnosed and treated him with diet, meditation, and herbs for the cardiovascular disorder that had been missed by the hospital tests. *Kahunas* were trained in the ability to sense their patient's energy fields by being taught to meditate at a very deep level, e.g., to meditate while carrying a 50-pound stone, barefoot across stony ground. *Kahunas* also used the dreams of the patient and the healer for diagnostic, and even treatment, information.[98]

In Chinese medicine a similar approach is used. Pulses are sometimes measured objectively, but they are most effectively measured in a meditative state. Dream diagnosis is described in *The Yellow Emperor's Book of Medicine*[99] (see also *The Tao of Dreaming*[100])

Greek physicians used pulses in much the same way as the Chinese. They also used dreams for diagnosis and treatment specification in Aesculapian temples. (Diagnosis through incubation in Aesculapian temples will be discussed in a later chapter.) *Unani Tibb* was derived from Hippocratic medicine and is still practiced in parts of Afghanistan and India. *Unani* physicians use pulses in a deep meditative state to diagnose the illness of their patients.

Many shamans read auras to diagnose illnesses, and some use pulse diagnosis. Regarding Inca shamans, Kalweit comments, in *Shamans, Healers, and Medicine Men*, "Besides being engaged in psychological diagnosis and therapy, [the shaman] also practices pulse diagnosis and coca-leaf reading and functions as a village midwife."[101]

Today research is being conducted that gives us new understanding of how traditional methods could be so successful. Research has been conducted at UCLA by Professor Valerie Hunt (discussed in the next chapter) with clairvoyant healer Rosalyn Bruyere reading auras. The contemporary Canadian healer Adam is a classic example of a healer seeing not only auras but a holographic image of the patient. This capability has also been reported of some advanced Qi Gong masters.[102]

The treatment methods of traditional/indigenous medicines include the correction of patient's imbalanced energy fields by various means. Tibetan physicians, in addition to lifestyle and diet modifications, use herbs to channel energy. Chinese physicians do the same, plus the addition of acupuncture. The Native American healer Frank Fools Crow strived to be a "hollow bone" to transmit healing energy. He also used herbs as he was guided.[103] Greek physicians used dream information to prescribe treatment (they also used patient's histories and diagnostic information derived from pulses and urine). They would prescribe diet, exercise, and lifestyle changes as they felt were required.[104]

2.21 Fractures

Hawaiian *kahunas* might use energy work (*lomi lomi*) to influence energy fields at the same time that they use prayer, meditation, diet, herbs, and counseling. An example of their effectiveness is found in their treatment of fractures. Papa Auwae found that simple fractures would take three days to heal; compound or multiple fractures would take five days. *Kahuna* Nana Veary healed her son's fracture overnight,[105] and we note

Max Freedom Long's report in the 1920s of a *kahuna's* healing a fracture in minutes. With Western medicine's approach, fractures often take weeks to heal.[106]

2.22 Cancer

Native Hawaiian medicine treated cancer with prayer, meditation, lifestyle and dietary changes, together with herbs. Papa Auwae's assistant, a hospital administrator, was diagnosed with stomach cancer and given six months to live by her oncologist. Papa's first instruction to her was to sit at the seaside and meditate, for days. He also treated her with diet and herbs. As reported earlier, the author knew her 14 years later.[107]

Mr. A, together with other healers, such as Rosalyn Bruyere (whose story was told in the film "Resurrection"), and Adam, direct energy to low energy locations, and to energy blockages, etc. The intent is to restore balance to the patient's energy field and to encourage self-healing. Thus, their intent is similar to the Chinese and Tibetan use of herbs and acupuncture.

Note that other forms of energy have also been used successfully in healing from antiquity: Music Therapy, Color Therapy, Magnetic Therapy. Mr. A states that a key issue is harmonious vibratory frequencies. These involve different frequencies of the electromagnetic spectrum. Note also the implications of quantum physics (to be discussed in later chapters).

2.23 Source of Wisdom

The access to a common wisdom by traditional/indigenous medicines brings us back to a question that we'll return to in a later chapter—Where is the information coming from?

The information is "out there," and the source of that information has been referred to by many names. Jung called it the Collective Unconscious. Edgar Cayce asked where his information was coming from and was told the Akashic Record, and scientist Ervin Laszlo refers to the Akashic Field. 19th Century physicists called it the Luminiferous Ether, and today quantum physicists refer to it as the Zero Point Field, the

The Origins of Traditional Indigenous Medicine

Quantum Field, the Quantum Hologram, or the Quantum Vacuum (which is a misnomer, as space is not a vacuum). Adam refers to it as the Universal Energy Field. It has been called the Mind of God, the Divine Matrix, and more.

It is clear that the information contained in this field *can* be obtained. Dowsers do it all the time, dowsing for water, geological (minerals) information, archeological information, medical information, and simply to answer questions. Map dowsing is particularly revealing, as it substantiates that there is a universal information field, accessible at a distance, to all.

2.24 Dreams and Intuitive Diagnosis

Patients' dreams regarding diagnosis and treatment have been used from Aesculapian temples to modern Hawaii. Intuitive diagnosis has been used by shamans in an altered state of consciousness, as well as by Rudolf Steiner and other healers in meditative visions and insights.

Dr. James Esdaile, a 19th century British physician who had learned hypnosis while stationed in India, found a patient who had had no medical training, but who, when hypnotized, could diagnose a patient's illness with complete accuracy.

The "Sleeping Prophet," Edgar Cayce, gave diagnostic advice to distant patients, and Caroline Myss was equally capable, with a diagnostic success equal to that of a physician with access to laboratory data. Adam, mentioned before, has had great success both with diagnosis and treatment. The Brazilian, John of God, is a medium through whom thousands have been healed (with the aid of his spirit helpers).

Others have had intuitive abilities of note, though not necessarily in a healing capacity. There are idiot savants who are capable of complete thinking, and scientists who have obtained profound insights in intuitive flashes, usually in a meditative state (Einstein, Kekulé, etc). Ancient navigators visualized the night sky of their destination. Charles Leadbeater saw visions of atomic structures which are only now being confirmed (nearly a century after descriptions were published by Leadbeater).[108]

2.25 Historical Record

The historical record, as we know it today, appears to be as follows: Sumer had the first recorded hospitals around 4,000 BCE. Egypt, which had a highly developed science and medicine, had a major influence on Greek and other medicines.

Tibetan medicine, which was derived originally from Asiatic shamans until the introduction of Bön Buddhism (apparently from Lemuria) into Tibet, is traditionally placed around 15,600 BCE. The spiritual nature of Tibetan medicine is described by Dorjee, et al, in *Heal Your Spirit, Heal Yourself*, as follows,

"Suffering and illness are related quintessentially to all the inner movements of our mind and senses, which had the power to block the life force flowing through a tapestry of channels in the body." Further, "This philosophy of medicine had unequivocally revealed that *spirituality* was the driving force behind all healing, to which treatment (however complex, knowledgeable and highly skilled) would always ultimately be secondary."[109]

Details of the development of the fetus, from conception to birth, have been known to Tibetan physicians for 2,000 years. Tibetan physicians stopped using surgery 1,000 years ago (Dorjee, et al), and in 750 CE a 45-year-long medical congress was held in Tibet to integrate the knowledge of Tibetan (Bön, Buddhist), Chinese, Nepalese, and Persian (Hippocratic) medicines. Out of that congress grew modern Tibetan medicine.[110]

In China, the initial phases of Chinese medicine were shamanic, then came recognition of the Tao and subsequent developments. See texts on the history of Chinese medicine for details of its development. Greek medicine will be discussed in a later chapter.

2.26 Traditional/Indigenous Medicines Today

Today there exist many forms of traditional/indigenous medicines. Indigenous healers are found throughout the globe: shamans, *kahunas*, medicine men and women, *curanderos*, witchdoctors, priests, and the list goes on. Hildegard's medicine is practiced in Germany; Steiner's Anthroposophic medicine is practiced both in Europe and in the U.S. Homeopathic medicine is enjoying a resurgence both in Europe and in the U.S. *Unani Tibb* is practiced in India and Afghanistan. Tibetan and Chinese medicines are practiced in many locations.

2.27 Summary

In summary, it may be stated that the issue of the pre-history of traditional/indigenous medicine is now undergoing a paradigm shift with the recognition that there have been well-developed civilizations long before ours, many apparently destroyed in cataclysms that began around 10,000 BCE. Those civilizations appear to have had advanced knowledge of medicine, psychology, and the connection between man and spirit.

Traditional/Indigenous medicines have been characterized by a common theme that *health is represented by harmony and balance, and that the function of healers is to restore that balance, thus aiding the body to heal itself.*

Traditional/indigenous medicines have obtained insight into medical knowledge through visions, dreams, prayer and meditation. They appear to have accessed some sort of cosmic information field in so doing.

Traditional/indigenous medicines' diagnostic methods used various methods of tuning into their patients, reading their energy, including measuring pulses, reading auras (energy bodies), and using dreams.

Traditional/indigenous medicines' treatment methods were focused on restoring the patient's harmony within him/herself, with his or her relationships, and with the environment, the cosmos, the Absolute. Given that balance, that harmony, the body will heal itself. Treatments commonly include diet, lifestyle changes, psychological shifts, often herbs, and occasionally surgery.

Most importantly, **traditional/indigenous medicines recognize mental, emotional and spiritual causes of illness as well as physical.**

Finally, traditional/indigenous medicines are still in use today, and they are often successful where Western scientific medicine fails. Western scientific medicine focuses on treating symptoms, and it does that well. Ancient and traditional/indigenous medicines went, and go, far beyond that—they focused on *healing* the patient.

Notes

35 Kuhn, Thomas *The Structure of Scientific Revolutions*, University of Chicago Press, 2012.
36 Fell, Barry, *America BC: Ancient Settlers in the New World*, Pocket Books, 1989.
37 Boland, Charles, *They All Discovered America*, Pocket Books, 1963.
38 Bobrowsky, Peter and Hans Rickman, editors, *Comet/Asteroid Impacts and Human Society: An Interdisciplinary Approach*, Springer, 2007.
39 Bauval, Robert and Thomas Brody, Ph.D., *Black Genesis: The Prehistoric Origins of Ancient Egypt*, Rochester, VT, Bear & Co., 2011.
40 Collins, Andrew, *Göbekli Tepe: Genesis of the Gods*, Rochester, VT, Bear & Company, 2014.
41 Hapgood, Charles, *Maps of the Ancient Sea Kings: Evidence of Advanced Civilization in the Ice Age*, New York, Chilton Books, 1966.
42 Ibid.
43 Le Plongeon, Auguste, *Maya/Atlantis: Queen Moo and the Egyptian Sphinx*, New York, Robert Rudolf Steiner Publications, 1973.
44 Ibid.
45 Plato, *Timaeus*.
46 Plato, *Critias*.
47 Plato, *Timaeus*
48 Collins, Andrew, *Gateway to Atlantis: The Search for the Source of a Lost Civilization*, New York, Carroll & Graf, 2000.
49 Ibid.
50 Flem-Ath, Rand and Rose, *When the Sky Fell: In Search of Atlantis*, New York, St. Martin's Press, 1995.
51 Casey, Edgar and Gale Casey Schwartzer and Douglas Richards, *Mysteries of Atlantis Revisited*, St. Martin's Paperbacks, 1988.
52 Bleeker, CJ, *Hathor and Thoth: Two Key Figures of the Ancient Egyptian Religion*, E.J. Brill, 1973.
53 Le Plongeon, Auguste, *Maya/Atlantis: Queen Moo and the Egyptian Sphinx*, New York, Robert Rudolf Steiner Publications, 1973.
54 Stacy-Judd, Robert B., *Atlantis: Mother of Empires*, Santa Monica, CA, DeVorss & Co., 1939.
55 Spence, Lewis, *The History of Atlanis*, University Books, Inc., 1968.
56 Wilson, Stuart & Joanna Prentis, *Atlantis and the New Consciousness*, Huntsville, AR, Ozark Mountain Publishing, 2011.
57 Allan, D. S. and J. B. Delair, *Cataclysm! Compelling Evidence of a Cosmic Catastrophe in 9500 B.C.*, Rochester, VT, Bear & Company, 1997.
58 Peniel, Jon, *The Children of the Law of One & the Lost Teachings of Atlantis*, Avada, CO, Network, 1997.
59 Ibid.

60 Wilson, Stuart & Joanna Prentis, *Atlantis and the New Consciousness*, Huntsville, AR, Ozark Mountain Publishing, 2011.
61 Melchizedek, Drunvalo, *The Serpent of Light: Beyond 2012*, Weiser Books, 2008.
62 Ibid.
63 Wilson, Stuart & Joanna Prentis, *Atlantis and the New Consciousness*, Huntsville, AR, Ozark Mountain Publishing, 2011.
64 Melchizedek, Drunvalo, *The Mayan Ouroboros: The Cosmic Cycles Come Full Circle*, San Francisco, Weiser Books, 2012.
65 Joseph, Frank, *The Lost Civilization of Lemuria: The Rise and Fall of the World's Oldest Culture*, Rochester, VT, Bear & Co., 2006.
66 Hancock, Graham, *Underworld: The Mysterious Origins of Civilization*, New York, NY, Three Rivers Press, 2002.
67 Joseph, Frank, *The Lost Civilization of Lemuria: The Rise and Fall of the World's Oldest Culture*, Rochester, VT, Bear & Co., 2006.
68 Allan, D. S. and J. B. Delair, *Cataclysm! Compelling Evidence of a Cosmic Catastrophe in 9500 B.C.*, Rochester, VT, Bear & Company, 1997.
69 Ryan, William & Walter Pitman, *Noah's Flood: The New Scientific Discoveries About the Event that Changed History*, New York, NY, Simon & Schuster, 1998.
70 Darquea, Javier Cabrera, *The Message of the Engraved Stones of Ica*, Ica, Peru, 1994.
71 Hauyta, Willaru personal communication, 2008.
72 Hand Clow, Barbara, *Catastrophobia: The Truth Behind Earth Changes in the Coming Age of Light*, Rochester, VT, Bear & Co., 2001.
73 Darquea, Javier Cabrera, *The Message of the Engraved Stones of Ica*, Ica, Peru, 1994.
74 Swift, Dennis, *Secrets of the Ica Stones and Nazca Lines*.
75 Joseph, Frank, *The Lost Civilization of Lemuria: The Rise and Fall of the World's Oldest Culture*, Rochester, VT, Bear & Co., 2006.
76 Wilson, Stuart & Joanna Prentis, *Atlantis and the New Consciousness*, Huntsville, AR, Ozark Mountain Publishing, 2011.
77 Ibid.
78 Nobel, Thomas, *Western Civilization: To 1715*, Houghton Mifflin, 1994.
79 Thanjan, Davis K., *Pebbles*, Morgan Hill, CA, Bookstand Publishing, 2010.
80 Andrews, Shirley, *Lemuria and Atlantis: Studying the Past to Survive the Future*, Woodbury, MN, Llewellyn Publications, 2004.
81 Morse, McKenzie Leigh, *Pollen from Laguna Verde, Blue Creek, Belize: Implications for Paleoecology, Paleoethnobotany, Agriculture, and Human Settlement*, Ph.D. dissertation, Texas A&M University, 2009.
82 Joseph, Frank, *Before Atlantis: 20 Million Years of Human and Pre-Human Cultures*, Bear & Company, 2013.
83 Marin, Diego, and Ivan Minella and Erik Schievenin, *The Three Ages of Atlantis: The Great Floods That Destroyed Civilization*, Bear & Company, 2013.
84 McNeil, William F., *Visitors to Ancient America: The Evidence for European*

and Asian Presence in America Prior to Columbus, Jefferson, NC, McFarland & Company, Inc., Publsihers, 2005.
85 https://en.wikipedia.org/wiki/Year
86 Jensen, E.A, *Manipulating the Last Pure Godly DNA: The Genetic Search for God's DNA on Earth*, Trafford Publishing, 2012.
87 Day, Richard A., *Nibiru Rediscovery, A Lopsided Mars and Ancient Longitudes*, Bloomington, IN, AuthorHouse, 2012.
88 Stokes, Jerry, *Changing World Religion, Cults & The Occult Today*, self-published e-book, 2007.
89 Andrea, Alford A., ed., *World History Encyclopedia*, Santa Barbara, CA, ABC-CLIO, LLC, 2011.
90 Lüders, Hans O., ed., *Textbook of Epilepsy Surgery*, London, Informa Healthcare, Telephone House, 2008.
91 Plato, in both *Timaeus* and *Critias*.
92 Kalweit, Holger, *Shamans, Healers, and Medicine Men*, Boston, Shambala Publications, 1992.
93 Mehl-Madrona, M.D., Ph.D., Lewis *Coyote Healing: Miracles in Native Medicine*, Rochester, VT, Bear & Co., 2003.
94 Auwae, Henry personal communication, 1998.
95 Kalweit, Holger, *Shamans, Healers, and Medicine Men*, Boston, Shambala Publications, 1992.
96 Otto, Herbert Arthur, *Dimensions in Wholistic Healing: New Frontiers in the Treatment of the Whole Person*, Chicago, Nelson-Hall, 1979.
97 Dorjee, Pema, Janet Jones, and Terence Moore, *Heal Your Spirit, Heal Yourself: The Spiritual Medicine of Tibet*, Watkins Publishing LTD, 2005.
98 Auwae, Henry personal communication, 1998.
99 Veith, Liza, *The Yellow Emperor's Book of Medicine*, (Chapter 2)
100 Kalweit, Holger, *The Tao of Dreaming*, (Chapter 2)
101 Kalweit, Holger, *Shamans, Healers, and Medicine Men*, Boston, Shambala Publications, 1992.
102 Laskow, M.D. Leonard, M.D., personal communication.
103 Drake, Michael, *Shamanic Drumming: Calling the Spirits*, Talking Drum Publications, 2012.
104 Kalweit, Holger, *Shamans, Healers, and Medicine Men*, Boston, Shambala Publications, 1992.
105 Auwae, Henry personal communication, 1998.
106 http://www.wisegeekhealth.com/how-long-do-broken-bones-take-to-heal.htm
107 Auwae, Henry personal communication, 1998.
108 Phillips, Stephen, *Extra-Sensory Perception of Quarks*, Theosophical Publishing House, 1980.
109 Dorjee, Pema Janet Jones, and Terence Moore, *Heal Your Spirit, Heal Yourself: The Spiritual Medicine of Tibet*, Watkins Publishing LTD, 2005.
110 Ibid.

Chapter 3
Shamanism

3.1 Shamanism

In sharp contrast to the materialism we have grown up with and which will be discussed in Chapter Five, not only the ancients, but Eastern & Indigenous peoples throughout the globe recognized an invisible reality behind the visible (and measurable) reality perceived through our five senses and studied by science. Psychotherapist Sandra Ingerman and paleoanthropologist Hank Wesselman, in their book, *Awakening to the Spirit World*, make this theme clear: "In the majority of cultures, the universe is viewed as being made up of two distinct realms: a world of things seen and a world of things hidden, yet no distinction is drawn between them. A shaman understands that these two worlds present themselves together as two halves of a whole."[111]

Perspective makes all the difference. In the materialism of Western Science vs. the invisible world of Indigenous science—*Cosmology is crucial.*

The existence of an invisible world underlying our physical world is a theme found throughout history and prehistory. The mystery schools and the religions of the world refer to such differing yet connected worlds. Plato's Cave provides an example of the real world, the Cave allegory suggesting that our perceived reality is but a shadow of an underlying reality[112] (see Chapter Five).

The wise men and women of Indigenous cultures are shamans. Shamanism is steeped in prehistory; evidence of shamans has been found that is *at least* 77,000 years old, and probably much older.[113] We know that prehistoric humans recognized an invisible world and its interconnectedness. The shamans' investigation of that world, and its relationship to the three-dimensional world we perceive with our five senses, provided the first insights that gave birth to an understanding of what we know today as the spiritual world. Often shamans were not only the healers and priests of their communities, but also the scientists of their cultures. Their insights were later codified into the religions of our globe, with mystery schools playing an important role in that development.

John Perkins defines *shaman* as "one who journeys to other worlds and uses the subconscious, as well as waking reality, in order to effect change."[114]

With this definition, many revered men and women in history qualify as shamans: Thoth (Hermes Trismegistus), Pythagoras, Socrates, Plato, Hippocrates, Zoroaster, Shakyamuni Buddha, Jesus of Nazareth, Plotinus, St. Francis of Assisi, St. Hildegard von Bingen, Meister Ekhart, Ralph Waldo Emerson, Black Elk, Frank Fools Crow, Crazy Horse, Walt Whitman, physicists Sir James Jeans and John Archibald Wheeler, Thomas Edison, Nikola Tesla, Albert Einstein, and Oxford physicist Roger Penrose. These and many others have proposed the existence of parallel but unseen worlds. In *Shamans, Healers and Medicine Men*, Kalweit quotes the twentieth century inventor and mystic Nikola Tesla commented a century ago that, "on that day when science begins to investigate non-physical phenomena, it will make greater progress in a decade than in all the centuries it has existed."[115]

A similar understanding was revealed in a dream to the Oglala chief and mystic Crazy Horse in the 19th century, "the real world is behind this one, and everything we see here is something like a shadow from that world."[116]

Today we have physicist David Bohm's Implicit Universe, discussed in a later chapter, suggesting the same thing.[117]

3.2 Etymology of the Term "Shaman"

Etymology of Shamans, Medicine Men and Women: The term "shaman" is Siberian in origin, but the designation has been generalized in recent usage. The term has become used to include Indigenous healers, priests, witch doctors, sorcerers, *kahunas, naguals,* and a variety of other culture-specific names. The term has also been used to include those whom Native Americans prefer to designate as medicine men or women. We have honored the Native American preference in this book, but it must be recognized that shamanism is found throughout the globe, by whatever name.

3.3 The Invisible World

Indigenous cultures throughout the world recognize the fundamental truth that there is an invisible world equally as important as is the world perceived by our five senses. It is the task of the shaman to be a mediator between, the physical world of Earth and Nature, and the world of the invisible.

Shamans use their access to the spirit world to heal, to aid their communities in their quest for food, and to see into the future (prophesy) for potential hazards to their communities and for solutions to those threats. Thus, when the Anasazi of Arizona and New Mexico were threatened by drought or enemies, their shamans led them into a different dimension; they vanished from their former dwellings.

Canadian physicist David Peat adds, "Indigenous science teaches that the world of the senses is only a fraction of a vastly greater reality. Dreams are often the doorways into these other worlds."[118]

The existence of an invisible world parallel to our own has for many years been proposed by physicists and philosophers alike. Reference was made earlier to Plato's Cave, to Crazy Horse's dream, and to Bohm's Implicit Universe. The list of scientists and thinkers who have suggested the existence of such worlds is extensive. Biologist and philosopher Teilhard de Chardin, physics Nobel laureate Brian Josephson, Princeton physicist John Archibald Wheeler, his doctoral student Hugh Everett III (who showed that a parallel universe would fit the mathematics of quantum physics), philosopher Ralph Waldo Emerson, Oxford physicist Roger Penrose, and many others have proposed the existence of parallel but unseen worlds.

British physicist Sir James Jeans commented, "Thus the material world ... constitutes the whole world of appearance, but not the whole world of reality; we may think of it as forming a cross-section of the world of reality."[119]

3.4 Shamanic Journeying

These philosophers and scientists are describing a universe long known to mystics and to Indigenous cultures and their shamans. The shaman visits this unseen universe in his or her shamanic journeying, journeying that is equivalent to a deep hypnotic trance, a theta brainwave state that is abetted by the rhythmic beat of rattles, drumbeats, or chanting. This state, reached in deep meditation, is a state known in different cultures by many names: to the Australian Aborigines as they travel to the Dreamtime it is *"dadirri"* ("deep listening"); to the Celts it is *accessing the Otherworld*; to the Native Americans it is *accessing the Outer World*, and by other terms in other cultures.

A consequence of the insights obtained by shamanic methods is their ability to travel out of body as well as to heal the bodies of their patients. They do not require rockets to travel to the moon [they consider our rockets both slow and cumbersome], nor radiograms or CAT scans to see inside the bodies of their patients. The !Kung of the Kalahari in Africa work with energy to see into the bodies of their patients. The Q'ero of the Peruvian Andes observe the energy bodies (auras, 'luminous bodies') of their patients and use herbal medicine to restore their balance, thus facilitating the patients' self healing, i.e., to encourage immune system activity.

3.5 The Power of the Invisible

There are many examples of the power of this invisible world. Lakota medicine and holy man, Frank Fools Crow, provides a twentieth century example. Fools Crow was invited to the Standing Rock Reservation to conduct a sweat lodge ceremony. The community was greatly honored that he would conduct this ceremony, so a large sweat lodge was built to accommodate all who wished to participate. A fire was laid to heat the stones, but in their excitement the fire keepers forgot to light the fire. When Fools Crow arrived for the ceremony, the fire keepers, with great embarrassment, confessed their omission to Fools Crow. He reassured them, instructing them to bring the cold stones to him. They did so, and Fools Crow proceeded to place his hand on the cold stones, sing to the stones, and place the now hot stones in the lodge's pit. The energy of the invisible *can* be utilized, as Fools Crow showed.[120]

Today's science provides an understanding of phenomena such as those reported above. Nobel laureate Richard Feynman advised his physics students that there is enough energy (the Zero Point Energy, described in Chapter Five) in one cubic meter of so-called empty space to boil dry all the oceans of the Earth. As will be discussed in Chapter Five, the information carrying capacity of that "empty space" (the Zero Point Field) is capable of storing all the information since the Big Bang in an incredibly efficient manner. This is the source of information apparently received by shamans and mystics the world over. It is the source of the energy used in performing apparently miraculous healings, and in producing the phenomena observed by large groups in events such as the sweat lodge ceremony just described, as well as the *Shaking Tent* and *Yuwipi* ceremonies described in the following section. Frank Fools Crow tapped into that energy, as have many shaman healers.

3.6 Native American Ceremonies Involving Spirit Power

Two Native American ceremonies well demonstrate the power of the invisible spirits; the Lakota *Yuwipi* ceremony and the *Shaking Tent* ceremony. The *Yuwipi* ceremony has been well described in Dr. Lewis Mehl-Madrona's book *Coyote Healing*.[121] This ceremony is a special case of the intervention of spirits in a particularly public manner. In this ceremony the medicine man is wrapped in a blanket and bound securely with ropes in the presence of an assembly that can include both Native American and Caucasian onlookers. When the medicine man is thoroughly trussed, the lights in the room are extinguished (all windows and doors have previously been covered to ensure that total darkness is obtained). The medicine man goes into a trance, with drumming and singing. Blue lights (spirits) appear and may be seen by those present. Many will feel a touch or a breeze as the spirits go by. The spirits may perform healings and/or give messages to the assembly. When the ceremony ends and the lights are turned on, the medicine man is no longer bound, but is standing (or sitting, smoking his pipe), his previously binding blanket and ropes neatly folded and coiled upon the floor. As Dr. Mehl-Madrona describes, this ceremony was given in a vision to a Lakota medicine man in 1868 as a way of curing the smallpox that was decimating Native Americans. Following the ceremony, the smallpox epidemic no longer plagued the participants. They were cured.[122]

The *Shaking Tent* ceremony is another example of physical evidence of spirit activity; it is found among many Indigenous nations of North American. Spirits not only move the tent, (which can be a large tepee) but the spirits answer questions from participants and so inform the assembly. The Shaking Tent ceremony has been described in detail by German anthropologist Holger Kalweit.[123]

In a healing ceremony conducted by Cheyenne and Lakota medicine man, Frank Fools Crow, which was observed by both Native Americans and Caucasians, a large tumor was removed by a weasel from the forehead of the patient, the weasel having manifested from a strip of weasel fur that had previously bound Fools Crow's hair. When the tumor was removed, the weasel returned to bind Fools Crow's hair, once again.[124]

Shamanic cultures are highly civilized and, in general, are not at all interested in Western "civilization," with its wars and destruction of the environment—of nature. The Venerable E. Nandisvara N. Thero, PhD., is a former professor of comparative religion at Madras University and now is head of a Buddhist monastery in India. He has lived with and studied Australian Aboriginals, and he has written, "If culture is the measure of self-discipline as well as the level of consciousness, then the Australian Aboriginals are actually one of the most civilized and highly cultured peoples in the world today."[125]

3.7 Healing Fractures and Distant Healing

There are many instances in which Hawaiian *kahunas* have healed broken bones in times far shorter than can be obtained with Western medicine. On one occasion Papa Auwae was leading a group of medical residents on a hike on the island of Lanai to identify plants that he used in his healing practice. One of the residents fell down a steep slope and broke her tibia. She wanted a helicopter flown in to take her to her hospital, but Papa insisted on treating her fractured leg with traditional Hawaiian medicine. He set her leg, applied a poultice of herbs over the break, splinted the leg, and used techniques of Hawaiian *lomi-lomi* to "smooth" the energy of the leg. He asked another resident to cut a branch from a nearby tree for her to use as a crutch. She then walked out, until coming to a road, down which a jeep could take her to the airport. At that point she was flown to her hospital on Oahu. Papa's final instructions were to touch nothing on her leg for three days. She followed his instructions, and at the end of the three days she hurried to radiology to see what the condition of her leg might be. The radiogram showed no sign of a break.[126]

Another *kahuna* described to a friend of the author's the instance when her son broke his leg late one day. The hospital couldn't operate on the leg until the morning, so she requested that she be allowed to spend the night at her son's bedside. She did so, and she spent the night praying. In the morning there was no sign of the break—her son's leg had been completely healed.[127]

The above incidents occurred in recent years, but there is also an account by Max Freedom Long of a *kahuna* healing a broken limb in minutes in the 1920s. Many more incidents of rapid fracture healing could be recounted, but the rule of thumb for Hawaiian healing of fractures, using Papa Auwae's procedure, is this: three days for a simple fracture to heal, five days for multiple or compound fractures.[128]

The rapid healing of fractures is not limited to Hawaiian medicine but is found in other traditional medicines as well. Song was used as a healing tool long ago in ancient Greece (Pythagoras), and it is used today by both the Australian Aboriginals and the Kalahari Bushmen.[129] That the energy to accomplish this comes from the invisible world is well described by Oglala Sioux holy man Black Elk.[130]

The healings accomplished by holy men such as Black Elk and Frank Fools Crow are reminiscent of the event described below by the author's late wife, Phronda, who thought of herself as an urban shaman.

Healing of fractures is not limited to local healing. A colleague at the University of California at Davis had a graduate student who was struck by a car on a rainy San Francisco night. He ended up in a San Francisco hospital so seriously injured that his physicians did not expect him to walk again. The student's wife phoned the professor's then wife, Phronda, to tell her of the accident. Phronda was a member of a meditation and healing group, and the student's wife asked for her help. Phronda alerted her group to the situation, and they assembled nightly to send healing energy to the injured student. To the physicians' astonishment, the student recovered rapidly and left the hospital within weeks. The student did walk again. He had one complaint, however. He had healed so rapidly that there was a lot of scar tissue on his legs, so he suggested to Phronda that next time her group might use a little less power.[131]

3.8 Indigenous and Ancient Science

There are many examples of a highly sophisticated science in antiquity, and Indigenous science continues to this day. Perhaps the oldest are remnants of a lost culture with a highly sophisticated science, including medical science, as depicted on engraved stones collected in the Cabrera Museum in Ica, Peru.[132] (See Chapter 2, Section 2.8.)

Evidence of an advanced ancient science is not limited to Peru. In Australia there are cliff wall paintings perhaps 40,000 years old that depict a double helix, the structure of DNA molecules not discovered in the West until the 20th century. Clearly the Australian Aboriginals obtained this knowledge from somewhere, perhaps from the same spirit sources informing *Shaking Tent* participants.[133]

Returning again to the Americas, the Mayans were noted for the sophistication of their mathematics and their astronomy. The accuracy of their 3,000-year-old calendar (dating back to the Olmecs who preceded them) has only recently been equaled by Western science with the development of the atomic clock. Their astronomer-shamans recognized the 26,000-year cycle of the precession of the equinoxes. The Mayans were not alone in recognizing this precession. That knowledge is also found among Toltecs, Zapotecs, Olmecs, Incas, Hopi, Diné (Navajo), Cherokee, and other North American nations as well. The Mayan world view was quite similar to that of the Indigenous peoples of North America.[134]

The Mayan shaman-scientists also had an understanding of biological evolution unmatched by Western science until recently—the 1,300-year-old Coba stele records the different stages in the earth's and nature's evolution only recognized by Western science in the twentieth century (1950s).[135]

Mathematics was highly developed among Native Americans, whose sciences included astronomy as well as surveying and architecture. Indigenous mathematics stand in sharp contrast to Western mathematics in that Native Americans recognized a spiritual component of numbers, just as did Pythagoras.[136]

Indigenous science continues to this day. Contemporary visions of *ayahuasqueros* include depictions of DNA, chromosomes, and cell division only recently discovered by Western science.[137]

3.9 Interconnectedness with Nature

There is a strong nature connection among Indigenous peoples. As Oglala Sioux Holy Man Black Elk commented, "All life is holy, and we two-leggeds share in it with the four-leggeds and the wings of the air and all green things; for these are children of one mother and their father is one Spirit."[138]

Black Elk has described an interconnectedness known to many Indigenous peoples: The Druids of Britain and Europe spoke of the *Web of Wyrd* (Being) that connected all of nature. Hawaiians speak of the *Aka* threads connecting Hawaiians with all life. Chief Seattle spoke eloquently of how we are all connected, and the Iroquois speak of the "Longbody," an interconnection between tribe members. The individuals so connected may be living or dead, an implication of not only interconnectedness but also contact with the invisible world.[139]

An ancient Hindu scripture speaks of Indra's Net, again an interconnection between all. However, this interconnection is not limited to antiquity, but is quite present today. The Canadian healer Adam observes the auras of his patients, and he has noted that, in a workshop or lecture, an emotional surge in one person's aura in the audience affects others' auras as well. Our emotions do affect those around us, even to the ends of the cosmos. Adam is not alone. Psychiatrist Dr. Brian Weiss's workshops often include a psychometry exercise, and he has observed many participants' interactions in those exercises.[140] Some years before their marriage, the author's wife put it this way, "Don't kick your cat unless you enjoy kicking yourself."[141]

Interconnectedness with nature makes possible the interaction with many aspects of nature. Perhaps best known among those interactions is "making rain" by Native American medicine men. This has been described many times in books, including Doug Boyd's *Rolling Thunder*[142] and Gregg Braden's *Secrets of the Lost Mode of Prayer*.[143]

Many have reported communication between different forms of life. For communication with animals, see Allen Boone's *Kinship With All Life* and his *Adventures in Kinship With All Life*.[144] For Indigenous people's communication with plants, see Elliot Cowan's *Plant Spirit Medicine*.[145]

There is good science behind this interconnectedness: Bell's Theorem (1965) postulated that we, and all of nature, are interconnected as a necessary consequence of quantum theory. Bell's Theorem has been proven experimentally by both John Clauser's group in Berkeley and, even more rigorously, by Alain Aspect's team in Paris (1982).[146]

3.10 Dreams as an Avenue to the Invisible

Dreams are a consistent avenue to the invisible, and they have informed shamans and lay persons, alike. David Peat recalls in Herbert's *Quantum Reality*, "Dreams are often the doorways into these other worlds." Dreams are often precognitive, as can be hypnotic trance, implying an interconnectedness transcending time and space.[147]

Dreams are often important in healing, as well. Cancer was relatively unknown in Hawaii until the advent of chemical fertilizers, herbicides, and pesticides on plantations. *Kahuna* Papa Auwae has described how the treatment of cancer was provided to him in a dream.[148] Dreams were similarly used in the Aesculapian temples of ancient Greece, as will be described in Chapter Six.

3.11 Elasticity of Time

The concept that time is not the simple clock time we are familiar with has been demonstrated at the Princeton Engineering Anomalies Research (PEAR) laboratory. Events have been foreseen by remote viewers in the laboratory up to five days before they were observed in the field [precognition], and events have been influenced by observers days after they were recorded. Consciousness proved to play a key role in influencing the experimental outcomes as well.[149]

Indigenous science has long understood that time is more accurately measured in cycles rather than in the linear fashion of our culture. Working with their sacred cycles, the Long Count enabled the Mayan shaman-scientists to recognize the evolutionary development recorded on the Coba stele, and it has permitted those same shamans to accurately forecast future events.[150]

3.12 Telepathy

One aspect of interconnectedness that is manifest in many Indigenous cultures is that of telepathy. Dr. Gary Holz observed communication via telepathy when he was with a tribe of Australian Aboriginals, and by the end of his stay with them he was joining in with their telepathic communication.[151]

Serge King, who had been trained by his uncle as a *kahuna*, went to Africa on a USAID mission. One day a local witch doctor emerged from the Bush to say that Serge's uncle (in Hawaii) had sent a telepathic message to the witch doctor asking him to continue Serge's training. Clearly, the distance from Hawaii to Africa had been no impediment![152]

Siri Khalsa, who had been assigned to West Africa as a member of the Peace Corps, described a related occurrence to the author. Discussing distant communication, Siri commented that he had learned details of the use of drums in sending messages. The drumbeat served the same function as does the ring of a telephone: "listen up!" Following the alert by the drumbeat, the intended recipient receives the actual message telepathically.[153]

Phronda Smith (neé Phronda Keala McDonald) who was born in Hawaii informed the author that, in old Hawaii, party invitations were sent telepathically—and woe be to the social standing of a recipient if he or she ignored the invitation![154]

Kalweit comments, "The principle of a telepathic communication network and the connection of all people through a telepathic link is common to all nature peoples. The universe is understood as a pulsating unity to which everyone, especially medicine persons, can open themselves." Note the implication of interconnectedness in this mode of communication.[155]

3.13 Precognition

Shamanic precognition is found everywhere. Anasazi and Essene shamans protected their communities by their precognition of drought conditions or hostile attacks. Old Testament prophets prophesied events in the future; Also, Noah built his ark well before the flood. Perhaps the most impressive of shamanic predictions, however, was that of the Mayan shaman-astronomers, who recognized the date of our alignment with the Galactic Center over a thousand years in advance of the event that occurred in 2012.

Reference has been made above to precognitive dreams. One such dream has particular significance to the author. Before we were married, my late wife (Phronda) was going through her old notebooks. One of the notebooks was a dream journal she had kept when taking a dream analysis class. A name unknown to her or her friends, at the time, had come to her in a dream and had been duly noted in her notebook. This happened three years before we met. The name she wrote down was "Robert E. Smith."[156]

Precognition is not limited to dreams. Some time ago my brother-in-law was working with hypnosis methods with his girlfriend, who was an excellent hypnotic subject. On one occasion, his girlfriend was very nervous about an upcoming job-related examination. Intending to minimize her anxiety, Michel hypnotized her and told her that she would be relaxed and confident while taking the exam. When she came out of the hypnotic trance, she said, "Now I can't take the exam—to do so would be cheating!" since she felt she had already taken the exam, and the rules were that one could not take the exam more than once. Counseled that she would not be cheating, she finally did agree to take the exam. She not only passed the exam, but she received the highest score of the group. Her comment afterwards was, "The exam sure was easier than the first time!"[157] Clearly there is a source of invisible but highly accurate information that can be used by many, shamans as well as others.

Perhaps the most famous case of precognition concerns the sinking of the *Titanic* in 1912. Fourteen years earlier, in 1898, the novel *Futility* was published, describing the sinking of the steamship *Titan*. The *Titan* was considered to be unsinkable, but it sank after striking an iceberg in the Atlantic. The details described in *Futility* and those of the sinking of the *Titanic* are remarkably similar.[158]

Much more recently, following the results obtained in the PEAR laboratory implying precognition, the Global Consciousness Project (GCP) was established throughout the globe with an array of random event generators and recorders. The random event generators' output was found to deviate from average in response to mass emotions, as in the case of Princess Diana's funeral. On 9/11/2001 the deviation was the greatest for the entire year. Most remarkable, however, was that the deviation peaked two hours *before* the first plane struck the World Trade Center. This is precognition on a massive scale![159]

Confirming the GCP findings were measurements taken of the geomagnetic field by the geostationary satellite poised above the Earth. Geomagnetic measurements are made by the satellite every thirty minutes, and those measurements showed a major change in response to the Twin Towers' destruction[160] and the mass emotional response to that destruction. Inasmuch as the geomagnetic field influences not only the weather and geological stresses, but both the physiology and psychology of all nature, including humans, the implications of this finding are profound.

3.14 Shamanic Healing

Shamans serve their communities. They assist their communities to hunt. On occasion, they may alert their community of the approach of an enemy and assist in their escape. Most commonly, however, they function as healers. Shamanic healing was described by Holger Kalweit in his *Shamans, Healers and Medicine Men,* as follows:

"Primeval medicine and primal healing methods travel the inner way, in a quest for wholeness and health beyond the ego. The medicine of the shaman knows no pills and shots, *does not seek to eliminate symptoms—that would go against nature* [Emphasis added]. Rather, it revives life and heals our relations with the world—for is illness not the clogging of our spiritual pores, a blockage of a global perception of the world, and 'illness' only in our limited sense? ... Shamanic therapy means the healing of an entire life rather than just healing failing functions and disruptive pains."[161]

In describing Navajo healing, Kalweit notes that many medicine men and women strive to attain inner balance for their patients, an inner harmony that facilitates the body's capability to heal itself. To the Hawaiian *kahuna,* this harmony is expressed as *lokahi,* harmony not only within the body and mind, but with one's relationships, with the environment, and with *Akua* (God).[162]

For the Navajo, sand paintings are used to bring the patient into harmony with all the cosmos, a juxtaposition of art with religion and with psychotherapy. As Kalweit points out, the resulting vision of a harmonious nature, heaven and humanity leads the patient to health. The entire community is engaged in singing, prayers are said, myths connect the patient with Source and give their lives new meaning. "They experience the unity of cosmos, mythos, society, and themselves. That is the prerequisite for healing—balance, abandonment of one-sided egoistic thinking."[163]

Shamans, in the course of attaining the goal described above, necessarily become master psychologists. Kalweit notes, "Shamanic psychotherapy is a therapy of the whole person, of the energies of the body. The shamans' healing power derives from other spaces, other times, other energy dimensions." And again, "Shamanic healing has many facets, which we may describe as (1) sociopsychological, group therapeutic, psychohygienic, (2) suggestive, psychoanalytic, psychocathartic; (3) transpersonal, ego-transcending; and (4) paranormal, spiritistic, transmaterial."[164]

Similarly, the Toltec *naguals* recognize the universe as a living being, both visible and invisible, the macrocosm reflecting the microcosm. Thoughts, dreams, and emotions are invisible, but we know they affect our physiology.[165]

John Perkins has led groups of MDs, including psychiatrists, as well as psychologists and other health care professionals, to learn from shamans in the Amazon and the Andes.[166]

David Peat comments, "Native healers have never fragmented their vision of health, for it is regarded as emerging out of the whole of nature and is one with the processes of renewal."[167]

Recall (Chapter 2) Papa Auwae often said, "Healing is 80% spiritual, 20% medicine."[168]

Hippocrates viewed symptoms as representing the body's healing process (e.g., the production of a fever in response to an infection). Hippocrates's way of stating this self healing of the body was to observe that "Vomiting cures nausea."

3.15 The Doctor Within

When Norman Cousins was the editor of the *Saturday Review of Literature,* he visited Dr. Albert Schweitzer at his hospital in Lambaréné, Gabon, Africa. While Dr. Schweitzer was showing Cousins around the hospital, a local witch doctor came to visit. Dr. Schweitzer introduced the witch doctor to Cousins with the respect due an honored colleague. After the witch doctor had departed, Cousins expressed his surprise at the deference shown the witch doctor, doubting that herbs and incantations could help the patient, especially as compared to *real* medicine. Dr. Schweitzer replied that the witch doctor knew the secret known to all good physicians since the days of Hippocrates, that if the physician could encourage "the doctor within" the patient, the patient would heal himself.[169]

In the mid-19th century, professor Claude Bernard (see Chapter Eleven), the "Father of Modern Physiology" and discoverer of the importance of homeostasis to health, focused on the *milieu interieur*. Bernard's view was that if the *milieu* were healthy, the body would heal itself. Cholera was epidemic in Paris at the time and was greatly feared by all, so when Bernard drank a glass of water laced with cholera germs before a meeting of the French Medical Academy, his physician audience was appalled. Bernard proved to be correct; his *milieu* was healthy, and the cholera germs had little effect.[170]

Bradford Keeney, in *Shaking out the Spirits,* cites the comments of contemporary Zulu shaman and healer Credo Mutwa as follows,

"When a person is attacked by cancer, he must never show fear or else he makes himself weak. Disease, being a living animal, is ahead when you are afraid. In the religion of the Great Mother, you must not call anything or anyone an enemy. If you do this, you make it stronger. We don't call the tribes we've been fighting for many years our enemy. We call it simply 'the other fellows' so that they never become stronger than we are. When you have cancer, you must never panic. You must fight your sickness with a great calm. You must, above all, realize that what kills you is not so much the actual disease itself as it is your own mind that is tempted to surrender to the disease. Take your mind and occupy it fully in a very exciting project or occupation. This will give the body time to heal itself. This I know. I have kept diabetes, tuberculosis and cancer at bay with this understanding."[171]

The role of the invisible was well illustrated when my class with Papa Auwae was assigned the task of preparing a tincture of Olena from a particular variety of ginger root. This tincture would be used to cure otitis media and sinus infections. The students obtained the ginger root and, at our next class meeting, followed a strict protocol, which included prayer, for the preparation of the Olena tincture. After we had all prepared our tinctures in front of the class, Papa carefully examined our results, sniffing the tinctures as well as scrutinizing them. One class member he admonished to use only half the normal dosage, as her energy had resulted in a particularly potent product.

Two men in the class were asked to repeat their preparation and, after Papa had examined the product of their second preparation, were told to repeat the procedure at home that night. The next morning Papa examined their tinctures, then dismissed them from the class, commenting that they could not be healers. Their medicines would harm, rather than cure, their patients. (We later found that one of the dismissed students was a drug counselor who had been sampling his clients' black tar heroin; the second was a native Hawaiian who had been dabbling in the black arts of sorcery.)

The Hawaiian term for the impact of those whose energy has a malignant effect on the medicine they're attempting to produce is *lima awa* ("bitter hand"), and the phenomenon is not restricted to the preparation of medicines. Cooks may exhibit *lima awa* as well, and more than one apprentice has been discharged from chef's school for just this reason. Papa Auwae had a niece who exhibited the same "bitter hand"—everything she attempted to cook turned sour.[172]

The above occasion provides an excellent example of the contrasting views of the shamanic world, and the perspective of materialistic medical science—the one with its recognition of the importance of the invisible, the other which views only the visible. Another example: A short time after the class in which the tincture of Olena was prepared, Papa Auwae was visited by two medical school professors of pharmocognosy. The professors wanted to learn of the herbal remedies used by Papa, and Papa's students were invited to participate. In the course of the ensuing discussions, students described the Olena preparation and the two students who had been dismissed. The professors were bewildered, and they suggested that the dismissed students must have made a mistake in following the protocol. The invisible energy of the dismissed students was foreign to their (materialistic) world view, and they couldn't comprehend what had happened.[173] The implications of this incident for the pharmaceutical industry and the food industry are profound.

3.16 Sensing Energy

Shamans are masters at sensing the energy bodies of their patients. *Kahuna* Papa Auwae used his hands, passing them near the body of the patient and so sensing disturbances in the patient's etheric body, often diagnosing his patient's problems well before those problems were detectable by our technologically sophisticated medical diagnostic tools. One patient known to the author had sensed that he had a cardiovascular condition that had gone undetected by a battery of hospital and laboratory tests. The patient was referred to Papa, who quickly confirmed the patient's sense that something was seriously wrong. Papa prescribed prayer and meditation, a strict diet, and some herbs, and the patient was healed. In the case of another patient, Papa used his hands to detect a brain tumor well before the presence of the tumor was detected in a Western medical laboratory.

Other shamans use their eyes to detect distortions in a patient's energy field, asserting that ailments are first detectable in the energy field before they manifest as physical symptoms. Often the cause of the illness can be detected in those energy fields ("auras") as well.

As medical anthropologist Alberto Villoldo describes, the Q'ero of the Andes observe these energy fields and thereby diagnose not only the patient's illness but the cause of that illness as well. Having diagnosed the patient's illness, the Q'ero shamans may, in addition to herbal remedies, use acupressure when they deem it appropriate.[174]

The utility of observing these energy fields has been confirmed at the University of California at Los Angeles by scientist Professor Valerie Hunt. Professor Hunt, used a shielded chamber, and computerized measurements of the surface potentials on a patient's body, worked with electrical engineer and clairvoyant healer Rosalyn Bruyere. Rosalyn, inside the chamber with the patient, was able to see the different levels of the aura, the etheric template, the mental, emotional and spiritual energy bodies. At the same time that Professor Hunt was measuring the electrical surface potentials of the patient, correlates of what Rosalyn was observing in their energy fields. Professor Hunt later remarked to the author, "Anyone can read auras if they have a million-dollar computer!"[175]

The Kalahari Bushmen not only observe the patient's aura, but they see into the patient's body, observing his or her internal organs and any pathology as a hologram. Their treatment methods involve ceremony, including prayer, singing and dancing, all methods of altering the body's vibrational energy and state of consciousness.[176]

The Canadian healer Adam not only senses auras, but, as do the Bushmen, senses holograms of his patients' organs and their pathologies. Adam is able to heal at a distance as well; he is on record as having healed a very serious cancer in a patient whom he had never met, thousands of miles away.[177]

There are many contemporary shamans. Adam and Rosalyn Bruyere have been mentioned above, but they are far from alone. Lewis Mehl-Madrona, M.D., Ph.D., obtained his medical degree at Stanford Medical School. He has the advantage of being of Cherokee and Lakota descent, and he has found his tribal elders particularly valuable in contributing to his education. He practices psychiatry, and he is the author of three books, *Coyote Medicine, Coyote Healing,* and *Coyote Wisdom.* Dr. Mehl-Madrona reiterates what others have observed, writing, "Historically, these treatments demand that personal and social transformation precede healing. Wellness is restored when body, mind, spirit, and community are in harmony. For physical, emotional, and spiritual unease—*disease*—are not separate phenomena within Native American medicine."[178]

Dr. Mehl-Madrona is in good company in pointing out the importance of community support in healing. Dr. Albert

Schweitzer, in his hospital at Lambaréné, has recognized the healing value of the patient's family's presence and loving care of the patient, allowing them to stay near the patient to support his or her healing. It is encouraging to note that the practice of permitting patients' families to stay with the patient has been adopted in some Western hospitals.

Dr. Mehl-Madrona adds that Ceremony engages the mind at all levels of consciousness, and repeatedly found that patients unresponsive to orthodox medical treatment are healed, sometimes overnight, when a healing ritual is performed.[179]

Dr. Mehl-Madrona is joined by Brian Weiss, M.D., in practicing psychiatry in an unusual manner. Dr. Weiss was a skeptic regarding the frequently reported phenomenon of past lives—until one day he was treating a patient with age regression and she suddenly reported being in a state prior to her physical birth (what the Essenes call the Interlife). He found her experience to be profoundly therapeutic, and since that time he has used past-life regression as a valuable therapy in treating many patients.[180]

Dolores Cannon and her husband, a career Navy man, were using age regression to treat sailors and their families with problems of substance abuse and addiction, patients who were referred to them by their base physician. They too were startled when one of the patients they were regressing reported a past-life experience. After her husband was retired from the Navy and their children were grown, Dolores resumed her work with past-life regressions, and she has regressed thousands of clients in the years since. Her primary interest is as an historian, and she has written many books describing her findings about historical events no longer in the written record. She has thus added to our knowledge of the prehistory of medicine.[181]

3.17 Physiological Control

Shamans have demonstrated the ability to control their physiology with their minds, sometimes piercing their bodies with arrows to demonstrate that control. Just a few years ago, Jack Schwarz, author of *Voluntary Controls*, *Human Energy*

Systems, The Path of Action, and *It's Not What You Eat but What Eats You,* demonstrated a similar ability, piercing through his arm with a knitting needle without pain, bleeding, or infection, after "sterilizing" the needle by rolling it on the floor under his foot, before audiences of physicians and scientists. The only time Jack ever incurred an infection was at a hospital where the chief surgeon was adamant that the needle be sterilized in an autoclave before Jack inserted the needle into his arm. Not wanting to create a disturbance, Jack acceded to the surgeon's demand, and an infection resulted![182] In related examples of the influence of the mind over physiology, numerous impassioned Christians have manifested the stigmata of Jesus' crucifixion, bleeding at their hands, feet, and forehead. The mind can have a tremendous influence over our physiology—it can make us ill, and it can heal us.

This influence of mind and spirit on physiology has long been demonstrated by medicine men and others participating in sun dances, gazing at the sun for days without injury. The impact of mind on physiology has been demonstrated many times in many cultures: individuals walking over beds of coals without adverse effect or, in contrast, sleeping naked on wintertime snow and ice without adverse effect. Tibetan lamas have warmed ice cold wet sheets covering their bodies in the dead of winter in the presence of Western scientists. Walking on beds of coals has been duplicated by Westerners, the secret being to enter the altered state of consciousness of the Indigenous peoples and their shamans.

3.18 Shamanic Training

Training to be a shaman is generally long and arduous, consuming many years under the guidance of an elder. Toltec apprentices study the three masteries: Awareness, Transformation, and Intent. The modern Toltec *nagual*, Don Miguel Angel Ruiz, has described many of the applications of Toltec teachings in his best-selling book, *The Four Agreements.*[183]

The reports of mystics down through the ages support descriptions of shamanic journeying.

St. Hildegard von Bingen, who had had no medical training, produced an entire system of healing, including a spiritual component, "dictated by God" in a vision.[184] Shamans often describe their insights as having been obtained from spirits, and not only do they communicate with spirits on their shamanic journeys, but spirits also guide them in their healing endeavors. Also they communicate with animals and plant spirits as well.[185]

3.19 Near-Death Experiences: Another Example of the Invisible

The phenomenon of Near-Death Experiences (NDE) has been a focus of study in recent years, and through those studies we have gained an increased understanding of the invisible world. Anita Moorjani, dying of cancer, in a coma and given only a few hours to live, has given an account of that world in her book, *Dying To Be Me: My Journey from Cancer, to Near Death, to True Healing*.[186] In her NDE Moorjani was shown the cause of her cancer and, with the cause recognized and released, she was able to heal herself. She healed in days, to the astonishment of her physicians. Anita reports, "I was shown how diseases start on an energetic level before they become physical. If I chose to go on into life, the cancer would be gone from my energy, and my physical body would catch up very quickly. I then understood that when people have medical treatments for illnesses, it rids the illness only from their body but not from their energy, so the illness returns. I realized that if I went back, it would be with very healthy energy. Then the physical body would catch up to the energetic conditions very quickly and permanently." [187]

And so it did—Anita returned to life, and her cancer was healed. The author is reminded of the teaching of Rosalyn Bruyere, who taught the same concept of energy fields as reported by Anita, and who provided overnight healing to a woman who had had an NDE that was so beautiful that her body had developed a serious food allergy, apparently hoping that she would return to the other side that had been so beautiful and loving. Once the cause of her food allergy was revealed, her body healed itself.

Dr. Eben Alexander, scientist, neurosurgeon, and profound skeptic about NDEs, had his views totally changed due to his own NDE, when his brain was being destroyed by a bacterial infection. His NDE is of particular value due to the close monitoring of his brain activity during his coma. Dr. Alexander has described his experience in his book, *Proof of Heaven: A Neurosurgeon's Journey into the Afterlife*.[188]

Dannion Brinkley has described his NDEs and the beautiful afterlife he observed after being struck by lightening, in his books *Saved By the Light, Secrets of the Light: Lessons from Heaven,* and *The Secrets of the Light*.[189]

Similar NDEs that provided healing have been reported by Dr. Raymond Moody and by Dr. Kenneth Ring, as well as by many others.[190]

Shamans frequently become clairvoyant after an NDE or a severe illness. Particularly enhanced capabilities have been found among those who survived being struck by lightning, as did Dannion Brinkley.

The lesson from each of these accounts is the same. *The invisible is quite real.*

Dr. Brian Weiss comments, "Mystical or spiritual phenomena present people with a glimpse of the other side—of the "real" world. They can occur through meditation, prayer, nature, near-death experiences, or in many other ways. ...[including] in dreams."[191]

3.20 On the Subject of Cause

The cause of an illness frequently is internal and invisible—emotional or spiritual. We are all, unfortunately, "domesticated" (conditioned) by our parental and school influences, as Don Miguel Ruiz explains in *The Four Agreements*.[192] Belief systems are a common cause of illness, and shamans are adept at addressing belief systems, as the next two examples demonstrate.

Dr. Gary Holz, an MIT-trained physicist, was a highly successful science entrepreneur but was faced with a dire medical prognosis. He had terminal multiple sclerosis, requiring the use of a wheelchair for his mobility, and his life expectancy was but two years. One evening, in his wheelchair, by "chance" he met an Australian naturopath. She suggested he contact an Australian Aboriginal shaman/healer. Against the advice of his family and friends, he went to Australia and contacted the healer. She soon ascertained that the cause of his illness was a belief system (that he was unworthy) which he had accepted from his father. She worked with Dr. Holz to change his subconscious belief and to engage him in a lifestyle that would heal him. At the conclusion of her work with him, Dr, Holz, no longer needing a wheelchair, flew back to the U.S., remarried, and proceeded to give workshops on health and healing. As anthropologist Holger Kalweit points out in *Shamans, Healers and Medicine Men*, healing does not come from the visible world, but rather from the invisible world.[193] Dr. Holz was healed through understanding the invisible cause of his illness. Dr. Holz and his wife, Robbie, subsequently published the story of his illness and his recovery in *Journey to the Heart: Secrets of Aboriginal Healing*.[194]

John Perkins, author of *Confessions of an Economic Hit Man; Shape Shifting; The World Is As You Dream I;* and other books, volunteered for the Peace Corps after graduating from business school. He was assigned to a remote Amazon village, but shortly after he arrived, he became deathly ill.

Perkins had grown up in New England in a very puritanical household, and he could readily envision his mother's reaction to the diet of squirming grubs and a beer made by the village women after chewing manioc root—'spit beer', as he put it—that was the diet in the village. John became so ill that he resigned himself to dying, for there was no way he could walk through the rain forest for two days, then take a bus over the Andes to the nearest physician. Happily, the village schoolmaster brought the local shaman to John, who said he could heal him. The shaman took John on a shamanic journey, and John recognized that the cause of his illness was not the food he'd consumed nor any external cause, but the belief system that he'd acquired from his mother. With that new understanding, plus a few herbs and a good night's sleep, John's body resumed its self-healing capability, and he was completely healed when he woke up the next morning.[195]

Shamans enter into an altered state of consciousness to obtain information useful for their community as well as to sense the energy body of a patient and to heal that patient. They heal an invisible *cause,* and the patient, perhaps with the assistance of ceremony (to communicate with the subconscious mind), diet and herbs, heals himself or herself. The shaman, as do several non-Western medical systems, restores harmony and balance to the patient. The body's self-healing capacity takes over, and the patient is healed (as was illustrated by Anita Moorjani's rapid healing from death's door, as well as Dr. Gary Holz and John Perkins being healed from terminal illnesses once *cause* was recognized and eliminated).

Shamanic healing works, and we can learn from the insights of those shamans.

Physicist David Peat comments, "The Indigenous people of the Americas and their Elders have much to teach us. It is just that we have forgotten how to listen or, rather, how to create that silence within ourselves into which knowledge can speak."[196] *Listen to your Inner Voice.*

3.21 Shamanic Malpractice

Not all shamans' actions are beneficent. Probably the best known negative effects are the actions of voodoo priests in cursing victims they wish to harm (e.g., by cursing them and sticking pins in dolls, which are images of their victim). Sometimes sorcerers will engage in battle using invisible energies to cause harm. A friend of the author was perceived to be a threat to a shaman in southeast Asia; the consequence was that the friend suffered a heart attack. He recovered from the heart attack, but the damage remained.

However, ceremony has been known to counteract such attacks. Dr. Larry Dossey, in his book, *Time, Space and Medicine,* describes a patient who was dying of unknown causes after such an attack. The resident in charge of the patient performed a ceremony that connected with and impressed the patient's subconscious mind and broke the spell. The patient healed himself and recovered fully.[197]

3.22 Shamans Today

Shamans are not a relic of the past. There are contemporary shamans in many guises, among them the many Indigenous shamans in Europe, Africa, the Near and Far East, Australia, Polynesia, and the Americas. There are many psychiatrists who may be considered to be shamans, especially those using past-life regressions in treating their patients; all are working with the invisible. There are many Intuitive Diagnosticians, Aura Readers, and Energy Healers (Healing Touch, Qi Gong masters, etc.) who would qualify as shamans, for they both perceive invisible information and use that information to serve their patients and their communities.

Dowsers are another group that not only detect information, but also use invisible energy to heal, to move underground streams, to recognize and use time warps (as did shamans of old), to move geopathic energies that would otherwise produce health problems, and to neutralize "evil" spirits. Many religious organizations have practitioners engaged in healing ministries. There are today mystics, clairvoyants, and psychometrists practicing these arts.

Many shamans are mediums, with their shamanic journeying extending to deceased individuals of significance to the shaman or to participants in a séance. Modern and well-known equivalents who have healed many are Brazil's Arigo, who followed the instructions of a deceased German physician as he healed patients, even though he himself had no medical training.[198] More recently we have Joao de Deus, in Abadiana, Brazil, who has healed thousands through his service as a medium for deceased physicians and saints[199] (Heather Cumming and Karen Leffler, *John of God: The Brazilian Healer Who's Touched the Lives of Millions*; Robert Pellegrino-Estrich, *The Miracle Man: The Life Story of Joao de Deus*). These are outstanding examples of the shaman within us, of *an ability common to us all.*

Though I have cited notable examples of mediums renowned for their healing records, there are many lesser-known mediums. In truth, mediumship is an ability common to many: information about those who have left their physical bodies seen in dreams, visions, or otherwise. It is the author's understanding that there is a remote tribe in Africa, many of whose members are accomplished mediums.

We are all potential mystics! We are all potential shamans!

3.23 Summary

There is much we can learn from the ancients and from contemporary shamans. Materialism is a false god. Many shamans succeed where Western medicine fails. Ovarian cancer results in the deaths of many despite the best that allopathic medicine can do. In contrast, John Perkins describes, in his book, *The World Is As You Dream It,* a woman was healed of an ovarian tumor by a shaman in the Andes.[200]

The invisible is just as real as the visible; they represent two aspects of Reality. The words of physicist David Peat bear repeating: "The Indigenous people of the Americas and their Elders have much to teach us. It is just that we have forgotten how to listen or, rather, how to create that silence within ourselves into which knowledge can speak."[201] *Listen to your Inner Voice.*

Consider also the implications of reports from NDEs: a universe that conforms to the experience of shamans, that is both an interconnected unity and a Oneness that is characterized by love. In *Miracles Happen,* regarding the lessons we can learn from past-life regressions, Brian Weiss notes, "The life lesson of choosing peace and compassion over war and violence is both common and important. We are here to learn about *love, kindness* and *cooperation.* We must renounce hatred and prejudice and overcome our fears."[202]

Notes

111 Ingerman, Sandra and Hank Wesselman *Awakening to the Spirit World: The Shamanic Path of Direct Revelation,* Boulder, CO, 2010.
112 Plato, *The Republic.*
113 Hancock, Graham *Supernatural: Meetings with the Ancient Teachers,* New York, The Disinformation Company, Ltd, 2007.
114 Perkins, John *The World Is As You Dream It: Shamanic Teachings from the Amazon and Andes,* Inner Traditions, 1994.
115 Kalweit, Holger *Shamans, Healers and Medicine Men,* Shambala, 1992.
116 Neihardt, John, *Black Elk Speaks: Being the Life Story of a Holy Man of the Oglala Sioux,* University of Nebraska Press, 1988.
117 Bohm PhD, David *Wholeness and the Implicate Order,* Routledge, 2002.
118 Peat, F. David, PhD, *Blackfoot Physics,* Weiser Books, 2006.
119 Jeans, Sir James Hopwood, *Physics and Philosophy,* Dover Publications, 1981.
120 Rodman, David & James Soto, Personal communications.
121 Mehl-Madrona M.D. PhD, Lewis, *Coyote Healing: Miracles in Native Medicine,* Bear & Company, 2003.
122 Ibid.
123 Kalweit, Holger *Shamans, Healers and Medicine Men,* Shambhala, 2000.
124 Mails, Thomas, *Fools Crow,* Bison Books, 1990.
125 Thero, PhD., Venerable, E. N. N. "The Dreamtime, Mysticism, and Liberation: Shamanism in Australia," in *The American Theosophist: The Ancient Wisdom in Shamanic Cultures.*
126 Auwae, Henry Personal communication, 1998.
127 Laskow M.D, Leonard Personal communication. 1989.
128 Freedom Long, Max *The Secret Science Behind Miracles,* Henry Auwae, Personal communication.
129 Pert, PhD., Candace *Molecules of Emotion: The Science Behind Mind-Body Medicine,*; Braden, Gregg *Secrets of the Lost Mode of Prayer,*; Keeney, Bradford *Shaking out the Spirits: A Psychotherapist's Entry into the Healing Mysteries of Global Shamanism.*
130 Neihardt, John *Black Elk Speaks: Being the Life Story of a Holy Man of the Oglala Sioux,* Ch. 17 "The First Cure", University of Nebraska Press, 1988.
131 Smith, Phronda personal communication.
132 *The Message of the Engraved Stones of Ica,* Javier Cabrera Darquea, M.D.; *Secrets of the Ica Stones and Nazca Lines,* Dennis Swift.
133 Narby, Jeremy and Francis Huxley, *Shamans Through Time: 500 Years on the Path to Knowledge,* Tarcher, 2001.
134 Jenkins, John Major, *Maya Cosmogenesis 2012*; Barbara Hand Clow, *The Mayan Code: Time Acceleration and Awakening the World Mind;* Adrian Gilbert and Maurice Cotterell, *The Mayan Prophecies: Unlocking the Secrets of a Lost*

Civilization.
135 Villoldo, Alberto and Erik Jendresen, *The Four Winds: A Shaman's Odyssey in the Amazon*, Harper Collins, 1990.
136 Peat, F. David *Blackfoot Physics*, Weiser Books, 2006.
137 Narby, Jeremy PhD. *The Cosmic Serpent: DNA and the Origins of Knowledge*, Tarcher/Putnam, 1999.
138 Neihardt, John *Black Elk Speaks: Being the Life Story of a Holy Man of the Oglala Sioux*, University of Nebraska Press, 1988.
139 Bates, Brian *The Way of Wyrd*, Hay House, 2013.
140 Adam, *Dream Healer: A True Story of Miracle Healings*; Adam *The Path of the Dream Healer: My Journey Through the Miraculous World of Energy Healing;* Weiss, Brian M.D.*Many Lives, Many Masters,*; Weiss, M.D., Brian and Amy Weiss *Miracles Happen: The Transformational Healing Power of Past-Life Memories,*
141 Smith, Phronda personal communication.
142 Boyd, Doug *Rolling Thunder: A Personal Exploration of the Secret Healing Powers of an American Indian Medicine Man*, Delta, 1976.
143 Braden, Gregg, *Secrets of the Lost Mode of Prayer*, Hay House (2nd edition), 2016.
144 Boone, Allen, *Kinship with All Life*, and Boone, Allen *Adventures in Kinship with All Life.*
145 Cowan, Elliot, *Plant Spirit Medicine*, Sounds True, 2014.
146 Herbert, PhD, Nick *Quantum Reality: Beyond the New Physics, An Excursion into Metaphysics and the Meaning of Reality*, Anchor, 1987.
147 Ibid.
148 Auwae, Henry Personal communication 1998.
149 Jahn, Robert and Brenda Dunne *Margins of Reality: The Role of Consciousness in the Physical Word*; Goswami, Ph.D., Amit *The Self-Aware Universe: How Consciousness Creates the Material World.*
150 Hand Clow, Barbara *The Mayan Code: Time Acceleration and Awakening the World Mind*, Bear & Company, 2007.
151 Holz, Gary and Robbie, *Journey to the Heart: Secrets of Aboriginal Healing*, iUniverse, 2011.
152 King, Serge Personal communication, 1985.
153 Khalsa, Siri personal communication.
154 Smith, Phronda personal communication.
155 Kalweit, Holger *Shamans, Healers and Medicine Men*, Shambala, 2000.
156 Smith, Phronda personal communication, 1983.
157 Smith, Maryse Bader personal communication.
158 Seifer, Marc *Transcending the Speed of Light: Consciousness, Quantum Physics, and the Fifth Dimension*, Inner Traditions, 2008.
159 Radin, PhD, Dean, *Entangled Minds: Extrasensory Experiences in a Quantum Reality*, Pocket Books, 2009.
160 Wood, PhD, Judy http://www.drjudywood.com/articles/erin/erin5.html,

2008.
161 Kalweit, Holger, *Shamans, Healers and Medicine Men*, Shambala, 2000.
162 Ibid.
163 Ibid.
164 Ibid.
165 Pert, PhD, Candace, *Molecules of Emotion: The Science Behind Mind-Body Medicine*, Scribner, 1997.
166 Perkins, John *The World Is As You Dream It: Shamanic Teachings from the Amazon and Andes,* Inner Traditions, 1994.
167 Peat, PhD, F. David, *Blackfoot Physics*, Weiser Books, 2005.
168 Auwae, Henry Personal communication, 1998.
169 Cousins, Norman, *Anatomy of an Illness: Reflections of Healing and Regeneration*, WW Norton, 1978.
170 Bernard, Claude, *Study of Experimental Medicine* (originally French, *l'Etude de la Medecine Experimentale*), 1865.
171 Keeney, Bradford, *Shaking out the Spirits: A Psychotherapist's Entry into the Healing Mysteries of Global Shamanism*, Station Hill Press, 1994.
172 Auwae, Henry Personal communication, 1998.
173 Ibid.
174 Villoldo, Alberto and Stanley Krippner, *Healing States: A Journey into the World of Spiritual Healing and Shamanism*, Simon & Schuster, 1987.
175 Hunt PhD, Valerie Personal communication.
176 Keeney, Bradford *Shaking out the Spirits: A Psychotherapist's Entry into the Healing Mysteries of Global Shamanism*, Station Hill Press, 1994.
177 Ibid.
178 Mehl-Madrona, MD PhD, Lewis, *Coyote Medicine*, Simon & Schuster, 1998.
179 Ibid.
180 Weiss M.D., Brian, *Many Lives, Many Masters*, Simon and Schuster, 1988.
181 Cannon, Dolores, *The Convoluted Universe, Books One through Three*, and other assorted books.
182 Schwartz, ND, Jack Presentation at Stanford Medical School, 1983.
183 Ruiz, Miguel *The Four Agreements,* Amber-Alan Publishing, 1997.
184 Wighard, Strefilow & Gottfried Hertzka *Hildegard of Bingen's Medicine*, Santa Fe, NM, Bear & Co., 1988.
185 Auwae, Henry Personal communication, 1998.
186 Moorjani, Anita, *Dying To Be Me: My Journey from Cancer, to Near Death, to True Healing*, Hay House, 2012.
187 Dyer, Wayne, *Wishes Fulfilled* [quote from Anita Moorjani, p. 125], Hay House, 2012.
188 Alexander, MD, Eben, *Proof of Heaven: A Neurosurgeon's Journey into the Afterlife*, Simon & Schuster, 2012.
189 Brinkley, Dannion, *Saved By the Light*; *Secrets of the Light: Lessons from Heaven,* and *The Secrets of the Light.*
190 Moody, Raymond, *Life After Life; The Life Beyond,* and Dr Kenneth Ring,

The Omega project: Life at Death: A Scientific Investigation of the Near-Death Experience.
191 Weiss M.D., Brian, *Many Lives, Many Masters*, Simon and Schuster Inc., 1988.
192 Ruiz, Miguel *The Four Agreements,* Amber-Alan Publishing, 1997.
193 Kalweit, Holger, *Shamans, Healers and Medicine Men*, Shambala, 2000.
194 Holz, Gary and Robbie, *Journey to the Heart: Secrets of Aboriginal Healing*, iUniverse, 2011.
195 Perkins, John *The World Is As You Dream It: Shamanic Teachings from the Amazon and Andes*, Inner Traditions, 1994.
196 Peat, PhD, F. David, *Blackfoot Physics*, Weiser Books, 2005.
197 Dossey, MD, Larry, *Time, Space and Medicine*, Shambala, 1982.
198 Fuller, John G., *Arigo: Surgeon of the Rusty Knife*, Devin-Adair Publishing, 1974.
199 Cumming, Heather and Karen Leffler, *John of God: the Brazilian Healer Who's Touched the Lives of Millions,* Pellegrino-Estrich, Robert, *The Miracle Man: The Life Story of Joao de Deus.*
200 Perkins, John, *The World Is As You Dream It: Shamanic Teachings from the Amazon and Andes*, Inner Traditions, 1994.
201 Peat, PhD, F. David *Blackfoot Physics*, Weiser Books, 2005.
202 Weiss, M.D., Brian and Amy Weiss, *Miracles Happen: The Transformational Healing Power of Past-Life Memories*, HarperOne (3rd edition), 2013.

Chapter 4
Mystery Schools—Ancient and Modern

4.1 Dmitri Nicholas

As an introduction to this chapter on mystery schools it is suggested that the reader consider a hypothetical candidate for graduation from a Hippocratic medical school in ancient Greece. Details of Hippocratic medicine will be discussed in a later chapter. Our hypothetical candidate we shall call Dmitri Nicholas. Dmitri is about to conclude 12 years of study. First he learned of anatomy, physiology, and botany. After that came pathology, considered to be a disharmony, an imbalance of the four humors. Diagnosis called for careful observation and intuition (to tune in to the patient, as Tibetan Medicine does today,[203] checking the pulses in a meditative state, as do Tibetan, Ayurvedic, and Chinese medicine today, considering urine—its color and odor. It may be noted that modern Tibetan medicine is very similar to Hippocratic medicine, suggesting that both tapped into the same Source. Therapy would include diet, fasting, lifestyle changes, exercise, counseling to obtain emotional balance, and use of herbals to balance energies and so to provide an optimal condition for self-healing.

Prognosis would require an understanding of all that Dmitri had learned from his studies, including the history of healing, of Thoth and Imhotep in Egypt, and of Greek medicine (Apollo, Aesculapius, Chiron) "tradition," implying an ancient understanding of herbal medicine, as well as the connection between body, mind, and spirit]). It may be noted that indigenous cultures' shamans understood all these issues.

Dmitri has studied the philosophy of Pythagoras, of Socrates, of Plato, and Heraclitus, who taught that "all is in flux." He has studied the importance of spirituality, learning to meditate as he trained to become a priest of Aesculapius, recognizing Oneness, that all beings are interconnected, and the importance of unconditional love for his patients.

Dmitri has learned what are known in the East as *Siddhis*, providing insight into the patient's problem (as does Tibetan medicine). He has been taught clairvoyance and the ability to sense energies (as do indigenous healers in many cultures, and as is taught in many martial arts.[204]

Dmitri now faces his final examination. He will descend into an underground labyrinth in a temple dedicated to Aesculapius, where he will remain, without food or water, for seven days and nights. Prior to entering the labyrinth, Dmitri will sacrifice a cock to Aesculapius. There will be poisonous snakes in the labyrinth, which he will avoid (in total darkness) by sensing their energies, or by befriending them by radiating love and respect. If Dmitri survives this examination, he will be required, upon his emerging from the labyrinth, to report on events that had occurred elsewhere in Greece (his examiners will have sent runners to report on those events). This will test Dmitri's ability at distant viewing, an art useful in the diagnosis of his patients, still practiced in Tibetan medicine today.[205] For details of the initiation procedure see Bruyere, *Wheels of Light*.[206]

Dmitri's medical education would be derived from his teachers' mystery school training, both academic and spiritual schools: Hippocrates and Plato would be paramount, with Socrates and especially Pythagoras being important. Zoroaster in Persia and Imhotep in Egypt also provided important teachings. It should be noted that these teachings would later be incorporated into the teachings of the Essenes, the Druids, Jesus, the Gnostics, and beyond.

4.2 Fundamental Theme

Mystery Schools owe their name to the Greek Mysterium, "secret thing," the esoteric or mystical tradition handed down from ancient times. Mystery schools provided the fundamental source for the religions of the world—both Jesus and Paul were mystery school initiates, and they each refer to the Mysteries in the New Testament[207] (see Freke and Gandy, *The Jesus Mysteries*, and McCannon, *Jesus*,[208] for details). The Mysteries were Esoteric and focused on the Inner World as opposed to the exoteric, the

Outer World of the five senses of ordinary three-dimensional material reality. Mystery school teachings would speak of the Mysteries to those prepared for such knowledge; however, they would teach the unprepared masses in parables.

The fundamental theme of the Mysteries was the permanence of life, that even in the face of physical death there is no ultimate death, only changes of state throughout an ever-renewing existence. An agricultural metaphor would be the progression from seed to fruit, which bears the new seed that must be buried to start the cycle anew. Many mystery schools taught the doctrine of reincarnation.

Caitlin and John Matthews have written, in *The Western Way,* "The mystery traditions—Western and Eastern—are concerned with keeping open the door between the worlds, of letting through and mediating energies from inner worlds to outer worlds, of co-operating with the Otherworld reality of which our world is a yet unrealized resonance."[209] Clearly the mystery schools are continuing the tradition of the shamans, and one can trace a direct linear connection between shamans and mystery schools.

There were many interconnections between mystery schools even though they might be separated geographically. Atlantis had connections to Egypt (the Kaloo) and thence to Zoroaster and to Mithras, which in turn influenced the Essenes, with their ties to the Druids. These in turn were closely connected to the Gnostics, with later ties to the Cathars and to the Rosicrucians.

There are many parallels between the mystery schools and Indigenous shamans, their healing methods providing a prime example. Mystery schools were based on the insights of mystics, and not all agreed. There were those who espoused dualism, as did Zoroaster. Most mystery schools, however, subscribed to the monism of Atlantis, and so this is the perspective of, for example, the Essenes, the Druids, the Gnostics, and the Rosicrucians. Christianity took a different view and adopted the dualistic perspective of Zoroaster, one of God opposing Satan.

The great minds of antiquity were all students and/or initiates of mystery schools: Pythagoras, Hippocrates, Socrates,

Plato, Zoroaster, Euclid, Plotinus, Democritus, Hypatia, Thales, Plutarch, Cicero, Zeno, Solon, Jesus of Nazareth, Paul of Tarsus, and many others. More recently were Leonardo da Vinci, Paracelsus, Roger Bacon, William Blake, Botticelli, Sir Isaac Newton, John Milton, Johannes Kepler, Copernicus, Thomas More, Jacob Boehme, Sir Francis Bacon and more. All were trained in the mystery schools of Egypt, Greece, Britain or Europe, and some in the East as well.

4.3 Goals of Mystery Schools

The goals of the various mystery schools were quite consistent. They were focused on Oneness with the All (whether that All was known as Source, God, Allah, Cosmic Mind, or many other names, and it included all mankind and nature). Survivors of Atlantis considered themselves Children of the Law of One. They recognized a Universal Consciousness, with the essence of the universe being *Unconditional Love* (Compare Anita Moorjani's insights reported in *Dying to be Me*[210]).

Henry Drake, of the Philosophical Research Society, quoted in Tobias Churton's *The Gnostics*, said of the mystery schools, "The end of the sacred sciences was the abstraction of the human soul from bondage to the senses and its preparation to receive *within itself* the light of vast truths.... The secrets of the Mysteries are obviously metaphysical, philosophical, and esoteric and relate to processes taking place within the fields of the human psyche during the practice of the spiritual disciplines."[211]

Mystery schools instructed students about the operation of divine law in the physical world, recognizing that nature was both visible and invisible, and that together they composed Reality. Their teachings were based on spiritual insights or experiences of liberating *gnosis,* or spiritual knowledge.

Along the way the mystery school student would learn awareness, spiritual insight, manifestation (including healing, psychokinesis, and levitation), telepathy, Out-of-Body travel, mediumship, clairvoyance, intuitive diagnosis, and above all, communication with the Mind of God (sometimes designated as the Akashic Record, the Zero Point Field, or other names). A fundamental precept was "What you sow, you shall reap." The techniques that were taught were similar to the training of a shaman: awareness, meditation, unselfish love, visualization (with *feeling*), affirmations (with *feeling*), journeying. Note that the *feeling* gives power to the visualization or affirmation in its communication with the subconscious mind. *Feeling* was taught as essential to effective prayer.

4.4 Healing in Mystery Schools

Mystery school healers attended to all aspects of their patients, to mind, body, and spirit. They were unselfish and endeavored to become selfless and giving, to eliminate the ego and *self consciousness*. Mystery school students worked to attain humility in everything they did and thought and were to heal patients *gratis.*

4.5 Initiation

In general there were three grades of initiation in mystery schools. First came initiation into the Lesser Mysteries after studies of The Divine Feminine, including studies of Nature, Science, the Healing Arts, and Morality. Second was initiation into the Greater Mysteries—The Divine Masculine: The Father returns periodically as the Divine Son. To be prepared for this level of initiation required studies of History, Geometry, Mathematics, the Divinities, and the Healing power of Sound. If all these had been mastered, the final initiation was Mastery, including Spiritual Service to all humanity; recognition of our Eternal Natures, of Life, Death, and Rebirth.[212]

Initiation in a mystery school was a highly significant event. It signified death of the old life (ego), and rebirth to new life. This rebirth was represented in the Essene community by baptism. The initiate was committing to the Divine and sacrificing to Unconditional Love. He or she was surrendering to grace, marrying the inner male with the inner female. Initiation could be life-threatening if the student was unprepared, as exemplified by Dmitri's final examination. As in the shaman's training, initiation sometimes involved a Near Death Experience.

4.6 Mystery Schools' Locations and Secrecy

Mystery schools were located in many different regions, and secrecy was an issue. Teachers used oral transmission from teacher to candidate. If written documents were ever used, they would use cryptograms and symbols, hiding the underlying message. As a result, many ancient documents, including some of *Dead Sea Scrolls,* were written in code. Part of the reason for secrecy was to keep mysteries from those who were unprepared; another reason was for the safety of the community, an individual, or the school from their disbelieving contemporaries. Pythagoras's school at Croton was burned by jealous neighbors; Qumran was destroyed by Roman soldiers.

There were mystery schools in Lemuria, whence they went to Tibet, Japan, Australia, the Pacific Islands, Atlantis, and the Americas. From Atlantis mystery schools went to Egypt (where Thoth, known in Greece as Hermes Trismegistus, "Thrice-Great Hermes," a spiritual leader in Atlantis, led his disciples), also to the Druids, the Basques, and the Mayans. From Egypt mystery schools spread to Greece and to the Middle and Far East.

Thoth (Hermes Trismegistus) was an Atlantian who foresaw the destruction of Atlantis and led his followers to Egypt; he was an important figure in history. Thoth bestowed knowledge upon humanity, including geometry, astronomy, mathematics, medicinal herbs, and healing, as well as spiritual philosophy. He taught the use of language, initially hieroglyphics, and later, with his wife, established the 26-letter alphabet used in European languages today. Thoth endowed humanity with the natural laws of the physical world. He gave us the dictum, "As above, so below," indicating that the Microcosm reflects the Macrocosm.

Thoth established the first mystery schools outside of Atlantis, providing an understanding of the spiritual world. Both the Essenes and the Druids derived their origins from the Egyptian mystery schools and all attributed their teachings to the Kaloo, from the Old Land in the West. A large number of mystery schools in the centuries that followed were based on Hermetic principles. There is a significant connection between Egypt and the Druids: There was a migration of Egyptian leaders to Britain around 1500 BCE, and they claimed a common origin in Atlantis.

In spiritual accounts, Thoth is considered one of the four Sons of God, as is Jesus. However, there are other Egyptian mystery schools other than those associated with Thoth. The Isis Mysteries are one of the great Egyptian Mysteries; Isis is the Divine Mother, a Madonna with her son Horus. Mary Magdalene, before joining the Essenes, was a priestess of the Isis Mysteries.[213]

There are also the Osiris Mysteries. Osiris was born on the 25th of December; he was sacrificed and resurrected at Easter (*ergo*, Osiris provides many parallels to Jesus, including the Lord's Prayer)[214].

The Therapeutae ("Physicians of Souls") of Egypt had their primary base in Alexandria, and were known as "Jewish Pythagoreans," though their origins were probably much older than Pythagoras. The Therapeutae were an Egyptian branch of the Essenes and of the Great White Brotherhood; they had branches in Greece, Britain, Damascus, Galilee, Persia, and the Himalayas. They were among the masters of the Far East. Philo compared the Therapeutae to the Mysteries of Osiris; he commented that they provided the model for later Christian monks and nuns.[215]

4.7 Greek Mystery Schools

In Greece, important mystery schools were established that had a major influence on the West. The Elusinian mystery school was the classic and enduring Greek Mystery. The Dionisynian mystery school gave us the model of the sacrificed king. The Samothracian mystery school was perhaps less significant, but the Orphic mystery school has a significant impact to this day. Paul of Tarsus was apparently an initiate of the Orphic Mysteries, and, according to some sources, he later became a teacher to the Gnostics. Paul's association with the Mysteries is reflected in his letters to the Corinthians and so teaches us doctrines associated with mystery schools.[216]

4.8 Persia, Zoroaster, and Mithraism

In Persia, Zoroaster was the source of the Persian Mysteries, from which Mithraism derived. Mithras anticipated Jesus: Mithras was born in a cave on December 25th, watched over by shepherds. According to a Persian Mithraic text, at the end of his life, Mithras held a "last supper" with his disciples, at which time he stated, "He who will not eat of my body and drink of my blood so that he will be made one with me and I with him, the same shall not know salvation." According to some sources, Mithras was crucified and was resurrected three days later. One pair of authorities, Caitlin and John Matthews, has suggested that Mithras was a prefiguring of Christ.[217]

Mithraism was dualistic, with Ahura Mazda, representing the good, in contrast with Ahiriman, the negative force. It is significant that Jesus was said to be an initiate of the Mithraic Mysteries.[218] We note further, that Mithraism was the predominant Roman religion at the beginning of Christianity, and that Persia was, by Christian tradition, the land of the Magi present at the birth of Jesus.

4.9 The Essenes

The Essenes were found in Palestine and Lebanon, and had key connections to both the Druids and the Therapeutae. They were teachers of both Jesus and his cousin, John the Baptist. When Qumran was destroyed by Roman soldiers around 68 CE, remnants of the community moved to Egypt, where they joined the Therapeutae. However, the inhabitants of Qumran had foreseen this destruction, and key documents were removed long before the destruction occurred.

The Hebrew historian, Josephus, referring to the Essenes, commented, "They are eminent for fidelity and are the perfect Ministers of Peace.... They also take great pains in studying the writings of the Ancients and choose out of them that which is most for the advantage for their Soul and body." The Essenes were part of the Great White Brotherhood, which was established in Egypt previous centuries, at a time prior to the reign of Pharaoh Akhenaton, founder of a monotheistic religion in Egypt.

The name Essene denotes "secret" or "mystic," and is also translated as "the pious ones," "healers" or "holy ones." The Essenes studied Pythagorean, Egyptian, Persian, Buddhist, Hebraic, and Druidic teachings. They believed in the immortality of the soul, which they contrasted with the impermanence of the body. They believed in karma and reincarnation. They studied astronomy, medicine, mathematics, nature, and the sciences.

Historian Robert Siblerud writes that the Essenes practiced clairvoyance, telekinesis, levitation, laying on of hands, and restoring the dead to life. They had learned from the gurus of ancient India the arts of healing, herbs, languages, and esoteric philosophy. The Essenes practiced baptism as a symbol of rebirth, a practice later adopted by Christianity.

As indicated above, there was a close connection between the Essenes and the Druids. The Essenes lived in much the same way as did the Pythagoreans and the Buddhists. They were vegetarian, practiced communal living, and introduced meditation to their children at age two or three. This lifestyle caused Yale professor Washington Hopkins to write, "Finally, the life, temptation, miracles, parables, and even the disciplines of Jesus have been derived directly from Buddhism."

4.10 Hindu and Buddhist Mystery Schools

The Hindus of India were a source of many teachings. Some yogic masters taught the *siddhis*, though they warned their students not to be deterred by the *siddhis* on their path to enlightenment.

Buddhists in Tibet and Ladakh were a major influence on mystery schools. It is said that Jesus studied at a monastery in Ladakh, and there are many parallels between his teachings and Buddhism.

4.11 The Druids

Important mystery schools were taught by the Druids in both Britain and Europe. Druids were physicians, poets, and prophets, and they had an educational system superior to any on the European Continent. Druids had a Madonna, a Virgin Mother with a Child in her arms who was sacred to their Mysteries, and their solar lord died and was resurrected at Easter. Both the cross and the serpent (symbol of rebirth) were sacred to the Druids.

Druids celebrated the winter solstice, around December 25th as the birth date of the solar lord, when the Virgin gave birth to the Holy Son or Son of God, as was the case with Jesus, Mithras, Horus, and Osiris. The first Christian church was established in Britain by Joseph of Arimathea on land given by the British king and at the invitation of high ranking Druids.

4.12 The Gnostics

An extremely important mystery school in the West was established by the Gnostics, first in Alexandria and later in France, and we still find Gnostics among us today. The Gnostics followed the same three phases of initiation as other mystery schools, transmitting teachings orally in order to protect them from the unprepared. British historian Tobias Churton has written, "What the Gnostic knows is that this world is not his or her true home. While the world sleeps the Gnostic awakes.... The Gnostic knows that he or she is a spiritual being 'of one substance with the Father'; for what the orthodox say of Christ the Gnostic is free to say of himself."[219]

The term *Gnosis* implies Inner Spiritual Awareness and thereby direct access to God. The Gnostics were labeled heretics by the Roman Catholic Church, and were opposed especially by Bishop Irenaeus of Lyon. The Gnostics were persecuted by the Church during the second century CE. At that time the *Nag Hammadi* scrolls were buried and thus preserved for posterity, not to be found until 1945. As a result, much of what we know of the Gnostics, as well as the Essenes (*Dead Sea Scrolls*), has only recently been learned.

The last stronghold of the Gnostics was in southern France. There the Cathars, who were a later group of Gnostics, were massacred at the beginning of the 13th century by the armies of the Pope and of the king of France in the Albigensian Crusade. Nevertheless, Gnostic mystery schools have appeared here and there down to the present day. The author has been told of a Gnostic church in Palo Alto, California, and there have been Gnostic mystery schools in Mexico City (not currently active) and near Cusco in Peru.

4.13 The Kabbalah and the Quran

Other mystery schools have been based on the Kabbalah. These mystery schools have existed in Palestine, Arabia, and Greece. Though originally Jewish (and still a mystical aspect of Judaism), there were several schools of Christian interpretations of the Kabbalah, during the Middle Ages and down to the present.

The Quran gave birth to mystery schools among the Sufis and among the Dervishes of Arabia. Muhammad, prophet of Islam, grew up in a region of mystery schools, and his early writings reflect mystery school philosophies.

Beyond these two main lines of teaching, mystery schools spread, one being associated with Odin in Scandinavia and Europe.

4.14 Native American Mystery Schools

There were important mystery schools among Native Americans in North, Central, and South America. In North America we have the Hopi (with connections to Mayans, Atlantis and Lemuria), Diné (Navajo), Iroquois, Cherokee, and many mystery school philosophies, usually associated with medicine men or women.

In Central America we have the Mayans, who brought their mystery school from Atlantis. Fortunately, we have the Popal Vuh and other codices that give us an understanding of the Mayan philosophy. Drunvalo Melchizedek is a member of the Mayan Council of Elders and has written of their sacred ceremonies as well as their heritage and prophecies.[220]

In South America we had the Pre-Incas, the Incas, and the Q'ero, who escaped the Spanish Conquistadors by moving to the high Andes and are now divulging the teachings that have been kept secret through the centuries.

4.15 The Alchemists

The Alchemists of Egypt, Arabia, and later in Europe, were concerned with "spiritual chemistry." Alchemists, commonly known only for transmuting base metals into gold, had as their primary goal the spiritual transmutation of man. Sir Isaac Newton was one of the great alchemists, though we know him better today for his contributions to mathematics (calculus) and for his *Principia Mathematica,* containing the laws of physics that we use to this day.

4.16 The Rosicrucians

The Rosicrucians constitute a mystery school, primarily in Europe, but found throughout the globe today. The Rosicrucians are a spiritual movement combining spiritual philosophy with science. Rosicrucians trace their origins back to the Egyptian mystery schools. Modern Rosicrucianism, however, was founded at the beginning of the 17th century, based in part on the inspiration provided by the iconoclastic Swiss physician, theologian and mystic, Paracelsus, who will be discussed in a later chapter. As a consequence, there was a close relationship between the Rosicrucians and medicine, emphasizing the connection between medicine and spiritual knowledge. They taught that the cross symbolized the human body and the rose represented the individual's unfolding consciousness.[221]

The founders of the Brotherhood of the Rosy Cross were rebelling against the authoritarian universities of the day, with their dependence on the classics. Rosicrucians were also rebelling against both Roman and Protestant Churches, fighting "Papacy, Galen and Aristotle," for their rigidity of dependence on authority. They felt the Reformation had failed. Rosicrucians, like Gnostics, taught direct access to God; indeed, they were spoken of as a *Gnostic Brotherhood*. They believed in the principles found in Matthew 7:7, "Ask and ye shall receive; seek and ye shall find; knock and it shall be opened unto you."

Rosicrucians were very secretive, and they recognized the importance of the invisible as well as the visible. For a long time, they maintained invisibility as a protection, for they were opposing the establishment. Being outcasts themselves, Rosicrucians were tolerant of other religions, including both Judaism and Islam.

4.17 The Bible

It is of interest to note the Bible's relationship to mystery schools. There are multiple aspects of this relationship. Jesus had a mystery school education and initiations, which will be discussed below. Paul was an initiate of the Orphic Mysteries, a relationship reflected in his first letter to the Corinthians. Also significant in the English-speaking world, Sir Francis Bacon was a Rosicrucian, a cryptographer, and the general editor of the King James translation of the Bible. The book of Revelation is a Mystery document; and there are many Mysteries hidden in the King James Bible.

4.18 Freemasons

The Freemasons trace their history to Pre-Deluge Egypt. Later they were active in Palestine and Europe, and are prominent today. Freemasons were founded in mysticism, though today their service functions are often paramount. There is, among their teachings, an emphasis on moral conduct.[222]

4.19 Knights Templar

The Knights Templar trace their history back to the Djedi Knights of Atlantis, Persia, and Egypt, to the Crusades, the Holy Grail, and the Round Table of King Arthur's Britain. The "Star Wars" depiction of the Djedi Knights is, in fact, quite accurate. The modern history of the Knights Templar begins with Crusades, where they were guarding Christian pilgrims to Jerusalem. The Knights Templar were allegedly disbanded after 14th century persecution by the king of France, but, in fact, they are still to be found today.

There are other lesser known modern mystery schools still to be found today: Theosophy, Anthroposophy, New Thought churches, and many others.

4.20 History of Mystery Schools

The history of mystery schools appears to originate in Lemuria, with diasporas occurring both before and after Lemuria's destruction. From Lemuria, emissaries and refugees went to the Gobi Desert, to Tibet, to Australia, and to the Pacific islands (Easter Island and New Zealand, where there is a sub-tribe of the Maori [the Waitaha] with an ancestral memory of fleeing from Lemuria). In Japan, the Ainu are apparently descendants of Lemurians. The West Coast of North America is apparently a remaining land from Lemuria, and there are credible stories of Lemurian descendants living within Mt. Shasta. There are reputedly connections between the Mayans and Lemuria, and in South America connections between the pre-Inca culture and Lemuria. The Lemurians' culture was highly spiritual, and that spiritual focus is reflected in their descendants.

Clearly a source of mystery schools was Atlantis, where many from Atlantis departed both before and after its destruction. Many went to Egypt and, thence, to Tibet and elsewhere. Others went to Britain and founded the Druids and their mystery schools. The Basques in the Pyrenees appear to be descendants of Atlanteans, as do the Berbers and the Mayans.

From Egypt, colonists went to Tibet, Babylon, Persia, and India. In each case, mystery schools were a hallmark of the culture.

4.21 Notable Mystery School Leaders

There are multiple examples of prominent mystery schools' leaders: Hypatia was a scholar, a scientist, and a teacher of neo-Platonic philosophy in Alexandria. She proved and taught the pagan origins of the Christian faith and so gained the hatred of Cyril, Bishop of Alexandria. She was murdered by a group of Christian fanatics in 415 CE.

Another notable example of a mystery school founder and influential philosopher was Pythagoras. We find in him many parallels to the life of Jesus. In each case, it had been prophesied before his birth that the child would be a son, and a benefactor to mankind. Both families were traveling when their son was born. Both Pythagoras and Jesus were known to the multitudes as a *Son of God*. Both taught the importance of loving others, including your enemies. Both were killed bringing their teaching careers to an end.

The mystery school of Pythagoras was "dedicated to Horus/Apollo, the god of light and healing," according to Josephus. Pythagoras was himself a mystic, and the Pythagorean teachings were important to the Essenes, the Druids, and to the mystery schools that followed.

The education of Pythagoras was intensive. He was first initiated into the Greek mystery schools. Then, following the advice of the preeminent Greek philosopher Thales of Miletus, Pythagoras traveled to Egypt, where he spent 22 years at Memphis and Thebes studying mathematics and astronomy with Egyptian priests. He was initiated into the Mysteries of Isis at Thebes. In all, Pythagoras was initiated into fourteen mystery schools in Greece, Egypt, in the Near and Far East, and in India. By one tradition he is said to have conversed with Lord Buddha and the child Sri Krishna. This tradition appears reasonable, for the dates are appropriate.

Pythagoras was a healer. He healed with sound, herbs, aromas and color. He taught that harmony was the key to health, and he healed body, mind, and spirit alike. He was an inspiration and major influence on Hippocrates, who learned from Pythagoras that harmony of body, mind, and spirit was the key to health.

Pythagoras was a teacher. He founded the first coeducational university, and his requirements for admission were rigorous. His most famous student was Plato, who learned much from him even though Plato lived years after Pythagoras's death.

Pythagoras was a scientist, his most important discoveries being in astronomy. He recognized that the earth was spherical, that the rotation of the earth produced day and night, and that the earth moved around the sun. In this recognition Pythagoras anticipated Copernicus, who acknowledged Pythagoras' priority two thousand years later. Unfortunately, Aristotle did not accept Pythagoras' heliocentric astronomy, and Aristotle's views were later adopted by St. Thomas Aquinas and became Church dogma.

Pythagoras was a mathematician. He is best known for the Pythagorean Theorem in geometry. He considered numbers to be the basis of the universe.

Pythagoras was a musician. He discovered the mathematical basis of music, and he used both voice and lyre to inspire and to heal. He was a composer as well as a musician. He recognized the "music of the spheres," only recently recorded by NASA.

Pythagoras recognized that secrecy was critical. As a result, we have no direct records of his teaching, only reports of his students. Pythagoras was killed by a mob.

Pythagoras viewed God as the Supreme Mind, a Mind distributed throughout the universe. He considered God to be the Cause of all things, the Intelligence of all things, the Power within all things. He taught that the nature of God was composed of the substance of truth.

Initiation into the Pythagorean Mysteries was a multiple day drama. It took place in an underground labyrinth. Initiation signified the death of the ego and a rebirth as a realized man or woman.

The historian Tricia McCannon writes, "Pythagoras' teachings were highly revered, not only by the Druids and the Greeks, but by the Essene sect of which Jesus and his family were a part. In fact, early Christian sects recognized Pythagoras as a true prophet and Herald of the Good Realm, and drew on the philosophy, science, and metaphysics taught in the ancient Orphic, Pythagorean, Platonic, and Neo-Platonic mystery schools."[223]

Most significant to our Western culture is the life of Jesus of Nazareth. There are many parallels between the life of Jesus and the life of Osiris, including the Lord's Prayer. There are also many parallels with the lives of Pythagoras, Mithras and the Solar Lord of the Druids.

Jesus spent the first years of his life in Alexandria, a center of scientific, philosophical and spiritual knowledge, taught by Therapeutae, a branch of the Great White Brotherhood and of the Essenes. He began his education by the Essenes at age eight, first at Qumran and later at Mount Carmel. Jesus' university education began at age 15 in Britain, where there were cultural centers, libraries, and universities taught by Druids. The Druids had close ties to the Essenes, recognizing the importance of a balance between physical, mental, emotional, and spiritual bodies. They also cultivated the gifts of prophecy, healing, and opening the third eye. Most relevant was a mystery school that included studies of the Kabbalah, also natural philosophy, astronomy, mathematics, law, medicine, poetry and oratory. It normally required 20 years to complete this education, but Jesus was an exceptional student.[224]

Jesus later traveled to the Near and Far East for further studies. There is today a monastery in Ladakh that has a record of the young Palestinian Jesus who was a student there 2,000 years ago. Jesus traveled widely with his uncle, Joseph of Arimathea, and he was fully conversant with the cultures of Alexandria, Athens, Rome and Persia.

Jesus was renowned for his healing "miracles." When he healed, he never said "God made you whole" or "I healed you," but he would often comment, "Your belief (in some translations "faith") has made you whole." That faith had eliminated the invisible *cause* of the sickness, and the self-healing capacity of the individual had done the rest.

4.22 Origin of Mystery School Teachings

An important question is: "How are mystery schools all teaching similar things?" One common factor would be their common origin in Lemuria and Atlantis. Another possible explanation is that the mystery schools' founding mystics all had access to the same library of knowledge, whether that Common Source is known as the Quantum Hologram, the Akashic Record, the Zero Point Field, the Mind of God, or by another name. This would appear to be the source not only tapped into by mystics, but by the "sleeping prophet," Edgar Cayce, and by shamans, intuitives, and many dowsers.

4.23 Modern Mystery Schools

As we have seen, there are many modern mystery schools. Included would be the Gnostics, found in England, the Americas, and in Europe. The Knights Templar are found in America and around the globe. There are Druids in Britain and America. Kabbalists are found in Israel, in America, and in Europe. Rosicrucians are found around the globe; they are service-oriented as well as metaphysical. Masons are also found globally; they too are service-oriented and fraternal as well as metaphysical.

Contemporary mystery schools that are not secret would include the martial arts, which use invisible energies in detecting their opponents' moves. The philosophies of the mystery schools can also be found in New Thought churches and other Hermetic schools.

A very important category of mystery schools are the Indigenous peoples and their shamans. Examples would include the Australian Aborigines, the Inca shamans, the Amazonian shamans, and the North American medicine men and women.

Notes

203 Dorjee, Pema, Janet Jones and Terence Moore, *Heal Your Spirit, Heal Yourself: The Spiritual Medicine of Tibet*, Watkins Publishing LTD, 2005.
204 A friend of the author's studied Aikido, and the final exam for the course require the blindfolded student to face three attackers and to defend herself by sensing the energy of the attacks.
205 Dorjee, Pema, Janet Jones and Terence Moore, *Heal Your Spirit, Heal Yourself: The Spiritual Medicine of Tibet*, Watkins Publishing LTD, 2005.
206 Bruyere, Rosalyn, *Wheels of Light: A Study of the Chakras*, Sierra Madre, CA, Bon Productions, 1989.
207 Freke, Timothy and Peter Gandy, *The Laughing Jesus: Religious Lies and Gnostic Wisdom*, Harmony, 2006.
208 McCannon, Tricia, *Jesus: The Explosive Story of the 30 Lost Years and the Ancient Mystery Religions*, Hampton Roads, 2010.
209 Matthews, Caitlin and John. *The Western Way: A Practical Guide to the Western Mystery Tradition, Vol. 2, The Hermetic Tradition*, Arkana, 1988.
210 Moorjani, Anita, *Dying to Be Me: My Journey from Cancer, to Near Death, to True Healing*, Hay House, 2014.
211 Churton, Tobias, *The Gnostics*, Orion Publishing Co., 1996.
212 McCannon, Tricia, *Jesus: The Explosive Story of the 30 Lost Years and the Ancient Mystery Religions*, Charlotteville, VA: Hampton Roads, 2010.
213 Leloup, Jean-Yves, The Gospel of Mary Magdalene, Rochester, VT, Inner Traditions, 2002.
214 Budge, E. A. Wallis, *The Gods of the Egyptians*, Dover Publications, 1969.
215 Philo Judeaus of Alexandria, David Winston translator, *Philo of Alexandria: On the Contemplative Life, The Giants, and Selections*, Mahwah, NJ, Paulist Press, 1981.
216 I and II Corinthians, *The Bible*, pretty much any edition out there.
217 Matthews, Caitlin and John Matthews, *Walkers Between the Worlds: The Western Mysteries from Shaman to Magus*, Rochester, VT, Inner Traditions, 2004.
218 Ulansey, David, "The Mithraic Mysteries", *Scientific American*, Vol. 261, No. 6, 1989.
219 Churton, Tobias, *The Gnostics*,
220 Melchizedeck, *The Mayan Ouroboros*.
221 Churton, Tobias, *The Invisible History of the Rosicrucians: The World's Most Mysterious Secret Society*, Inner Traditions, 2009.
222 Pike, Albert, *Morals and Dogma of the Ancient and Accepted Scottish Rite of Freemasonry*, Charleston, 1871.
223 McCannon, Tricia, *Jesus: The Explosive Story of the 30 Lost Years and the Ancient Mystery Religions*, Charlotteville, VA: Hampton Roads, 2010.
224 Cannon, Dolores, *Jesus and the Essenes*, Ozark Mountain Publishing, 2000.

Chapter 5
The Material and the Invisible, or Is What We See All There Is?

5.1 The Origin of Materialism

Four hundred years ago (2,000 years ago if one considers Aristotle's logic a forerunner of materialism) a series of events occurred that led to a materialist science, including medical science, and a materialist culture. Let us provide some background and so set the scene.

The origins of healing practices have been traced from Lemuria to Atlantis to Egypt and the East and to Greece. Shamans and the Mystery Schools and their connection with healing were addressed in the preceding chapters.

Key to our understanding of the development of ancient healing practices is Pythagoras—mystic, scientist, healer, honored by many in the ancient world, including the Essenes and the Druids, and both a student and a founder of Mystery Schools. Pythagoras fully understood the importance of the spiritual, the invisible.

Although he lived later than Pythagoras, Plato is today the best-known student of Pythagoras' teachings. The importance of the invisible is well illustrated in Plato's allegory of the Cave. In that allegory, Plato describes a group of people sitting in chairs and bound, facing the back of the cave. Reality is outside the cave, and those bound in the chairs can see only the shadows cast by the outside light onto the back wall of the cave. Reality is outside; only the shadows of that reality are seen by the people in the cave. What the viewers observed was only the shadow of the True Reality.[225] David Bohm's Implicit and Explicit universes reflect a modern physicist's expression of the same concept.[226]

Hippocrates was also a student of Pythagorian teachings and was greatly influenced by them. Considered the Father of Western medicine, Hippocrates will be discussed in a later chapter. He was and still is renowned today as a physician and scientist, and he was a priest as well.

The Material and the Invisible

Pythagoras was an astronomer, and he recognized that the earth revolved around the sun. When, two thousand years later, Copernicus came to the same conclusion, he recognized that Pythagoras had understood the heliocentric makeup of the solar system long before.

Unfortunately, Aristotle disagreed with Pythagoras: Aristotle believed the heavens were unchanging. St. Thomas Aquinas found Aristotle's views appealing and accepted them. As a result, Aristotle's opinion became Church dogma, and to believe otherwise was considered heresy. With Aristotle's views being accepted by the Church as dogma, Copernicus wisely did not publish his findings until shortly before his death in 1543. For committing the heresy of believing Copernicus was correct, philosopher and mystic Giordano Bruno was burned at the stake by the Roman Inquisition in 1600. A few years later (400 years ago), Galileo was accused of the same heresy. Fully aware of Bruno's fate, Galileo denied his belief that Copernicus was correct, but he was nevertheless found guilty of being "Vehemently suspected of heresy." He was sentenced to house arrest for the remainder of his life.[227]

A few years later, the renowned French mathematician and philosopher René Descartes agreed with Bruno and Galileo that Copernicus was correct. However, recognizing the position of the Roman Inquisition and the fates of Bruno and Galileo, Descartes concluded that it would be politic not to publish his opinion. Descartes had been sickly as a youth and had developed an interest in medicine, and he found it expedient to strike a bargain with the Church: "You give me the body, and I will give you the mind and the soul." There was no hypocrisy in this bargain, for Descartes believed in a universe, including man, that functioned as a clockwork, and he believed that the body did not require a mind to function.[228] Descartes' views of a clockwork universe were reflected in his physics as well as his medicine, and those views laid the groundwork for today's materialism in both our science and our culture.

Descartes' views were followed fifty years later, in 1687, by those of Sir Isaac Newton, who laid down the mathematical rules for the interaction of separate bodies in his *Principia Mathematica*. Newton's laws work very well, and we use them constantly, (for example, computing trajectories to send rockets to the moon). Science came to think of the universe as reflecting the interaction of separate objects. Newton's influence further reinforced Descartes' materialism.

Thus, science recognizes a "billiard ball" universe (separate interacting objects). Scientists conduct experiments which have outcomes that they can see and/or measure. If their instruments are unable to measure something, then that thing is not considered real. As a consequence, the invisible universe of the ancients—of the Egyptians, of Pythagoras, Plato, Socrates and Hippocrates—is "not real" to materialist scientists.

The materialist perspective in the West was followed and reinforced in 1859 with the publication of Charles Darwin's *On the Origin of Species*. Darwin's theory of evolution, and the interpretation of "survival of the fittest" that followed, contributed to materialistic science and culture, including medical science. It may be noted that Chaos Theory (the recently developed theory of non-linear systems, systems found throughout nature) demonstrates that our universe is far from being the clockwork universe of Descartes or the billiard ball universe of Newton. Cooperation, rather than competition, is the way Nature truly works. (For a lucid and scientific discussion of this issue, see Gregg Braden's *Deep Truth: Igniting the Memory of Our Origin, History, Destiny, and Fate*.[229])

Darwin's highly influential theory was followed less than 30 years later by an experiment that abolished 19th century physicists' quest for the *luminiferous ether,* the invisible field that physicists had believed permeated the universe and connected all things. Michelson-Morley's 1887 experiment, using the limited instrumentation of the day, was interpreted as demonstrating that no such field was present, that objects were truly unconnected. Note that in 1986 scientist E. W. Silvertooth repeated Michelson-Morley's experiment using the far more sensitive instruments of today's science and proved that the interpretation of Michelson-Morley's results as demonstrating that objects were truly separate and unconnected was false. The universe is in fact interconnected, as today's science has proven, again and again.[230]

The influence of Descartes, Newton, Darwin, and Michelson-Morley have led not only to a materialistic science but to a materialistic culture with consequences that prompted His Holiness the Dalai Lama to write, "Yet even in the most developed countries we do not find a corresponding increase in peace and happiness; if anything, there is even greater anxiety and stress. Fear stimulates the need for terrifyingly destructive weapons systems, while greed gives rise to damage and pollution of the environment, putting the very existence of humanity at risk.

"These trends are symptomatic of the dangers of pursuing external progress alone. What is missing is a corresponding inner development. To redeem the balance, our new frontier should be inner worlds, not outer space. If the mind is explored with the same stringent scrutiny applied in other branches of science, it will certainly be of immense benefit not only to individuals but to society as a whole."[231] The Dalai Lama's perspective is reflected in Gary Zukov's *The Seat of the Soul*.[232] The significance of the Dalai Lama's comments are reflected in today's dismal health statistics.

5.2 Commonality of Traditional Medicines

Before addressing the invisible, first let us review the commonality of traditional medicines. It is apparent that traditional medicines, across time and space, say much the same thing. A first example is acupuncture and acupressure, found in China, Japan, among the Incas, but also formerly in Tibet, *and* in Europe, evidenced by the so-called "Ice Man," found in a Swiss glacier and dated around 8,000 BCE.

Chakras are associated with India but are also found in Navajo and Inca medicines. Among the Incas chakras are known as *Ojos de luz*. Recognition of auras is found among many Indigenous cultures, including the Hopi, the Inca, the Maya, the

Maori, among Tibetan physicians, mystics, and many modern spiritual healers.

Many commonalities are found among Traditional Medicines, including the definition of health and disease. In Egypt we find emphasis placed on the importance of balance and harmony between man and the cosmos. In Greece the term *eucrasia* suggests the importance of harmony, of the balance of the four humors. The harmony of body, mind, and spirit is a requisite for true health.

In Tibetan medicine, per Tibetan physician Dr. Pema Dorjee, the goal is to balance the three basic humors, recognizing the "essential need for balance, harmony." Dr. Dorjee further comments, "spirituality is the driving force behind all healing."[233]

In Ayurvedic medicine the goal is to balance the three humors, the body's energies. Chinese medicine strives for the balance of yin and yang and of the five elements. Hawaiian medicine has as its goal *lokahi*—harmony within the individual, within the patient's relationships, with the environment, and with God, *Akua*.

Among various Indigenous cultures, shamans proceed with the assumption that *"All is spirit."* Health is defined as the attainment of inner balance, inner purification from imbalance. Shamanic healing does not seek to eliminate symptoms—that would go against nature. The shaman's intent is to heal the entire life, not just the dysfunction or the symptoms.

Diagnostic procedures among traditional medicines also have much in common. All use a meditative state to gather information. Many traditional physicians use the measurement of pulses to gather diagnostic information. In ancient Greece the use of pulse diagnosis was similar to its later use in China, Tibet, and India.

The Tibetan physician, in a meditative state, would tune into his patient in. He used pulses, observation, the energy of the patient, plus palpation. The Tibetan physician strives to go beneath signs and symptoms always cognizant that the root of all suffering is in the mind.

Recently, Dr. Lissa Rankin reviewed the scientific literature and found studies that reflected the Tibetan point of view, that the root of suffering is in the mind. Dr. Rankin published her findings in a book pointedly entitled *Mind Over Medicine.*[234]

For the Chinese, Ayurvedic, Tibetan, or Japanese physician, pulses are best measured in a meditative state. The *Unani Tibb* (Greek medicine healing the physical, mental and spiritual realms) medicine found in Afghanistan and portions of India similarly assessed pulses in a deep meditative state.

Many traditional medicines used dreams to tune into the subconscious mind of their patients. In Tibet both the physicians' dreams or visions and also the patients' dreams were used. The Chinese used dream diagnosis in classical Chinese medicine.[235] Dreams played an important role in Greece, where incubation in Aesculapian temples was an important part of healing practice. In Hawaii the dreams of both the patient and the *kahuna* were used.

Many traditional medicines used detection of auras for diagnostic purposes. The physician might see the patient's aura or sense the energy of the aura, usually with his or her hands. This is true of Tibetan and Hawaiian medicine; the author's teacher, Papa Auwae, used his hands to sense the energy field and thereby diagnose the patient's problem. Inca shamans read auras to diagnose a patient's illness.

Today research has confirmed the value of auras for diagnostic information. As stated in earlier chapters, Dr. Valerie Hunt at UCLA has conducted such research with aura reader Rosalyn Bruyere. Jack Schwarz has diagnosed both present and past illness in the aura, seeing "tree rings" in the invisible (to most) etheric body indicating past disease or injury. The Canadian healer Adam sees both auras and holographic images of his patients.[236]

Medical intuitives such as Carolyn Myss and Caroline Sutherland are noted for the accuracy of their diagnoses, even though they may be many miles distant from their patients. Dr. James Esdaile, who learned hypnosis while stationed in the

Punjab in the 1840s, found a subject who was capable of diagnosing a patient's illness when in a hypnotic trance.

Most traditional medicines use treatment methods calculated to bring the energy of the patient back into balance, thus facilitating the patient's self-healing. The healer would recommend changes in the patient's lifestyle and his diet. Hippocrates was noted to have said, "Leave thy drugs in the chemist's pot if thou can heal the patient with food." Herbs were used to channel energy as required. Shamans, through shamanic journeying, would gain information as needed to heal the patient. Amazonian natives, in answer to an ethnobotanist's inquiry about the healing power of a plant, responded, "Ask the plant!"[237]

Acupuncture and acupressure were and are used by Greek, Chinese, Tibetan (in the past), American, and European healers. Counseling was often required if an emotional or spiritual cause of the illness was present—careful history taking would be important in such cases.

Specifics of treatment modalities varied. In Tibetan medicine, in addition to lifestyle, diet, the use of herbs to channel energy, and counseling as appropriate, the relationship between patient and doctor was recognized as being crucial, and the importance of spirituality was fully recognized: "*Spirituality* is the driving force behind all healing.... Spiritual support lay as an all-embracing power at the foundation of all ancient cultures. These cultures were linked so inextricably with this divine power, that every fragment of their existence was totally aligned with this divine power, that every fragment of their existence was totally aligned with spirituality. Physicians from these cultures encouraged spiritual practice for their patients as an essential aid to healing."[238]

In Greece the primary treatments were lifestyle, diet, exercise, herbs as necessary, rarely chemicals or surgery. The Chinese used the same methods as did the Tibetans, plus acupuncture.

The Native American medicine man Frank Fools Crow said his goal was to be a "hollow bone" for the spirits' healing. Fools Crow used herbs, and sometimes a form of hypnosis.

Healers such as Rosalyn Bruyere direct energy to low energy locations, energy blockages, etc. Her intent is to restore balance to the patient's energy field. Thus, Bruyere is healing in a manner similar to that of the Tibetans and Chinese.

A Hawaiian *kahuna* might use energy work (*lomi lomi*) to influence the patient's energy fields at the same time that she or he used diet, herbs, and counseling. The use of prayer was important before approaching the patient. Essential to effective healing is the advice to the healer, to *'Always give hope!'* Fractures have been discussed previously, and it should be noted that Max Freedom Long's report in the1920s of a *kahuna* healing a fracture in minutes is likely accurate. Such healing is confirmed by contemporary Slim Sperling's experience, where he brought about healing of a fracture with focused energy in 20 minutes. It should be noted that orthopedic surgeon Dr. Robert Becker has similarly used electrical energy to accelerate fracture healing.

The Hawaiian approach to cancer was to use prayer, meditation, lifestyle, diet, and herbs. The story was related previously of the hospital administrator, diagnosed with stomach cancer and given six months to live. Her first instruction was to sit at the seaside and to meditate, for days. The author knew her 14 years later.

Medicine was far from the only similarity between ancient cultures. Laszlo comments, "Although each culture added its own embellishments, Aztecs and Etruscans, Zulus and Malaya, classical Indians and ancient Chinese built their monuments and fashioned their tools as if following a shared pattern."[239]

5.3 Interconnectedness in the Invisible

A feature found in most traditional cultures is a recognition of the interconnectedness between humans and with all nature. This is a recurring theme in traditional medicines, the sense that we're somehow connected to the universe and to each other. This is depicted in Australian cliff art, around 20,000 years old, as well as art in many Egyptian temples.

The Hindu Vedas are believed to be more than 7,000 years old. They depict Indra as the supreme ruler of the gods in Vedic times. Indra's Net is notable in its description of the universe:

There is an endless net of threads throughout the universe.
The horizontal threads are in space.
The vertical threads in time.
At every crossing of threads there is an individual.

In Greece the existence of an *ether* was recognized as a universal field of energy that connects everything. Hawaiians recognize the *aka* threads that unite everything. The Celtic Druids similarly refer to the *Web of Wyrd,* the Web of Being.

The Native American Chief Seattle described a "Web of life; we are all interconnected." The Iroquois refer to the "longbody," a web interconnecting tribe members both living and dead.

Mystics of all religions recognize this interconnectedness, and the contemporary healer Adam sees interacting auras.[240] Science is now verifying the existence of this interconnectedness (entanglement), as will be discussed later.

Laszlo observes, "At the quantum level, reality is strange and it is nonlocal (entangled); the whole universe is a network of time and space-transcending interconnection.... Their nonlocality respects neither time nor space: it exists whether the distance that separates the particles and the atoms is measured in millimeters or in light-years, and whether the time that separates them consists of seconds or of millions of years."[241]

Entanglement applies on a macro scale as well as on the micro. German biophysicist Marco Bischof has summarized his views: "Quantum mechanics has established the primacy of the inseparable whole. For this reason, the basis of the new biophysics must be the insight into the fundamental interconnectedness *within* the organism as well as *between* organisms, and that of the organism *with the environment."* (Emphasis Bischof's).

Laszlo emphasizes this point: "... At the roots of reality there is an interconnecting, information-conserving, and information-conveying cosmic field. For thousands of years, mystics and seers, sages and philosophers maintained that there was such a field; in the East they called it the Akashic Field.... Today, at the new horizons opened by the latest scientific discoveries, this field is being rediscovered."[242]

5.4 Spiritual Component in Healing

There is a spiritual component of healing implicit in much of the above, a theme repeated throughout history. Thoth (Hermes Trismegistus) was the founder of both Egyptian religion and medicine. Hippocrates was a priest of Aesculapius as well as a great physician. Pythagoras, Socrates, and Plato were both spiritual teachers and healers. The spiritual focus of Tibetan medicine has been mentioned earlier.

Fools Crow and Black Elk were considered holy men as well as medicine men. They are not alone among their people. The American physician, Dr. Lewis Mehl-Madrona, a graduate of Stanford Medical School, commented that he learned more from his Cherokee and Lakota elders than he did from many of his medical school professors.[243]

Perhaps the healer with whom most of us are familiar is Jesus of Nazareth, but we do well to recognize that the Buddha was a healer as well as a holy man, as was Mohammed and other Muslim holy men and healers. Quetzalcoatl, Kulkukan, and Viracocha were all holy men revered in the Americas, and they were healers as well.

The Australian Aborigines spend much time in meditation, as do their healers. Taoist sages are the originators of Chinese medicine. Early Christians performed many healings, as did St. Hildegard von Bingen in the Middle Ages, whose medicine is practiced today in Germany and which includes a major spiritual component.

More contemporary is the Anthroposophic medicine of Rudolf Steiner, who felt that health depends on energy balance, and that distortions in one's energy arise from imbalance in soul and spirit. Today John of God in Brazil uses spiritual energy as he heals thousands (Technically, John of God is a medium who serves as a channel for healing energy.)

5.5 What Is the Information Source?

Given this similarity in traditional medicines, we return to the central mystery,

How can all traditional medicines be so similar? What is the information source?

In some cases there appears to be a geographical connection: as in Hawaiian medicine's connection to Egypt, Greece, and India,—regions through which Hawaiians migrated on their way to the Pacific Ocean, as indicated by their genealogy chants. The Hawaiian language is linguistically connected with North Africa. There also appears to be a connection between Tibetans and Navajos, in their respective religions and languages. Is navigation the answer? Clairvoyance? Telepathy? Same Source?

Most commonly, traditional medicines are "revealed" in visions, dreams, Near Death Experiences, the insights of spiritual leaders, mystics, prophets, sages and shamans. *What is the source of their common insights?*

One might hypothesize that DNA is the source of the visions, that shamans and others take their consciousness down to the molecular level and gain access to information originating in DNA, that which shamans call "animate essences" or "spirits." Per Narby, "This is where they see double helixes, twisted ladders, and chromosome shapes."[244] The next step is to infer that the knowledge contained in DNA, in turn comes from the Akashic Field described below.

We should note that the ability to envision microscopic events is not limited to shamans. Theosophists Charles Leadbeater and Annie Besant, using yoga techniques thousands of years old, accurately described elements down to the molecular level, and even to the atomic and subatomic level, at the end of the 19th century. They accurately depicted not only all the atomic elements but the subatomic particles (e.g., quarks)—all a hundred years before physicists verified the existence of these particles.[245] Nevertheless, the question still remains: *What is the ultimate information source?*

5.6 The Science

The scientific advances of the past 50 years have revealed that we live in an *informed universe.* We now know that the universe is made up of not only matter and energy, but also *information.* But let's look first at the historical precedents for our new understanding.

Thoth (Hermes Trismegistus) taught "As above, so below," a fundamental tenet of Ancient Egyptian spiritual knowledge. This understanding existed somewhere between 5,000 and 12,000 years ago, if not earlier. The Hindu philosopher Patanjali, some 2,300 years ago, called the source "above" the Akashic Record: *Akasha* is a Sanskrit word meaning "ether": all-pervading space. Originally signifying "radiation" or "brilliance" in Hindu philosophy; *akasha* was considered to be the first and the most fundamental of the five elements, the others being *vata* (air), *agni* (fire), *ap* (water), and *prithivi* (earth). *Akasha* embraces the properties of all five elements. It is the womb from which everything we perceive with our senses has emerged and into which everything will ultimately re-descend. The Akashic Record, also called The Akashic Chronicle, is the enduring record of all that happens, and has ever happened, in space and time.[246]

Mystics of various cultures have called this field The Mind of God. Vedanta mystic Swami Vivekananda describes it as "the infinite ocean of knowledge and power that lies behind mankind."[247]

We note that the term Akashic Record was given to Edgar Cayce, the Sleeping Prophet, when he asked the source of the information he tapped into when doing readings in a sleeping trance state. It was in this trance state that he responded to clients' health needs and provided past life or other historical information. For a discussion of the use of the Akashic Record to gain access to past life information, see Sherri Cortland's *Spiritual Toolbox.*[248]

According to Mayan tradition, around 1,000 years ago (earlier, if Mayans came from Atlantis) the Maya described 13 Tones as the energy frequencies in our lives and in creation. For example, Tone Four is that associated with balance and healing.

The Twelfth Tone is describing what Patanjali called the Akashic Record, the Mayans calling it the *Library of All Knowledge*. The Twelfth Tone has the energy of Wisdom and promotes understanding. Tone Twelve creates by adding the memory of each and every one of our experiences, along with the knowledge gained from them, to this Universal Library. This Library is sometimes called the *Vast Mind of God*.[249]

English biologist Rupert Sheldrake has long been interested in how DNA information about the production of proteins is translated into different biological forms. In the course of his research, he has developed the hypothesis of formative causation, the formation of *morphic fields*—fields that contain information about structure and forms, whether that field is morphogenetic, behavioral, or social (i.e., ant and bee colonies, flocks of birds, schools of fish, or packs of wolves, anywhere the group acts as one)—again an information field. The morphic field concept further provides a perspective on such phenomena as telepathy and precognition.[250]

International journalist, author, and movie industry pioneer J. Allen Boone has extended communication from humans to animals (intuiting the thoughts behind the words), finding that animals had much to teach him if he were able to greet them with respect, love, and understanding. Boone found that even "dangerous" animals, snakes and insects were companionable fellow beings if given the respect, love and understanding, subjectively as well as objectively, that animals desire. Boone refers to the field in which such communication occurs as the Mind of the Universe, the divine consciousness, the omniactive intelligence.[251]

This field is not limited to inter-human or to human-animal communication. Eliot Cowan, in *Plant Spirit Medicine,* describes human-plant communication that enables Indigenous peoples throughout the world to ascertain which plants are appropriate to heal a particular patient's illness.[252]

Nineteenth-century physicists described a "Luminiferous Ether" that has many of the characteristics of this field. Carl Jung called this field of information the "Collective Unconscious", and

The Material and the Invisible

French theologian Teilhard de Chardin called the field the "noosphere", envisioning a mental envelope that encompasses the earth like a threaded fabric, connecting all minds, all consciousness together in a web of luminescence.

Astrophysicist, founder of the Institute of Noetic Sciences, and Apollo 14 astronaut Edgar Mitchell observed, after returning from the moon, that information is a fundamental part of the universe. This observation conforms with the Indigenous peoples' ability to know of events outside of their sensory range.

Physicist and Einstein protégé David Bohm has referred to the reality underlying this field as the "Implicate Order."[253] Canadian psychiatrist and mystic Richard Bucke called it "Cosmic Consciousness,[254] as does quantum physicist Amit Goswami. Systems philosopher Ervin Laszlo, calls it the "Akashic Field."

This field has also been called the "Field of Loving Awareness," the "Field of Information," or simply, "The Field." Scientist Gregg Braden has recently called it the "Divine Matrix."[255]

5.7 Characteristics of The Field

Modern physics is now getting a sense of the makeup of The Field.[256] Schrödinger's Equation, one of the fundamental descriptions of quantum physics, includes a background term that is commonly subtracted out as being a constant factor not important in applications of the Equation (so-called "renormalization"). This factor describes the subatomic energy fluctuations of "empty space," sometimes called by the misleading term, "Quantum Vacuum". A more informative term now used by many physicists is the "Quantum Plenum", as space is far from empty—indeed, it is "an interconnecting, information-conserving and information-conveying cosmic field. For thousands of years, mystics and seers, sages and philosophers maintained there is such a field; in the East they called it the Akashic Field. However, the majority of Western scientists considered it a myth, for it cannot be measured (yet). Today, at the new horizons opened by the latest scientific discoveries, this field is being rediscovered. The effects of the Akashic Field are not limited to the physical world." As Laslo asserts, "The A-field (as we shall call it) informs all living things—the entire web of life. It also informs our consciousness."[257]

Superstring theorist Michio Kaku calls this field the "Quantum Hologram," a term that describes its properties well. Physicists are coming to recognize that, though perhaps not important in quantum applications such as the design of computer chips, the factor "renormalized" out of Schrödinger's Equation describes a fundamental and extremely important aspect of our universe.

Theoretical physicist Amit Goswami has suggested that consciousness is even more fundamental than are either matter or energy. Professor Goswami refers to this field as "Cosmic Consciousness", and points to the significance of its properties of non-locality, discontinuity, and downward causation—the opposite of the upward causation posited by those limited in their world view to material realism. The downward causation posited by Goswami originates from considerations of quantum measurement, which result in the following:

(1) Consciousness is the ground of all being.

(2) Matter, vital energies, mental meaning, and supramental archetypes are all quantum possibilities of consciousness.

(3) We choose, not in the ordinary state of consciousness that we call ego, but in a nonordinary state of consciousness that is variously known as unitive, nonlocal, or cosmic consciousness, a state in which we experience ourselves as one with everyone else.

(4) In an event of quantum collapse, consciousness splits itself into what we experience as subject-object awareness, subject experiencing an object as separate from it.

(5) Past experiences cloud our cosmic nature to an apparent individuality, the ego, via a process that can be called conditioning.[258]

Goswami's view of this field as fundamental is joined by scholars such as Ervin Laszlo, who refers to it as the Akashic Field. Laszlo comments that through the ages mystics and seers have affirmed that consciousness is fundamental in the universe. Seyyed Hossein Nasr, a medieval Islamic scholar and philosopher, wrote, "[T]he nature of reality is none other than consciousness."[259] Sri Aurobindo concurred: "[A]ll is consciousness—at various levels of its own manifestation....This universe is a gradation of planes of consciousness."[260] Scientists have occasionally joined the ranks of the mystics. Sir Arthur Eddington noted, "[T]he stuff of the universe is mind-stuff...the source and condition of physical reality."[261] And the Nobel Laureate biologist George Wald said "Mind, rather than emerging as a late outgrowth of the evolution of life, has existed always."[262]

Other physicists have studied this field both theoretically and experimentally. In addition, neurosurgeon and former Harvard Medical School faculty member Eben Alexander, M.D., may have had a direct experience of what may be this same field during a Near Death Experience (NDE) that he describes in *Proof of Heaven: A Neurosurgeon's Journey into the Afterlife.* Dr. Alexander, a skeptic about reported NDEs prior to his own experience, reports that he experienced a universe of Oneness that was characterized by Love.[263]

Experiments conducted at the Princeton Engineering Anomalies Research (PEAR) laboratory provide information about the properties of this field, by whatever name. These properties include the ability of the mind to affect the output of random event generators, and to obtain information regardless of temporal or spatial constraints. The ability to influence a machine output was also independent of space and time but was affected by consciousness and emotion.[264]

Because this field is that which remains when all molecular motions cease and all classical forms of energy vanish, at the temperature of Absolute Zero, the field has been called by physicists the Zero Point Field (ZPF)—described by Lynne Mc Taggart as "the very underpinning of our universe was that of a heaving sea of energy—one vast quantum field."[265] The ZPF has been studied extensively by physicists Harold Puthoff, Bernard Haisch, and others. It has been described as a unifying concept of the universe, which showed that everything was in some sort of connection and balance with the rest of the cosmos. As was mentioned above, Laszlo has described this field as an interconnecting, information-conserving and information-conveying cosmic field.[266]

The ZPF has two characteristics that are of great importance to our question regarding the source of the common insights of traditional medicines.

(1) The ZPF is made up of waves, and it stores information by wave interference patterns, with no reference to space or time. (further explained in Sect. 5.9). This is an incredibly efficient way of storing information. It has been estimated that the field would store all the information in the Library of Congress in a volume the size of a sugar cube. Thus, the ZPF is capable of containing all thoughts, actions and events since the Big Bang and even before.

(2) The ZPF contains incredible amounts of energy. Nobel Laureate Richard Feynman has commented to his physics students that a cubic meter of empty space contains enough energy to boil dry all the earth's oceans.[267] Princeton theoretical physicist John Wheeler has calculated that the energy density of empty space is far greater than the energy associated with all the matter in the universe. This energy may be the source of the healing energy used by many healers. Healers state that they are only a channel (John of God, Lakota holy man Fools Crow) for that energy.

NASA is presently conducting research with the goal of harnessing the energy contained in the Field for use in interstellar travel.

As described earlier, (Chapter 3) on one occasion Frank Fool's Crow was to preside at a sweat-lodge ceremony at the Standing Rock Lakota reservation. Upon discovering the fire keepers had not lighted the fire, (hence the stones were not heated), Fool's Crow asked that they bring him the cold stones. He placed his hands on them, sang to them, heated them instantly and the heated stones were placed in the lodge's pit. That takes a lot of energy![268]

5.8 Accessing the Zero Point Field

We can all access this information field. Apollo 14 astronaut Edgar Mitchell, when in deep space and in a higher state of consciousness, found he could enter into deep communication with the universe. Mitchell identified that communication as being with "the holographically embedded information in the quantum zero-point energy field."[269] According to Mitchell, all things in the universe have a capacity to know, a perspective echoed by Allen Boone's experiences mentioned earlier.

Dowsing, an art that goes back into antiquity, is another means of accessing the Field. Cave paintings in Egypt depicting the use of dowsing tools have been carbon dated to at least 9,000 BCE, and it may be inferred that the art of dowsing was known long before that date.

The renowned California dowser, Walt Woods, provides us with an instructive definition of dowsing: "Mother's intuition with a read-out device."[270] Often, dowsers operate in an altered state of consciousness, a state in which they have access to The Field. Children, whose brain waves normally reside in the delta, theta, and alpha frequencies as they grow older, are particularly adept at dowsing. Even as adults we can relax and reach at least an alpha state and thus have access to the Field.

In a somewhat similar vein to Fools Crow's heating of stones, many dowsers have been known to move underground streams to a more convenient location, by accessing the energy of the Field, ensuring a water supply to a well. A friend of the author, an experienced dowser, had a daughter whose well in rural Arkansas had run dry. The daughter was most astonished when her father, using map dowsing, moved an underground stream to her well, and the well began flowing again.[271]

That same dowser provided another example that the Field is not constrained by space limitations. The daughter of a University of California psychologist and faculty member owned an antique harp that was stolen. The mother, a confirmed skeptic about such matters as dowsing, after failing with conventional means (contacting the police, contacting likely pawn shops, etc.) to recover her daughter's harp, reluctantly followed a friend's advice to contact the author's friend, who lived in Arkansas. The dowser quickly determined where the harp was located and, following the dowser's instructions, the mother soon retrieved the harp. For details of this incident see Professor Elizabeth Mayer's book.[272]

Another dowser friend of the author, who lived in San Francisco, had her car stolen from in front of her apartment. She contacted the police, who gave her little hope of seeing her car again. She phoned her daughter, and had her daughter drive while she used her dowsing tools to determine how to find her car. At every intersection she would ask her dowsing tools for instructions: Turn right? Turn left? or Go straight ahead? In 20 minutes, much to the astonishment of the police, she found her car.[273]

As waves are functions of frequency rather than time, the ZPF can hold all information, regardless of the time the information occurred. Events that occurred even before the Big Bang can thus be encoded and preserved, in the Field.

5.9 The Hologram

Interference patterns define a "hologram," and an important property of a hologram is that each part of the hologram contains all of the information of the entire hologram. Consequently, access to any part of the Zero Point Field provides access to *all* the information ever stored in the Field.

Due to the essential identity between Patanjali's Akashic Record and the ZPF, some are now referring to the ZPF as the Akashic Field. The impact of this Field was described by Targ and Katra as follows: "*Any event that occurs is immediately available anywhere as information. That is, each portion of space contains information about all others.*"[274] This is what would be expected in a holographic universe, and it informs us enormously as to prospects for telepathy, distant healing, and tapping into the record of past and future events.

It should be noted that experiments during the past forty years in distant viewing (supported during the Cold War by the CIA) have provided strong evidence that time and space do not have the limitations we commonly associate with materialist (objective) reality.[275] Laszlo summarizes this new/old concept as the informed universe, rooted in the rediscovery of ancient tradition's Akashic Field as the vacuum [ZPF]-based holofield. In this concept the universe is a highly integrated, coherent system, much like a living organism. Its crucial feature is information that is generated, conserved, and conveyed by and among all its parts. Further, in this theory, the underlying physical reality is a holographic field in which everything is connected with every other thing. He goes on to describe its impact upon evolution as a strongly interconnected system that builds on the information it has already generated. And he comments, "The ancients knew that space is not empty: it is the origin and the memory of all things that exist and have ever existed."[276]

Russell Targ reminds us that "nothing is secret," including events in the past and future.[277] Further, *everything is interconnected* at a quantum and macro level, probably via the holographic universe. We note that Karl Pribram's work suggests that we have a holographic memory, perhaps that memory's being stored in the Akashic Field.[278] David Bohm's concept of a *holographic universe* (the Implicate Order) is also consistent with concepts of an Akashic Field.[279]

Thus, we now have a pretty well-defined candidate, the Zero Point or Akashic Field, for the store of information that mystics, shamans, and practitioners of traditional medicines, across time and across space, have tuned into, consistently coming up with the same answers.

We live in an informed universe, which gives us not only a new view of the world, but also a new view of life and of mind. It permits our brains and minds to access a broad band of information, well beyond the information conveyed by our eyes and ears. We are, or can be, literally 'in touch' with almost any part of the world, whether here on Earth or beyond in the cosmos.[280] Good examples of this capability are given by Mayer, by Jahn and Dunne, by and Targ and by Katra. Drunvalo Melchizedek also describes the amazing story of a blind woman employed by NASA to report on outer space objects that they couldn't observe optically.[281]

Whether it entails distant viewing, dowsing for information, moving underground streams of water, healing, or shamanic journeying, there is a field of information and energy available to us at all times. The commonality of traditional medicines now makes good sense. The Quantum Hologram is very real, by whatever name.

We have found that all healing appears to be self-healing. As was observed by internist Dr. Jerry Cohn, "We keep the patient happy while nature cures her."[282] Healers of whatever type assist the patient to heal him/herself. And we always remember Papa Auwae's assuring us that, "Healing is only 20% medicine, and is 80% spiritual."[283]

5.10 Conclusion: The Material and the Invisible

We began this chapter with a review of how a series of events 400 years ago led to a materialistic science and a materialistic culture. Now we are in the midst of another paradigm shift, a new science that is returning us to a perspective akin to that of the Ancients, of Indigenous peoples, their science and their shamans.

A leader in this transformation is Amit Goswami, PhD., a theoretical physicist who is the author of the textbook, *Quantum Physics,* and many other books, including *The Self-Aware Universe: How Consciousness Creates the Material World*.[284] Goswami is Professor Emeritus of Physics at the University of Oregon, member of the Advisory Board of the Institute of Noetic Sciences, and is now at the Holmes Institute in Los Angeles. Goswami posits that *consciousness* is the ground of being; that consciousness is more fundamental than are either matter or energy. In so positing, Goswami joins the highly respected mathematician, John von Neumann, together with Princeton professor and Einstein's colleague, John Archibald Wheeler, and other prominent physicists, who recognized that we live in a participatory universe.

Goswami summarizes the principles (assumptions about the nature of being) of materialism, (*material realism*, as scientists refer to it) in *The Self-Aware Universe*, as follows:

1. Strong objectivity—objects are independent of and separate from the mind. (The tree falls in the forest even if no one watches it.)

2. Causal determinism—all motion can be predicted given the laws of motion and initial conditions of the objects.

3. Locality—that one object affects another *only* by connecting with it in some physical way, and never does this occur at more than the speed of light.

4. Physical or material monism—all things in the world, including mind and consciousness, are made of matter (energy).

5. Epiphenomenalism—mental phenomena can be explained as a secondary phenomenon of matter (brain).[285]

As Goswami points out, *each of these assumptions has been proven to be false*, and thus material realism is *not* an accurate description of our universe. Quantum physics has repeatedly shown that these assumptions do *not* reflect the real world.

Nevertheless, material realism continues to be the philosophical basis of Western scientific medicine. We can overcome this mistake by recognizing the wisdom of the Ancients, of Pythagoras, Socrates, Plato and Hippocrates, as well as the mystics and the Indigenous shamans of the world.

Notes

225 Plato, *The Allegory of the Cave*, translation by Benjamin Jowett, Los Angles, Enhanced Media Publishing, 2017.
226 Bohm, David, *Wholeness and the Implicate Order*, London, Routledge & Kegan Paul, 1980.
227 Heilbron, J.L., *Galileo*, Oxford, Oxford University Press, 2010.
228 Descartes, Rene, *Discourse on Method*, Hackett Publishing Company, 1999.
229 Braden, Gregg, *Deep Truth: Igniting the Memory of Our Origin, History, Destiny, and Fate*, Hay House, 2011.
230 Silvertooth, E.W., "Motion Through the Ether," *Electronics & Wireless World*, 1989.
231 Dalai Lama, Forward to Joel and Michelle Levey, *Living In Balance: A Dynamic Approach for Creating Harmony & Wholeness in a Chaotic World*, Divine Arts, 2014.
232 Zukov, Gary, *The Seat of the Soul*, New York, Simon and Schuster, 1989.
233 Dorjee, Pema, Janet Jones and Terence Moore, *Heal Your Spirit, Heal Yourself: The Spiritual Medicine of Tibet*, Watkins Publishing LTD, 2005.
234 Rankin, Lissa, *Mind Over Medicine*, Hay House, 2014.
235 Guiley, Rosemary, and Sheryl Martin, *The Tao of Dreaming*, Berkley Trade, 2005.
236 Adam, *Dreamhealer, A True Story of Miracle Healings*, Plume, 2006.
237 Cowan, Eliot, *Plant Spirit Medicine*, Sounds True, 2014.
238 Dorjee, Pema, Janet Jones and Terence Moore, *Heal Your Spirit, Heal Yourself: The Spiritual Medicine of Tibet*, Watkins Publishing LTD, 2005.
239 Laszlo, Ervin, *Science and the Akashic Field: An Integral Theory of Everything*, Inner Traditions, 2007.
240 Adam, *Dreamhealer: A True Story of Miracle Healings*, Plume, 2006.
241 Laszlo, Ervin, *Science and the Akashic Field: An Integral Theory of Everything*, Inner Traditions, 2007.
242 Ibid.
243 Mehl-Madrona, Lewis, MD PhD *Coyote Healing: Miracles in Native Medicine*,
244 Narby, Jeremy, The *Cosmic Serpent*, Bear & Company, 2003.
245 Leadbeater, Charles, and Annie Besant, *Occult Chemistry*, 1905. See also, Bird, Christopher *The Secret Life of Plants*, Harper Collins, 1973.
246 Laszlo, Ervin, *Science and the Akashic Field: An Integral Theory of Everything*, Inner Traditions, 2007.
247 Vivekananda, Swami, *Living at the Source: Yoga Teachings of Vivekananda*, Shambala Dragon Editions, 2001.
248 Cortland, Sherri, *Spiritual Toolbox*, Ozark Mountain Publishing, Inc., 2013. See also: Newton, Michael, PhD, *Journey of Souls: New Case Studies of Life Between Lives, Destiny of Souls: Case Studies of Life Between Lives, Memories of the Afterlife: Life Between Lives,* and *Stories of Personal Transformation.*

249 Burgan Ph.D, Louise (Mayan scholar, professor at Butte College, CA) personal communication, 2010. It should be noted that this Library is described by Michael Newton's subjects in his book *Destiny of Souls.*
250 Sheldrake, Rupert, PhD, *Morphic Resonance: The Nature of Formative Causation*, Park Street Press, 2009.
251 Boone, J. Allen, *Kinship With All Life*, HarperOne, 1976, and *Adventures in Kinship With All Life*, Tree of Life Publications, 1990.
252 Cowan, Eliot, *Plant Spirit Medicine*, Sounds True, 2014.
253 Bohm, David, PhD, *Wholeness and the Implicate Order*, London, Routledge & Kegan Paul, 1980.
254 Bucke, Richard Maurice, MD, *Cosmic Consciousness. A Classic Investigation of the Development of Man's Mystic Relationship to the Infinite*, Dutton, 1991.
255 Braden, Gregg *The Divine Matrix: Bridging Time, Space, Miracles, and Belief*, Hay House, 2008.
256 McTaggart, Lynne *The Field: The Quest for the Secret Force of the Universe*, Harper Perennial, 2008.
257 Laszlo, Ervin, *Science and the Akashic Field: An Integral Theory of Everything*, Inner Traditions, 2007.
258 Goswami, Amit, PhD, *The Self-Aware Universe: How Consciousness Creates the Material World*, TarcherPerigee ,1995.
259 Seyyed, Hossein Nasr, *Knowledge and the Sacred*, State University of New York Press, 1989.
260 Ibid.
261 Eddington, Arthur, quoted in Ramesh, Chidambaram, *Thought-Forms and Hallucinations*, Chennai, Notion Press, 2014.
262 Wald, George, "Life and Mind in the Universe," in *Cosmos Bios, Theos*, ed. Henry Margenau, La Salle, IL, Open Court, 1992.
263 Alexander, Eben, MD *Proof of Heaven: A Neurosurgeon's Journey into the Afterlife.* NY, Simon and Schuster, 2012.
264 Jahn, Robert G., and Brenda J. Dunne, *Margins of Reality: The Role of Consciousness in the Physical World*, ICRL Press, 2009.
265 McTaggart, Lynne, *The Field: The Quest for the Secret Force of the Universe*, Harper Perennial, 2008.
266 Laszlo, Ervin, *Science and the Akashic Field: An Integral Theory of Everything*, Inner Traditions, 2007.
267 Professor Richard Feynman PhD and Nobel Prize winning physicist who taught at Caltech. The author was a student there and heard him say this many times, 1947–1951.
268 Rodman, David, personal communication.
269 Mitchell, Edgar, quoted by Laszlo, Ervin, *Science and the Reenchantment of the Cosmos*, Rochester, VT, Inner Traditions, 2006.
270 Woods, Walter, personal communication.
271 McCoy, Harold, personal communication.
272 Mayer, Elizabeth Lloyd, *Extraordinary Knowing: Science, Skepticism, and*

the Inexplicable Powers of the Human Mind, Bantam, 2008.
273 Ashley, Karen, personal communication.
274 Targ, Russell, and Jane Katra, *Miracles of Mind: Exploring Nonlocal Consciousness and Spiritual Healing*, and Jahn, Robert G., and Brenda J. Dunne, *Margins of Reality: The Role of Consciousness in the Physical World*.
275 McMoneagle, Joseph, *Remote Viewing Secrets: A Handbook*, Hampton Roads Publishing Co, 2000.
276 Laszlo, Ervin, *Science and the Akashic Field: An Integral Theory of Everything*, Inner Traditions, 2007.
277 Targ, Russell, and Jane Katra, *Miracles of Mind: Exploring Nonlocal Consciousness and Spiritual Healing*, New World Library, 1999.
278 Pribram, K. H., *Languages of the Brain: Experimental Paradoxes and Principles in Neuropsychology*, Englewood Cliffs, NJ: Prentice-Hall, 1971.
279 Bohm, David, PhD, *Wholeness and the Implicate Order*, Routledge & Kegan Paul, 1980.
280 Laszlo, Ervin, *Science and the Akashic Field: An Integral Theory of Everything*, Inner Traditions, 2007.
281 Melchizedek, Drunvalo, *Living in the Heart*, Light Technology Publishing, 2003.
282 Cohn, MD, Jerry, personal communication.
283 Auwae, Papa, personal communication, 1998.
284 Goswami, Amit, PhD, *The Self-Aware Universe: How Consciousness Creates the Material World*, TarcherPerigee, 1995.
285 Ibid.

Chapter 6
The Development of Medicine in the West

6.1 Sumer

There is evidence of an advanced state of medicine and surgery in Sumer, presumably medical arts inherited from Atlantis, with hospitals being known to have existed as early as 4000 BCE and references being found to physicians as early as 5000 BCE.[286] This is about the time of the historical record of the establishment of medicine in Egypt, though Thoth was said to be the founder of Egyptian medicine at a much earlier date. Egyptian medicine had a direct effect on Greek medicine and thus on Western medicine. There is also evidence of an advanced science in Sumer, of mathematics, astronomy, and chemistry. Expertise in these sciences would in turn have supported medical science.

6.2 Egypt

The immediate predecessor of Greek medicine was that of Egypt, and there is clear evidence of ties between the two. Egyptian physicians were scientists who considered the macrocosm and microcosm closely interrelated.[287] In the words attributed to Thoth, known in Egypt as the World-Teacher and known to Greece as Hermes Trismegistus, "As above, so below."

The first Egyptian dynasty is dated by astronomical calculations at 4240 BCE, which would antedate Chinese medicine, though some traditions date Thoth's founding of Egyptian cosmological concepts as early as ca. 40,000 BCE. In any case, Thoth was the founder of both Egyptian medicine and religion, teaching of "the Light that lighteth every man that cometh into the world. When man becomes one with the Light, which was God, then he becomes one with the whole of which he was part, and then he can see the Light in everyone, however thickly veiled, pressed down, and shut away. All the rest is not;

but the Light is. The Light is the life of men."[288] We note the implication of an interconnectedness of man in Thoth's statement.

With Thoth's concept of man's relationship to the cosmos, it is not surprising that the Egyptian scientist/priests interrelated human anatomy and function with religious concepts. Thus, for example, the Egyptian word for the innermost nasal recess is the same as the word for the inner sanctum, the most sacred part of a temple. What's the connection? Perhaps because when one resonates sounds in that cavity, particularly the sound M, it produces a shift in consciousness due to the presence of sympathetic and parasympathetic nerves in that region. In any case, Egyptian medical texts embrace not only the analytical science that we study today, but also a metaphysical view related to the Art of Medicine that our modern medical science does not encompass.

Imhotep, in 2600 BCE, became the archetypical Egyptian architect and physician,[289] as did the Greek Æsculapius in later years, and after Imhotep's death he was elevated to the status of a demigod. Temples, schools of medicine, and clinics were established in his name.[290]

There are many examples of the advanced state of Egyptian medicine. When medical papyri were initially translated and found to suggest the use of crocodile dung to treat certain infections, this was considered to be a reflection of the "primitive" state of ancient Egyptian medicine. Many years later it was discovered that a crocodile's intestinal tract contained antibiotic flora, and that crocodile dung contained antibiotics that were indeed appropriate for the treatment of those infections. It might be noted that in South America, condor dung has similar antibiotic properties, as both crocodiles and condors are scavengers.

Another example of an advanced state of Egyptian medicine was found in the Smith Papyrus, dated to the Middle Kingdom. In this papyrus is found a detailed discussion of the effects of different head injuries, including the neurological consequences of those injuries. This papyrus thus implies that Egyptian physicians had an accurate understanding of the functions of the different parts of the brain, together with their interactions, in some cases going beyond the knowledge of present day neurologists and neurophysiologists.[291]

As a result of the sophistication of Egyptian medicine, the Egyptians enjoyed the highest level of health of any civilization in the ancient world. This high level of health appears to be related to their understanding of the relationship between man and the cosmos, that *when man was in tune with the cosmos, health reigned. When man was out of tune, the body became unhealthy or diseased.* Because of the interconnections between man and the cosmos's rhythms, man could be brought back into tune. The processes whereby this attunement was accomplished were an important aspect of Egyptian medicine.[292]

Thus, we find, early in Egyptian medicine, recognition of the importance of balance and harmony with the cosmos. As mentioned previously, Egyptian medicine also recognized that a primary cause of disease was unhealthy mental attitudes.[293]

6.3 Greece[294]

Greece borrowed much knowledge of medicine from Egypt, but what is known as Greek medicine began with Æsculapius. The history of Æsculapius is steeped in mythology beginning with his birth. Apollo, the Sun god who came to be thought of as the supreme divine healer, and the mortal princess, Coronis, were the parents of Æsculapius. Although impregnated by Apollo, Coronis favored another mortal. Apollo became enraged upon learning of this, and he slew Coronis. However, when Coronis's body was on the funeral pyre, Apollo relented and determined to save his son. He withdrew the infant Æsculapius from Coronis's womb, and the child was born.

Apollo asked the mystic centaur Cheiron, famed for his scientific attainments and his knowledge of the medicinal properties of plants, to raise and become the teacher of Æsculapius. Cheiron watched over Æsculapius and trained him in the healing arts.

Æsculapius, the great healer, became the hero from Thessaly, which was the original home of Greek medicine. Long after his death, Æsculapius was, raised to immortality and joined the pantheon of the Greek gods.[295]

It was Æsculapius's knowledge of herbal medicine that became the foundation of Greek medicine. According to the *Iliad*, Æsculapius died in 1237 BCE, prior to the Trojan War. He was reputably killed by a thunderbolt from Zeus for encroaching on the privileges of the gods by raising a mortal from the dead. The sons of Æsculapius were the prototypical physician and surgeon in the Trojan War.[296]

Æsculapius was raised from his hero-status and became the god of medicine in the 6th century BCE, symbolizing all that is best in medicine. *He represented divine intervention in healing*, whether that intervention took the form of diagnosis in dreams or "miraculous" healing.[297] He was the compassionate healer who both performed healing in dreams and gave instructions for healing in dreams, as can happen in many traditional medicines.

Æsculapius used herbal medicine, drugs, diet, surgery, and, very importantly, *incubation* (dream sleep) to heal. He treated both body and soul, but he would only treat the pure in heart.

6.4 Æsculapian Temples and Incubation

The Æsculapian Temples were the centers of healing in ancient Greece. These were the temples where Æsculapius was believed to dwell, and his priests, who were also physicians, treated the patients in the temple. A primary aspect of the healing process was *incubation*, healing through the use of dreams.[298]

Incubation proceeded as follows: The suppliant [patient], or a kinsman representing him, would retire to the shrine of the god or hero, and would sleep in the portico of the temple, or near the image of the divinity. Only the pure were permitted to approach the god, and such temple-sleep, or incubation, was always preceded by rites of purification and by abstinence from food and wine for varying lengths of time. These ceremonies were designed to increase the tendency to dreaming and to enhance the clarity of the vision. This use of temple-sleep was also found in Babylonia and Egypt, but in those countries temple-sleep came into use some time after Æsculapius had become the symbol of healing.[299]

After temple-sleep, patients often reported being visited by sacred snakes, which were considered to have magic powers associated with prophecy, dreams, and healing. This visitation by a sacred animal, or by a priest or priestess, was an example of the "direct method" of healing. In these cases the presence of the divinity, the laying-on of hands by the attending priest or priestess, or the visitation brought about the healing.[300]

The "indirect method" of healing was as follows: In the "indirect method," healing occurred through following the directions received in the dream. This was the more common method of healing, and the remedies prescribed varied widely from mild purgatives, roots, herbs, diets, fasts, baths, and rubbings with ointments, to gymnastics and a general regimen. These measures were usually applied with some "magical" formulas or incantations, which would engage the subconscious mind in the healing process. Purification and fasting were normal procedures, and the visions or dreams could provide prescriptions to the patient, or through the medium of a priest, relative, or friend.[301]

It may be noted that a connection to this procedure can be found in traditional Hawaiian Medicine. Dreams by either the *Kahuna La'au Lapa'au* or the patient can be used to diagnose the patient's needs, including the prescription of appropriate *la'au* (herbs). According to *Po'okela La'au Lapa'au* Papa Auwae, recurrent dreams are given the most weight in such situations.[302]

It is also worthy to recognize the long record of highly successful diagnoses and prescriptions by the "Sleeping Prophet," Edgar Cayce.[303] Each of these processes, from the Æsculapian temples' use of incubation to the use of dreams by shamans and prophets, appear to be some sort of tapping into a store of knowledge that is both universal and, in the case of particular patients, quite individual.

After the time of Jesus, a rivalry arose between Christianity and Greek medicine. The early Church fathers considered Æsculapius the forerunner of Jesus, the only major difference being that Jesus would treat sinners as well as the pure in heart. As a result, Æsculapius was considered Jesus' biggest rival among the pagan gods, and note the similarity between Jesus and the pagan gods who preceded him.[304]

6.5 Hippocrates

The Hippocratic Oath is probably the best known of all the recollections of Hippocrates known to modern day Western physicians. That Oath goes as follows:

> I swear by Apollo, the physician, by Æsculapius, by Hygeia, and Panacea, and I take to witness all the gods, all the goddesses, to keep according to my ability and my judgement, the following Oath:
>
> To reckon him who taught me this Art equally dear to me as my parents; to share my substance with him, and relieve his necessities if required; to look upon his children in the same footing as my own brothers, to teach them this Art if they shall wish to learn it, without fee or stipulation; and that by precept, lecture, and every other mode of instruction, I will impart a knowledge of the Art to my own sons and those of my teachers, and the disciples bound by a stipulation and oath according to the law of medicine, but to none others. I will follow that system of regimen which, according to my ability and judgement, I consider for the benefit of my patients and abstain from whatever is deleterious and mischievous. To please no one will I prescribe a deadly drug, nor give advice which may cause his death. Nor will I give a woman a pessary to procure abortion. With purity and with holiness I will pass my life and practice my Art. I will not cut for stone, even for patients in whom the disease is manifest; I will this operation to be performed by practitioners of this art. In every house where I come I will enter only for the good of my patients, keeping myself far from all intentional ill-doing and all seduction, and especially from the seduction of women or men, be they free or slaves. All that may come

to my knowledge in the exercise of my profession or outside of my profession or in daily commerce with men, which ought not to be spread abroad, I will keep secret and will never reveal. If I keep this oath faithfully, may I enjoy my life and practice my art, respected by all men and in all times; but if I trespass and violate this Oath, may the reverse be my lot![305]

Hippocrates played a pivotal role in the development of Western Medicine. He was the father of systematic medicine. As one who treated the whole person—body, mind and spirit—Hippocrates embodied holistic medicine, and he is often considered the father of holistic medicine. The latter statement does not signify that Hippocrates was the founder of holistic medicine, since what we usually term "holistic" medicine can be found long prior to Hippocrates in Egyptian and Æsculapian medicine, as well as in shamanic and other traditional medicines, including Chinese, Ayurvedic, and Tibetan. Nevertheless, there is no doubt that Hippocrates is today our model of an holistic physician.[306]

What is often forgotten about Hippocrates is that he was a *priest*-physician. Recognizing the unity of mind, spirit and body, he wrote, "There is no need to make such a division in nature, for all things are alike divine, or all are alike human."[307]

In truth, Hippocrates was not only the founder of modern Western medicine. He, together with his contemporaries, Plato and Socrates, represented the culmination of a long history of shamanic and mystery school healing, of traditional medicines. Hippocrates, Socrates and Plato represent the juncture, the tipping point, between ancient and modern medicine, medicine found today primarily in the remnants of traditional medicines. There were intellectual descendants of Hippocrates, Socrates, and Plato in the centuries that followed (e.g., Paracelsus and Hahnemann), but the shift to allopathic medicine began shortly after the time of Hippocrates.

Hippocrates brought together a school of physicians who together developed a body of writing known as the Hippocratic Corpus and which provided the basis for not only Greek, but much of Oriental medicine and some of Western medicine in the centuries that followed. The Hippocrates school also set the ethical standard for medicine through the Hippocratic Oath. There is a similar oath used by Hindu physicians. The Hippocratic Oath also has much in common with the Admonition of Sun Si-Mo in Chinese medicine.

6.6 The Historic Hippocrates

The historic Hippocrates was descended from both Æsculapius and Hercules. He was born on the Island of Kos in 460 BCE; and he died there in 377 BCE. He was the eighteenth descendent of Æsculapius on his father's side and the twentieth descendent of Hercules on his mother's side, giving him a most noble heritage.[308]

Hippocrates lived at the time of the blossoming of Greek philosophy. He was a contemporary of the philosopher Anaxagoras, who was a bridge between Pythagoras and Socrates. He was a student of the work of both Heraclitus and Pythagoras, who had lived around 30 years prior to Hippocrates. He was a personal friend of Socrates, who lived from 469 to 399 BCE. Plato, Socrates' student, was a contemporary of Hippocrates.[309]

The fame of Hippocrates was so great that he was worshipped in his own time. He was made an honorary citizen of Athens after he contained the plague of 430 BCE, when he was 30 years old. In 411 BCE (19 years later) the Greek general Alcibiades destroyed Kos for insubordination to the Athenian Alliance. Alcibiades was then ordered by Athens to rebuild the city for Hippocrates.[310]

The king of Persia, Artaxerxes, offered Hippocrates as much gold as he wanted to fight an epidemic in Persia. However, the Greeks were hostile to Persia, so Hippocrates responded, "Thank you, Artaxerxes, for the honor and confidence placed in me. However, it is impossible for me to help a declared foe of my country. Consequently, both the gold and the disease are yours to keep."[311]

Artaxerxes was so infuriated at this reply that he sent a message to the people of Kos ordering them to surrender

Hippocrates or their entire city would be so devastated that it would be impossible afterwards to distinguish the inhabited areas from the surrounding deserts and the sea. To this message the inhabitants of Kos replied, "Artaxerxes, the people of Kos will never do anything unworthy which would offend their divine ancestors and Hippocrates, who is the glory of this island. We shall not hand him over to you, no matter if this decision were to entail the most terrible consequences. The gods will not abandon us."[312]

The gods were indeed with the people of Kos. Artaxerxes became apoplectic (can refer either to a stroke or to a ruptured aneurism, either causing loss of consciousness and paralysis) when he read this insulting reply, and he died instantly.[313]

6.7 Education of Hippocrates

The education of Hippocrates was wide-ranging. He studied medicine with his father, Hereclides, a celebrated physician and a priest of Æsculapius. Later, in Athens, Hippocrates studied with the physician Herodicus, and he was taught philosophy by Georgias of Leontini and Democritus of Abdena, the founder of atomic theory.[314]

After completing his education, Hippocrates returned to Kos, where he took his vows to Æsculapius, becoming a priest-physician as his father had been. Hippocrates then spent twelve years visiting all the renowned medical centers, the Æsculapia, of the world of his time. He was one of the first Western medical scientists, pursuing whatever avenues of empirical enquiry became available. In his Æsclapeion at Kos, some 6,000 herbs were known and used. There were many investigations of the effects of herbs on different patients and their illnesses.[315]

From Heraclitus (544-484 BCE), who deposited his papyri as a gift to the gods at the Æscalepean at Ephesus, Hippocrates learned that *all wears out,* that "Everything flows and nothing abides; everything gives way and nothing stays fixed."[316] Thus, all is in flux, in continuous transformation.

6.8 The Influence of Pythagoras

Pythagoras (580-490 BCE) was a great influence on Hippocrates, Socrates, and Plato, and on Jesus of Nazareth, through his education by the Essenes and Druids. Today we know Pythagoras primarily for the Pythagorean Theorem in geometry. However, Pythagoras was a renowned philosopher, a scientist, a healer, founder of an important mystery school and *much* more. He was a student of all the celebrated Greek philosophers of his day, initiated into the Orphic and thirteen other mystery schools, from Egypt to the Near East to India.[317]

Pythagoras spent twenty-two years in Egypt, Memphis and Thebes, where the priests taught him mathematics and astronomy. He then spent twelve years in Babylon, and he also studied in Persia and Chaldea, where he studied astrology, astronomy, and the science of numbers. Pythagoras made many travels to the Orient, especially the Near East. He is said by one tradition to have conversed with Lord Buddha and to have known the child Sri Krishna.[318]

In mathematics Pythagoras studied and made important discoveries about the geometry of planes and solids. In astronomy, Pythagoras recognized that the earth was a sphere, and that the rotation of the earth produced day and night. He also recognized that the earth rotated around the sun. In this, Pythagoras preceded Copernicus two thousand years later, and Copernicus attributed his understanding of heliocentricity to Pythagoras. Unfortunately for many, Aristotle rejected Pythagoras' understanding of the solar system, and the Roman Church accepted Aristotle's views.

Pythagoras founded a philosophical, or mystery, school in Croton in southern Italy, where he spent the rest of his life secluded with his disciples. Pythagoras was a healer, and he conducted research on music, aroma and color therapies.[319]

Pythagoras had a major influence on Hippocrates, who learned from Pythagoras that *health, as wholeness, means that body and soul must be examined together, that there are spiritual laws that humans ignore at their peril, that human will ensures and completes the harmony between body, mind and soul*, and that *harmony means thinking correctly and living correctly.* Here, *harmony* was the key term—harmony of body, mind, and spirit is required for true health to exist.[320]

Note the implication that *a philosophy that does not perceive body and mind as one whole creates disharmony*. We should also note that the idea of harmony pervaded all of Greek culture, so it was not new to Hippocrates. Nevertheless, Hippocrates was significantly influenced by Pythagoras's emphasizing the importance of this concept.

Hippocrates succeeded in integrating the divergent Heracletean and Pythagorean views. One insisted that everything was in flux and constant transformation, the other that there is a pre-established harmony. Hippocrates recognized a Dynamic Harmony, a concept much needed today in our scientific focus on static models rather than those that have prevailed in the East, where change is a recognized part of existence. As an example of the East-West contrast, consider the *I Ching*, the "Book of Changes," illustrating this fundamental concept in Chinese philosophy.

Socrates was a friend of Hippocrates, representative of the philosophical strength of the era in which Hippocrates flourished and taught. Socrates' student, Plato, was also a student of Pythagoras' teachings and joined Hippocrates in representing all that was the best of mystery schools' teaching.

Plato was fully aware of the importance of the invisible world and the healing power of the mind. When he opened his school in the Lyceum, he became seriously ill of a fever brought about by the school's location near a swamp. His students wanted to move the school, but Plato assured them that a wise man could heal himself from any environmental influences. He cured himself with his mind and lived to age 81, still in the Lyceum, with no recurrence of the fever. He taught his students that *man possesses within himself the power to heal the diseases of the body, that in the end every man is his own priest and his own physician*.[321]

One historian wrote of Hippocrates, "[He] was the wholeness of the human condition; he clearly realized that philosophy is not an intellectual game but the foundation in which our well-being is imbedded."[322]

6.9 Hippocratic Corpus

The Hippocratic Corpus, written around 100 years after Hippocrates' death, is a body of 50-70 books collected in Alexandria in the third century BCE and known as the Corpus Hippocraticum. It is not known whether Hippocrates actually wrote any of these books, but clearly they describe the work of his school and so provide a description of Hippocratic medicine. Observations were recorded, and libraries contained the repositories of the knowledge so collected and refined. In this exposition of Hippocratic medicine, the author is emphasizing the views of the earliest books of the Hippocratic Corpus (Group I, Kos), the Empiricist books. Other volumes (Group III, Cnidian) formed the basis of the Rationalist medical approach, one that emphasized *logos,* reason, rather than observation.

Several books in the Hippocratic Corpus dealt exclusively with *diet*, which played a crucial role in Hippocratic medicine. One book in the Corpus related *climatic conditions* to disease, also recognizing the influence of *social institutions* on disease. Today we find this understanding of the effects of the environment—dietary, physical, relationships, and emotions—to be an important cause of illness; the entire field of epigenetics reflects our most modern scientific research.

Similarly, surgical books in the Hippocratic Corpus are quite modern in their descriptions. The sophistication of the Hippocratic Corpus does not end there. *On the Sacred Disease* (epilepsy) anticipated modern thought by making a strong case for natural causes for this disease, previously thought to have been of supernatural origin.

- *On the Nature of Man* addresses the theory of four humors as it describes both anatomy and physiology. This book made it clear that *balance* was the key; as is the goal with Chinese medicine's Five Elements and Tibetan medicine's Three Humors.

- *The Law and The Physician* deals with the professional attitude and the ethics of the physician.

We note the elements found in common in all the Hippocratic books:
1. A naturalistic approach.
2. A great emphasis on the value of *observation* of the disease process, on the practical rather than the theoretical. It is in the stress on observation, the *empirical* approach, that Hippocratic medicine used the inductive method (reasoning from the particular to the general) to provide the beginnings of scientific medicine.
3. Groups I and IV of the Hippocratic Corpus are those representing true Hippocratic thought, a scientific approach to medicine.
4. In all, the Hippocratic Corpus, (in particular Groups I and IV,) provides an excellent summary of the teachings of Hippocrates, of the approach to the medicine and healing of Hippocratic medicine.

The Hippocratic physician may be characterized as following these precepts:
1. Nature provides the cure for illness.
2. "Leave thy drugs in the chemist's pot if thou can heal the patient with food."[323]

The Hippocratic physician was primarily interested, not in diagnosis, but in prognosis and treatment. This, again, is the *empirical* rather than the *rational* approach to medicine and healing. Part of the emphasis on prognosis can be attributed to the unprotected social status of the Greek physician. It was important that he succeed in healing his patient, or his livelihood would be in jeopardy.

The Hippocratic physician was concerned with the body as a whole rather than dividing it into parts. In this he reflected the philosophical viewpoint of his friend, Socrates, who commented that one cannot heal the body without healing the soul. *Hippocratic treatment was the treatment of an individual, not of a disease, and the treatment of the whole body, not of any part of it.*

Treatment followed the axiom that treatment of *holon tou somatos*—the whole person—is absolutely primary.

Hippocratic treatment was based on the fundamental assumption that nature (physis) had a strong healing force and tendency of its own, and that the main role of the physician was to assist nature in this healing process (rather than to direct it arbitrarily).

Health was defined as a state of harmonic mixture of the humors (eucrasia), and disease was a state of disharmony (dyscrasia). Note the similarity of Hippocratic medicine to traditional medicines.

The main ally of the physician in assisting nature in the process of healing was diet. Only if diet failed were drugs used, and surgery was resorted to only as a last resort.

The key elements of Greek medical thought were expressed in terms of patterns, relationships and synthesis, as did Chinese views of the day. As Hippocratic writing stated in De veteri medicina in the 4th century BCE, "All thought that is founded on observation leads to truth, every skill owes its original results to the observation of every phenomenon, reflected on and then reduced to general principles."[324]

An element of Hippocratic medical thought that is common to all traditional medicines is the importance of breath. There was a recognition of the relationship between breath, pneuma (outside the body, air) and vital energy, spirit. This relationship is mirrored in many traditional cultures. In the Hindu culture we find a similar relationship between breath and vital energy, Prana. In Arabic this relationship is expressed as Ruh and also Nafs, and in Hebrew as Ruach.[325] Confirming a linguistic relationship between Egypt and Hawaii, we find, expressing both breath and spirit, Ba in Egypt and Ha in Hawaii. In China we find Qi, and in Japan, Ki.[326]

Comparing Greek and Oriental medicine, pneuma equates with both Qi and shen, describing a spiritual (vital) force that creates and maintains all physiological energies.

Other parallels between Greek and Oriental concepts are found as well:

1. Spirit: In Greece, *Spiritus vitalis;* In China, *shen.*
2. Fluids: In Greece, *Chumoi;* in China, *jin ye.*
3. Blood: In Greece, *Haima;* in China, *xue.*[327]

The goal of the Hippocratic physician was to bring about the delicate, dynamic state of individual harmony according to each person's *physis*—their innate, natural condition. To the Greek physician, this balance is based on a person's particular constitutional *krasis*, or mixture of fluids. The individual's balance represents a *eucrasia*, a positive mixture of the four fluids. Preventive treatment is aimed at rebalancing a person's inborn constitutional condition. This goal was termed *kata physis*, and it was the highest form of therapy.

The method of treating disharmonies (syndromes) was, barring emergencies, to advise lifestyle and dietary adjustments, exercise and changes of attitude—in addition to prescribing herbal medicine for rebalancing the whole individual in all his/her capacities. Greek medicine, as has Chinese and Tibetan, developed herbal prescriptions that addressed the whole *energetic state of imbalance rather than being limited to relieving the symptoms caused by the imbalance.*

6.10 Training the Hippocratic Healer

The training of the Hippocratic healer has been addressed in Chapter Four, but it is worthwhile to review that training here. A medical student's initial training was little different from that of medical training today, *except* that the training of the Hippocratic medical student involved philosophical studies as well as what have been considered medical subjects in the West. The ultimate training, however, required that the candidate become highly skilled in what today we consider paranormal capabilities, abilities that would provide accurate insight into the cause of his patient's illness in addition to his training in academic and technical skills (There is a similarity to Tibetan and other traditional medicines' training of physicians.)[328]

The requirements for a Hippocratic medical student to graduate go far beyond that demanded of today's medical students and are more akin to that of a shaman's apprentice. At the Æsculapian temple at Epidauros, for example, there is a labyrinth under the chapel. Our fictional student, Dmitri, in Chapter 4, faced this trial. An inner sanctuary, the labyrinth, existed under a keystone in the chapel floor. The initiate would be dropped into the labyrinth through the hole made by the removal of the keystone (capstone). The capstone would then be replaced. Underground, there was a series of concentric passageways cut in such a way as to form a maze, and within that maze were poisonous snakes. The initiate was required to live in that underground maze for nine days in total darkness with no food or water—and to avoid the snakes or to relate to them in a mutually respectful manner. (Means of establishing a rapport with "dangerous" animals, including snakes, are discussed in Allen Boones' *Adventures in Kinship with all Life*.)[329] If the initiate survived, when he was brought out he was to report what had occurred in and around the country (runners had been sent to report on distant events) while he was in the labyrinth. Thus, staying alive was only the first part of the test. Proper use of inner sight and psychic awareness was an additional part of the challenge.[330] (Distant viewing, required of Hippocratic medical graduates, has been the subject of research at the Stanford Research Institute and at Princeton University, as well as at the CIA and military intelligence units, in recent years. For a discussion of procedures, see Joseph McMoneagle's *Remote Viewing Secrets: A Handbook*.)[331]

In sum, the training of the Hippocratic physician encompassed far more than the focus of modern Western medicine on material matters, physical symptoms and their management. Hippocratic medicine did use herbs and even chemicals at times (for example, purgatives), but it used those herbs to assist in restoring harmony. The Hippocratic physician relied far more on assisting nature through the use of diet and changes in lifestyle to correct the *causes* of disease. The Hippocratic physician used dreams in the Æsculapia, and he was required to develop the insight suggested by the initiation ceremony in addition to his knowledge of symptoms and *materia medica.* He followed the precepts of Hippocratic medicine and treated the whole person—body, mind, and soul.

Hippocratic medicine derived much from Egyptian medicine, and much of its spiritual content from the ancient mystery schools. Æsculapius was a healer-priest who was elevated to the status of the god of healing. Hippocrates was a healer-priest who healed the whole person with diet, lifestyle changes, and herbs. His focus was on restoring balance in the patient, and he recognized that our philosophical and spiritual foundation is the basis of health. Note well the consistent connection between spirit and healing. Most great spiritual leaders have also been healers or teachers of healing, whether Buddha, Jesus, Æsculapius, Mohammed, Thoth, Imhotep, or Quetzalcoatl, Kukulcan or Viracocha.

Hippocrates, together with Socrates and Plato, represent a tipping point between the wisdom of the past and today's materialistic medicine-a medicine that is focused on symptoms rather than the cause of illness, and accepts a limited concept of health as being the absence of symptoms. Hippocrates learned from the ancients, and, in turn he was followed by physicians such as Paracelsus, Hahnemann, and today's holistic physicians. We do well to honor the wisdom of Hippocrates and his treatment of the whole person.

6.11 Greek Medicine After Hippocrates

In the centuries following Hippocrates, Greek medicine continued its systematic inquiry into the nature and treatment of illness. It continued to be influenced by Greek philosophers, and it spread both to Rome and to the East. The path through Rome led, with an interruption of 1,000 years, to modern Western medicine. (Timeline in appendix). The real preservation of Greek medicine, and its influence on both Western and Eastern medicine, however, went via a "detour" through the Near East, where Greek medicine was preserved during the Dark Ages and then reintroduced to Europe. At the same time, Greek medicine became an important influence on the medicine of the East.

6.12 Aristotle

The first break with Hippocratic medicine came about through the influence of Plato's student, Aristotle, (384-322 BCE) who was born 7 years before Hippocrates died (377 BCE) and was the tutor of Alexander the Great (356-323 BCE). He played a key role in the development of the Rationalist approach to medicine through his philosophical beliefs. These beliefs were highly influential in Europe, especially during the Middle Ages and Renaissance, and many Aristotelian concepts still prevail today.

Aristotle was both a philosopher and a physician, and his philosophical views were actually in conflict with his medical views. His early writings, which were under the influence of his teacher, Plato, emphasized *logos* (reason), and this later formed the metaphysical basis for Rationalist thought. As he grew older, however, Aristotle began increasingly to value experience. As the son of a physician and as an individual who had received medical training himself, he recognized the value of observation and experience in medical practice. There is thus a contrast between Aristotelian metaphysics, which supports the Rationalist views of Group III of the Hippocratic Corpus (and later, of Galen,) and Aristotle's own views on the practice of medicine.

Aristotelian philosophy followed Plato in the conviction that the visible world is only the reflection of another world lying beyond it. Consider Plato's allegory of the Cave, where the inhabitants saw on the wall of the cave the shadows cast by the "real" events outside the cave. Aristotle recognized the invisible, but he interpreted that invisible world differently than had his teacher. Plato called this invisible world the abode of *Ideas*. Aristotle converted "Ideas" into *"Forms"* as he worked to establish the connection between the Idea and the visible object. To him there was a cause and effect relationship between the invisible forms and physical objects—the objects are "caused" by the underlying and invisible forms. Aristotle then placed primary importance on the use of thought to understand the underlying forms, as the world of forms was considered the "real" world in that it is the permanent and rational world, whereas the world of physical objects is always changing, as pointed out by Heraclitus's flux.

A corollary of this reasoning is that sense-perception, and therefore observation, is unimportant, inasmuch as the senses only perceive the external visible and changing world. Thus, Aristotelian logic proposed that there was a structure of form that, if understood, was far more meaningful than could be understood from empirical observations. This logic was taken up and used by the Rationalist physicians.

The Empirical tradition of the Hippocratic physician was based on his experience and observation of the patient's symptoms, and so the Empiricist stressed the development of symptomatic knowledge. The Rationalists, in contrast, looked for the entity (the *forms,* the diseases) that was assumed to be hidden behind the "veil" of the symptoms.

The Aristotelian dichotomy between the world of sense-perception and the underlying reality of forms became, in medicine, a dichotomy between the *organism*, with its sense-perceptible symptoms, and the *disease*, conceived of as an invisible *form*—an entity inherent in the organism. This view came to be taught in medieval medical universities and is often the view followed by Western medicine to this day.

This concept of the disease being the fundamental and invisible entity, the *form*, led to the ignoring of symptoms that were not considered to be linked to identifying the disease *form*. As a consequence; only the "genuine" symptoms were of interest, and others were considered of less importance and were therefore ignored.

Aristotle's conclusions *(1) Re Disease:* medicine does not deal with individual patients but with classes of disease. Only those symptoms related to an identified *form* (disease) were considered "real;" all other symptoms were considered due to chance. *Aristotle and the Rationalists thus treated diseases, not patients.* This is a practice that is found all too commonly among allopathic physicians today; it is exemplified by the physician's focusing on test results appearing on a computer screen rather than on the patient.

Aristotle's logic *(2) Re Treatment:* Aristotle used the *Principle of Contradiction* to define therapy. Thus, the Rationalist physician would reduce the complexity of a disease to certain elements considered fundamental to identifying that disease. He then would look for medicines that had the opposite qualities, to contradict the disease process. It is the *Principle of Contradiction applied to diseases that is the fundamental philosophical basis of allopathic medicine.*

It is important to note that therapeutics based on the Principle of Contradiction, or the Doctrine of Contraries, is exactly the opposite of the Hippocratic approach (Group I of the Hippocratic Corpus) of aiding nature's self-healing capacity through the use of similars *(secunda remedia)*, which later became the basis of homeopathic medicine.

6.13 Aristotle's Science

Aristotle's scientific views had a major impact in the years that followed. His logic was black and white, and that perspective still pervades much thinking today ("You're either for us or against us!").

Either A or Not A was Aristotle's perspective, a view that prohibited Neither A or Not A or Both A and Not A. Eastern logic was more flexible and included the latter two possibilities.

Aristotle's astronomical views were similarly fixed. He viewed the heavens as unchanging; in his view, the stars were fixed in their positions. Thus, medieval European astronomers, who had been trained in Aristotle's views, missed seeing a supernova that occurred in *ca.* 1000 CE and which was observed by Oriental astronomers.

6.14 Galen

The next major influence on Greek medicine was provided by Galen. Galen played a major role in illustrating the schism between Rationalism and Empiricism. Galen (129-199 CE) was the greatest thinker in Greek medicine after Hippocrates, and his thinking and writing was preeminent in Western medicine until at least the 17th century. Even that underestimates Galen's influence, for the American Medical Association was founded in 1846 on principles that specifically embraced Galen's theory, and even today that theory underlies much, probably most, of allopathic medicine.

Although this book has focused on the Empiricist aspect of Hippocratic medicine (Groups I and IV of the Hippocratic Corpus), there were also the Rationalists (Aristotelian, and Hippocratic Corpus Groups II and III), and later other branches of thinking in Greek medicine, as well. Galen, who had been highly educated in philosophy, as well as in all schools of medicine, attempted to bring together the conflicting views in Greek medical thought. He knew the Hippocratic Corpus very well, and he described himself as following Hippocrates. However, he was in fact following the Aristotelian-Rationalist (Group III) philosophy rather than the Empirical views (Group I) that appear most clearly to reflect Hippocratic thinking.

Galen was a prolific writer, producing over 30 books on medical subjects, of which 22 are still extant. He described his theories persuasively, and they persevered in the centuries that followed. Although Galen tried to include empirical thought in his writing, in the end it was his Rationalist views that prevailed. He preferred theory to observation, and to him it was the *Doctrine of Contraries* that was the basis of therapeutics. *Galen defined diseases, and then he prescribed the antidotes for those diseases.* Symptoms were only used to define the disease *form*, following the logic of Aristotle. Once the disease was defined, the antidote would presumably be known, and other symptoms that might lead to identifying the *cause* of an illness would be ignored.

Diet and climate, important to the Hippocratic Empiricists, was discarded by Galen in favor of drugs and often quite "heroic" treatments. Galen, and Rationalist doctrine, separated the body from its environment. This logic also separated the patient from the physician, for once the disease was identified, the treatment was by definition identified. The cause of the disease, the *form*, was invisible, and the physician had no interest in the process of the disease (in fact did not see disease as a process). The Rationalist physician had an approach that had real economic advantage, an advantage reflected in much of modern medicine. All the physician had to do was to diagnose and then to prescribe an antidote. They had no interest in prognosis, and their treatments often violated *Primum non nocere.* (First of all, do no harm.)

Just as Galen espoused the Doctrine of Contraries, so he rejected the use of similars. He was thus squarely in the tradition of what became allopathic medicine.

Galen's prolific literary output is difficult to analyze, many inconsistencies being buried in a torrent of words, disguised in long-winded treatises. Galen really stopped the scientific developments of the Hippocratic Empiricists, and his work destroyed Empiricism for centuries. He made "empiric" a derogatory term, denoting inability to apply intellect to medical problems. Medicine suffered a great loss thereby, and the scientific medicine of Hippocrates was stopped in its tracks.

Galen's Rationalism, despite its logical inconsistencies and lack of therapeutic value nevertheless became, due to Aristotle's influence, the medical orthodoxy of the Middle Ages and into modern times. This acceptance of Rationalism appears to have been based more on socio-economic factors than on any logical or intellectual basis. The Rationalist approach did not produce superior physicians, but it did enhance the prestige of the physician, as it was he who knew the theories of disease. Thus, this presumed intellectual superiority set him above the layman.

The Rationalist approach also enabled the practitioner to treat patients more rapidly and therefore earn more money. A present-day equivalent can be seen in the HMOs where MDs are allowed to spend only very limited time with each patient and to focus on diagnosing the disease (i.e., find the correct pigeon hole for the diagnosis, which then dictates the treatment). Being a Rationalist physician was also easier than being an Empiricist, for the Rationalist only has to have received his medical training/theories, whereas the Empiricist must use his experience to define appropriate treatment.

6.15 Diagnosis

Diagnosis by the Rationalist physician: Although Hippocratic physicians focused on prognosis rather than on diagnosis, diagnostic methods were gradually developed in Greek medicine. Greek physicians used pulse diagnosis, examination of the tongue, examination or inquiry about urine, stool, and phlegm as part of their diagnostic procedures.

Pulse diagnosis was studied extensively by Greek physicians in the years following Hippocrates. Galen describes 27 standard pulse qualities in *De pulsibus* (ca. 100 CE), the same number as Chinese medicine's Li Shi-Zhen 1,500 years later. Greek physicians considered the basic six pulses to be the Large and Small, Strong and Weak, Quick and Slow. These characteristics are similar to Chinese usages:

1. Galen's bowstring pulse (*pulsus nervosus*) is equivalent to the Chinese bowstring or wiry pulse (*xuan mai*)

2. Galen's surging pulse (*pulsus undosus*) is equivalent to the Chinese flooding pulse (*hong mai*)

3. Galen's vibrating pulse (*pulsus vibrans*) is equivalent to the Chinese tight pulse (*jin mai*)

Examination of urine was the other primary method of Greek diagnostics, as it is in Tibetan medicine.

Notes

286 Mark, Joshua J., "Health Care in Ancient Mesopotamia" *Ancient History Encyclopedia*, 2014, https://www.ancient.eu/article/687/health-care-in-ancient-mesopotamia/.
287 Sawandi, Tariq, "The Science of Egyptian Medicine", 2000, http://www.think-downloads.com/download/Ancient%20Times/Mid%20Eastern%20History/Egyptian%20History/the_science_of_egyptian_medicine.pdf.
288 Besant, Annie and C.W. Leadbeater, *Man: Whence, How and Whither*, Chicago, IL: The Theosophical Press, 1922.
289 Bard, R *Imhotep*,
290 Bailey, James E., "Asklepios: Ancient Hero of Medical Caring", *Annals of Internal Medicine*, January 1996.
291 Allen, James, *The Art of Medicine in Ancient Egypt*, NY: Metropolitan Museum of Art, 2005.
292 Sawandi, Tariq, "The Science of Egyptian Medicine", 2000, http://www.think-downloads.com/download/Ancient%20Times/Mid%20Eastern%20History/Egyptian%20History/the_science_of_egyptian_medicine.pdf.
293 Jayne, Walter Addison, *The Healing Gods of Ancient Civilizations*, University Books, Inc., 1962.
294 Ackerknecht, Erwin H., *A Short History of Medicine*, Johns Hopkins University Press, 1982.
295 Edelstein, E.J. and L., *Ascklepius: Collection and Interpretation of the Testimonies*, The Johns Hopkins Press, 1998.
296 Ibid.
297 Most, Glenn, 'A Cock for Asclepius', *The Classical Quarterly*, 43(1), 96-111, 1993.
298 Edelstein, E.J. and L., *Ascklepius: Collection and Interpretation of the Testimonies*, The Johns Hopkins Press, 1998.
299 Ibid.
300 Ibid.
301 Ibid.
302 Auwae, Papa Henry, Personal communication, 2000.
303 Sugrue, Thomas, *There is a River, the story of Edgar Cayce*, A.R.E. Press, Virginia Beach, VA, 1997.
304 Gandy, Timothy Freke & Peter, *The Jesus Mysteries: Was the 'Original Jesus' A Pagan God?*, New York, Three Rivers Press, 1999.
305 Ackerknecht, Erwin H., *A Short History of Medicine*, Johns Hopkins University Press, 1982.
306 Coulter, Harris, *Divided Legacy: A History of the Schism in Medical Thought*, Vol. I, Wehawken Book Co., 1975.

307 Singer, Charles, *A Short History of Science to the Nineteenth Century*, Oxford Press, 1943.
308 Ackerknecht, Erwin H., *A Short History of Medicine*, Johns Hopkins University Press, 1982.
309 Ibid.
310 Ibid.
311 Ibid.
312 Ibid.
313 Ibid.
314 Begbie, J. Warburton, "Hippocrates: His Life and Writings", *The British Medical Journal*, December 1872.
315 Ackerknecht, Erwin H., *A Short History of Medicine*, Johns Hopkins University Press, 1982.
316 Heraclitus, *Talk:* Wikipedia, https://en.wikipedia.org/wiki/Talk%3AHeraclitus.
317 Pythagoras Sources:
Cheney, Sheldon, *Men Who Have Walked with God*, New York, Alfred A. Knopf, 1945.
Hall, Manley P, *The Secret Teachings of All Ages*, New York, Jeremy P. Tarcher/Penguin, 2003.
318 Ibid.
319 Ibid.
320 Dorjee, Pema, Janet Jones, and Terence Moore, *Heal Your Spirit, Heal Yourself: The Spiritual Medicine of Tibet*, Watkins Publishing, London, 2005.
321 Hall, Manley P, The Secret Teachings of All Ages, New York, Jeremy P. Tarcher/Penguin, 2003.
322 Kunz, Dora, *Spiritual Healing*, Wheaton, IL: The Theosophical Publishing House, 1995.
323 Hippocrates, *The Medical Works of Hippocrates*, Blackwell, Oxford, 1950.
324 Ibid.
325 Translations from https://en.wikipedia.org.
326 Adams, James D, et al, *Traditional Chinese Medicine: Scientific Basis for Its Use*, Royal Society of Chemistry, 2013.
327 Cohen, Misha, *The New Chinese Medicine Handbook*, Fair Winds Press, 2015.
328 Hippocrates, *The Medical Works of Hippocrates*, Blackwell, Oxford, 1950.
329 Boone, J. Allen, *Adventures in Kinship with All Life*, Tree of Life Publications, 1990.
330 Bruyere, Rosalyn, *Wheels of Light*, Vol. I, Bon Productions, 1989.
331 McMoneagle, Joseph, *Remote Viewing Secrets: A Handbook*, Hampton Roads Publishing Co, 2000.

Chapter 7
The Spread of Greek Medicine

7.1 The Spread of Greek Medicine

From Greece the history of Western medicine after Hippocrates and Galen goes to Persia. The expansion of the Arabian empire, from the 7th century onward, was key to the preservation of Greek medicine during the Middle Ages. Many Greek texts that had been lost in the West were taken to the Middle East and translated into Arabic; they were later retranslated into Latin and reintroduced into Europe. Greek medicine became known in the Middle East as *Unani Tibb*, meaning Ionian, or "of the Greeks," designating "Medicine and healing of the physical, mental and spiritual realms."[332]

Following the collapse of the western Roman Empire in the 5th century, 300 years after Galen, almost all of the Latin and Greek literary legacy was lost, including most of philosophy and essentially all of medicine. The European focus was on the Roman Church, and monastic orders ran the "hospitals" of the day. The "hospitals," however, were not places of healing but simply places to take seriously ill people, who were expected to recover or die according to God's will.

7.2 Healing and Christianity

A brief divergence into Christian history is appropriate here. Jesus of Nazareth had been noted as a healer as well as a spiritual teacher, and he passed that legacy on to his followers. Thus, in the early centuries following Jesus' death, many healings were reported by the early Christians.

However, that tradition proved to be short-lived. The Roman Emperor Constantine legalized Christianity in 313 CE. He wanted a centralized church and he wanted that church to have an established dogma. This was accomplished at the Council of Nicaea in 325 CE. An orthodox dogma was established by a vote of the bishops, and views contrary to that dogma were declared heretical.

That dogma conflicted with the teachings of the Essenes—the Jewish mystery school established centuries prior to Jesus' birth, the community wherein both Jesus and his cousin, John the Baptist, were taught as children.[333] The Essenes taught their children to meditate at an early age as the path to inner wisdom, the way to know God.[334] The Essenes were very interested in healing, and taught that art as well. When the Romans destroyed the community at Qumran, the Essenes emigrated to Alexandria, where they became known as *Therapeutae*.[335]

It might be noted that there was a close relationship between the Essenes and the Druids in Britain. The Druids had established libraries and schools of higher learning in Britain during a period when the mainland of Europe was still in the Dark Ages and under the domination of the Roman Church.

Also, at Alexandria, were many early Christians who became known as Gnostics. The Gnostics were Christians who believed in direct access to God, and they were therefore considered heretics and persecuted by the Roman Church. The beliefs of the Gnostics were described by Oxford-trained theologian Tobias Churton in his book, *The Gnostics*: "The Gnostic knows that he or she is a spiritual being 'of one substance with the Father'; for what the orthodox say of Christ, the Gnostic is free to say of himself."[336] And later, "[The Gnostic] believes he is going right to the source and is wary that the Church is becoming or has become a middleman with special interests of its own, namely, the continuity of the Church structure."[337] It is clear why the orthodox Roman Church considered the Gnostics as heretics.

Among the Gnostics were many healers, continuing the example set by Jesus. The last of the Gnostics, the Cathars, were burned at the stake by the armies of the King of France, and centuries later by the armies of the Pope in southern France (most in 1210 and 1244 CE).

Much of what we know of the Gnostics was derived from the discovery of the Nag Hammadi Library at Hamra Dum in Upper Egypt by Muhammed-Ali al Samman and his brothers in 1945. The *Gospel of Thomas* is probably the most important book of the

Library in adding to our understanding of the work of Jesus; it is a major source of our understanding of Gnostic thought.[338]

With the establishment of a Church hierarchy, healing diminished. Not all of the Church leaders were healers, and the leaders were not pleased to have low-ranking monks healing when they could not. The Church considered the soul to be far more important than the body, so care of the body and medical treatment were considered of little value. Mortification of the flesh was equated with saintliness. Thus, with the support of the Roman Church, Holy Roman Emperor Justinian closed the medical schools at Athens and Alexandria in 529 CE.

As a result, medicine as a craft virtually disappeared in Europe, with only the wise women of the countryside (in later centuries burned at the stake as witches by the Inquisition) serving their communities as healers. In the 7th century the Church banned surgery by monks as being a danger to their souls. In 1130 the Council of Clermont officially banned the practice of medicine by monks as being too disruptive of their monastic lives.

Following the return of Greek medicine to Europe (see below), the Church's view of healing did not change. In 1215 CE, Pope Innocent the Third condemned surgery and those who practiced it. In 1418 CE, the dissection of the human body was declared to be sacrilegious.

A Greek manuscript of the *Corpus Hermeticum* was brought to Florence from Macedonia in 1460. Nevertheless, the medicine of Greece, including the advances made by Hippocrates, was not considered of value by the Roman Church during the Middle Ages.

7.3 The Arabian Detour

In contrast, Greek medicine came to Arab countries, brought by Christians who had been driven out of the Byzantine Empire. Most of these were excommunicated Nestorian Christian scholars, including physicians, who emigrated from Byzantium as early as 431 CE, just prior to the collapse of the Western Roman Empire. These scholars translated the Greek writings—

philosophical, scientific, and medical—first into Syriac or Hebrew, and then into Arabic.[339]

The first major center of such translations was in Persia in the 6th century, and by the 10th century all the important Greek writings had been translated in the major Near Eastern capitals: Damascus in 707 CE, Cairo in 874 CE, and Baghdad in the 800s CE. The caliphs sent emissaries to collect Greek scientific works. The Arab translators had translated all the Greek medical texts, including those of Hippocrates and Galen, into Arabic by the end of the 9th century.[340]

The Muslim medical practice followed the (Hippocratic) theory of humors, that a person was healthy when the humors were in balance, and that sickness was due to humoral imbalance and could be corrected by the healing arts.

The first modern hospital was established in Baghdad in 805 CE. Known as the *bimaristanm*, it was devoted to the promotion of health, the cure of disease, and the expansion and dissemination of medical knowledge. Pharmacies were developed, following the Islamic teaching that "God has provided a remedy for every illness."[341]

Arabic medicine was built on Greek medicine, the first great Arab medical writer being the Persian Al Rhazi (860-932 CE), considered the "Arabian Galen." Al Rhazi was considered Islamic medicine's greatest clinician, and deemed the father of pediatrics due to his work on the diseases of children. Al Rhazi advocated reliance on observation. He was a strong proponent of experimental medicine and of the beneficial use of medicinal plants. He wrote of medical theories, of diet and drugs, and their effects on the human body, the effect of environment on health, and on many other areas.

7.4 Avicenna

The greatest Persian physician and medical writer, however, was Ibn Sina (980-1063 CE), the "Arabian Hippocrates." Ibn Sina became known in the West as Avicenna, and his encyclopedia of medicine, the *Canon of Medicine*, became the leading medical textbook in both the Eastern and Western worlds for centuries. It is still, a thousand years later, considered a fundamental text by many physicians.[342]

Ibn Sina was an incredible individual, an all-purpose man who excelled in everything he did. He has been described as being to the Arab world what Aristotle was to Greece, and Leonardo da Vinci was to the Renaissance. He was preeminent not only in medicine but in philosophy, science, music, poetry, and statecraft. He had memorized the Qur'an by the age of 10, studied law, mathematics, physics, and philosophy, and at the age of 16 turned to medicine. By 18 he was a famous physician, and at age 20 he was appointed physician to the Persian court.

Avicenna wrote 20 books on theology, metaphysics, astronomy, philology (linguistics, literature) and poetry, and 20 more on medicine. His *Canon of Medicine*, containing over 1,000,000 words, was a codification of all existing medical knowledge, including, Greek, Middle Eastern, and Indian medicine. As had Hippocrates before him, Ibn Sina (Avicenna) stressed the importance of diet and the influence of climate and environment on health.

The tie between Avicenna and Hippocrates is reflected in the comment by a modern author, "While (Avicenna's) conception of the physical, emotional, and spiritual aspects of health is vast in scope, he once condensed his system into a single statement (echoing Hippocrates), 'Food is the best medicine'."[343]

Avicenna followed the same theory of humors found in Hippocratic, Oriental and most other traditional medical systems. He described some 760 medicinal plants in the *Canon*, and he laid out the basic rules of clinical trials still followed today.

Avicenna was well aware of the importance of the mind on health and its capability for distant healing. He wrote, "The imagination of a man can act not only on his own body but even others and very distant bodies. It can fascinate and modify them; make them ill, or restore them to health." Our modern recognition of healing at a distance, is informed by our understanding of the physics (Quantum Physics; the Field) underlying distant healing.[344]

7.5 Greek Medicine's Return to Europe

The Greek medical works returned to Europe 1,000 years after Galen, by way of the Middle East and North Africa. This was accomplished through the translation from Arabic into Latin of what had become Arab medical classics.

These translations occurred primarily at Salerno and Toledo in the 11th and 12th centuries, both of which were on the border between Christian Europe and the Islamic world. Salerno became Europe's first great medical facility of the Middle Ages, and Salerno was, of course, close to Arab Sicily. It should be noted that at some point, perhaps in translation, the *Canon* came primarily to reflect Galen's thinking, in contrast to Hippocratic thinking and much of what prevailed in *Unani Tibb*.

7.6 Unani Tibb

The fundamentals of *Unani Tibb* medicine are clearly derivative of Hippocratic thought. Avicenna has been described as the Prince of Physicians, and he has been considered by many to be the most influential physician in history. His literary output was almost unbelievable, and his *Canon of Medicine* is without doubt the most encyclopedic treatise on medicine ever written. Avicenna continued Hippocrates' work, and *Unani Tibb* clearly continues the medical approach espoused by Hippocrates.[345]

Unani Tibb medicine continues to be a thriving medicine today, being practiced, taught, and researched in 25 countries of Europe, Asia, and the Near East, as well as in the United States, and is practiced most extensively in Afghanistan and India[346], and it is found in many other areas as well.

Unani Tibb medicine is recognized by the World Health Organization (WHO). The first World Conference on *Unani Tibb* Medicine, sponsored by the WHO, was held in India in 1987. An Institute of *Unani* Medicine exists in the United States, promoting both the teaching and practice of *Unani Tibb* medicine.

The spread of Hippocratic medicine to Asia and the Pacific is the story of *Unani Tibb*. Persia had ties with both China and India, although for geographical reasons the contact with India, and hence the connection between *Unani Tibb* and Ayurvedic medicine, is the more prominent. An International Medical Congress was held in the 8th century in Tibet that lasted 45 years, bringing together medical scholars from Persia (*Unani Tibb*), Nepal, India, China, as well as Tibetan Bön (Buddhist) medicine. It is thus not surprising that we find a somewhat closer parallel between Greek and Tibetan Medical diagnostic methods than between Greek and Chinese methods. All use pulses for diagnosis, but both Tibetan and Greek use urine, which is not an important part of Chinese medicine.

Although classical Chinese medicine is not as closely tied to Greek medicine as is Ayurvedic medicine, there was a college of *Unani Tibb* medicine (thus, Hippocratic medicine) established in Beijing by a group of Muslim practitioners in the 12th century. This was, of course, about the same time that the Greek texts were being translated from Arabic back into Latin in Europe. Many ties exist between Greek medicine and Ayurvedic medicine, again with an emphasis on diet, seasonal changes, proper exercise and conduct, an origin in humoral theory, and an emphasis on a person's connection both with the environment and with spiritual influences. Ayurvedic medicine also shows its ties to Greek medicine through the use of dreams and of pulses in diagnosis, with the more advanced Ayurvedic physicians also using their "inner sight" as a part of the diagnostic process.

An interesting related story is the spread of Greek medicine to the Pacific. According to Hawaiian genealogy chants, Hawaiian ancestors moved from Egypt to Greece during the era of prominence of Greek medicine, then moved on to India and thence to the Pacific. It is thus not surprising that many of the principles of Hippocratic medicine are reflected in the herbal medicine (*La'au Lapa'au*) of Hawaii, including the use of dreams for diagnosis.

Additional evidence for the connection between Egypt and Hawaii is linguistic: several Hawaiian words show a clear connection to Egyptian terms. This connection has been further reinforced with the discovery of linguistic ties between Hawaiian and an ancient Berber language in North Africa. The Berber tradition also describes the emigration of Egyptians to the Pacific.[347]

7.7 Hildegard von Bingen

In medieval Europe, 1,000 years after Galen, and at the time Greek medical texts were being retranslated from Arabic into Latin, Hildegard von Bingen represented a continuation of Hippocrates's approach to healing. A mystic who wrote down what she saw in her visions, Saint Hildegard (1098 – 1181CE) became the Abbess of a Benedictine convent at age 38, and later founded her own convent near Bingen. Hildegard wrote books on theology, philosophy, devotion, nature, medicine, psychotherapy, and prophecy, and she composed music that is enjoying a renewed popularity today.[348]

Hildegard never practiced medicine—her books were written from her spiritual visions. Nevertheless, her medical texts provide an excellent treatise on not only managing the symptoms of disease but also addressing their spiritual roots. Her healing methods were at the causal level. Hildegard's is today considered to be an outstanding example of a revealed medicine. Her medicine has been described as "a comprehensive system of healing for body, mind, and spirit," a truly holistic medicine that stressed the importance of harmony among the elements.

She wrote of the harm of suppressed emotions, and she was highly aware of the role of the subconscious mind. She wrote of psychotherapy long before its importance was recognized by the medical profession.

Hildegard's medicine was a four-humor or four-element medicine that was consistent with Hippocratic medicine. She wrote of an energetic medicine that made effective use of natural medicines, primarily using herbs, and also gems and some animal parts. She was well aware of the importance of diet, and one commentator said, "Diet was essential to her healing system and she sets forth sound principles for a balanced diet."[349]

Hildegard's medicines were only the first step, however. To Hildegard, "True healing cannot be arrived at by outer action alone; it requires contacting that inner consciousness and organic intelligence which is the real healing power... It requires opening up to the spiritual force in us and in the world around us." Hildegard reflected the wisdom of the great healers of the past, knowing that the healing power is within.

(Compare the above with Dr. Albert Schweitzer's comments regarding the "doctor within" in Chapter Three.)

Hildegard's medical works were ignored for centuries. They were almost completely forgotten for 800 years. Fortunately, her medical manuscripts were discovered about 100 years ago, and they have subsequently been studied and found to be highly effective. There is a clinic successfully using Hildegard medicine in Germany today, and Hildegard's medicine has been termed "The Healing Art of the Future."

7.8 Anthroposophic Medicine

In modern times the vision of Hippocrates has been found in Anthroposophic Medicine—a term coined by Steiner. Rudolph Steiner was an Austrian who lived from 1861 to 1925 CE. He attended the Technical University in Vienna, focusing on mathematics and science. He also tutored students in the classics. From the age of nine Steiner had spiritual insights and clairvoyant vision.[350]

After receiving his doctorate, Steiner was recognized as an authority on Goethe's scientific work. He became a respected lecturer on Goethe as well as on his own spiritual insights. Steiner became the president of the German section of the Theosophical Society. However, he eventually left the Theosophists, for their concern was primarily with Indian religion, while his interest was related to his own insights and their applications.

Steiner later founded the Anthroposophic Society. He was interested in agriculture, education—the Waldorf Schools were founded by him—and many other areas, including medicine. He established a school in Switzerland where Anthroposophic Medicine was taught. Anthroposophic Medicine is used today in several clinics in Switzerland and elsewhere.

Steiner taught that health depends on a general balance throughout the body, and that distortions in this balance arise out of the distortion of balance in the human soul and spirit. In regards to remedies, Anthroposophic Medicine used not only cures effected by diet or lifestyle changes, but also used herbs and minerals to help restore balance within the patient to assist the patient's self-healing capacity. Steiner considered bacteria to be secondary phenomena, existing due to the spiritual or physical lack of balance in the patient or in some particular organ.[351]

Steiner noted that at the ancient Mystery temples there was a healing center nearby. One anthroposophic physician known to the author's wife, Maryse, used his hand to sense a patient's energy, using a dowsing technique to determine when an organ's energy was out of balance. The author's Hawaiian teacher, Papa Henry Auwae, used a similar technique to sense energy imbalances.

This chapter omits the story of Paracelsus and Hahnemann, who were also followers of Hippocratic practices, as they will be addressed in Chapters Eight and Ten.

Timeline of Western Medicine, Egypt to the Middle Ages

Event	Date	Interval
Egyptian medicine	4000 BCE	2,700 years
Aesculapius	1300 BCE	900 years
Hippocrates	400 BCE	500 years
Galen	100 CE	
Fall of the Western Roman Empire	476 CE	
Council of Nicaea establishes Christian orthodoxy	325 CE	

Greek Medicine's Detour via Persia

Greek medical writings to Persia	431 CE
Tibetan Medical Congress	ca. 750 CE
Al Razi	900 CE
Avicenna	1000 CE
Unani Tibb in Beijing	1100 CE
Greek medicine's return to Europe (Salerno) (Galen to Salerno—1,000 years)	1100 CE
Hildegard von Bingen (Revealed medicine)	1100 CE
Anthroposophic Medicine (Rudolf Steiner) (Revealed medicine)	1900 CE

Notes

332 Bowman, Marion, *Healing and Religion*, Hisarlik Press, 2000.
333 Schonfield, Hugh, *The Essene Odyssey: The Mystery of the True Teacher & the Essene Impact on the Shaping of Human Destiny*, Element Books, 1984.
334 Cannon, Dolores, *Jesus and The Essenes*, Ozark Mountain Publishing, 1992.
335 Wilson, Stuart and Joanna Prentis, *The Essenes: Children of the Light*, 2005.
336 Churton, Tobias, *The Gnostics*, New York, Barnes and Noble, 1987.
337 Ibid.
338 Meyer, Marvin *The Nag Hammadi Scriptures: The International Edition*, Harper One, 2007.
339 Tschanz, David, "The Arab Roots of European Medicine" in *Aramco World*, May/June 1997.
340 Ibid.
341 Ackerknecht, Erwin H., A *Short History of Medicine*, Johns Hopkins University Press, 1982.
342 Coulter, Harris *Divided Legacy: A History of the Schism in Medical Thought*, Vol. I, Wehawken Book Co., 1975.
343 Ibid.
344 Adam, *Dreamhealer: A True Story of Miracle Healings*, 2006.
345 Chishti, Haim G. M., *The Traditional Healer: A Comprehensive Guide to the Principles and Practice of Unani Herbal Medicine*, Rochester, VT, Healing Arts Press, 1988.
346 Kakar, Sudhir *Shamans, Mystics and Doctors*, Beacon Press, 1982.
347 Long, Max Freedom *The Secret Science Behind Miracles*, 1954.
348 Strehlow, Wighard and Gottfried Hertzka, *Hildegard of Bingen's Medicine*, Santa Fe, NM, Bear & Co., 1988.
349 Ibid.
350 Shepherd, A. P. *Scientist of the Invisible. Spiritual Science: The Life and Work of Rudolph Steiner*, 1954.
351 Bott, Victor, *Spiritual Science and the Art of Healing: Rudolf Steiner's Anthroposophical Medicine*, 1984.

Chapter 8
Paracelsus, the Middle Ages, and the Renaissance

8.1 Paracelsus and the Cultural Context of His Time

Paracelsus was a physician, alchemist, mystic, and theologian. He lived at the beginning of the Renaissance, a time when the Roman Church dominated all life in Europe. He became a major influence on the Rosicrucians more than 100 years after his death.

Medicine in Europe during the Middle Ages and into the Renaissance was a medicine heavily influenced by religious concepts. The Roman Church was extremely powerful, not only in religious affairs but in the medieval universities. Many ancient Greek writings, including those of Aristotle and Galen, and also Avicenna's *Canon of Medicine*, had been translated from Arabic into Latin and had returned to Europe. Those texts constituted the primary source of medical teaching in medieval Europe. Thomas Aquinas had adopted Aristotelian philosophy and science. Aristotelian philosophy and Galen's medicine had become accepted by the Roman Church as dogma, were taught in medieval universities and medical schools.[352]

Medical science as we know it today had not yet begun, but what began with the Hippocratic tradition of observation had been supplemented by the experimental work of the medieval alchemists. This was the background of the age when Paracelsus initiated a medical reformation at about the same time that Martin Luther was initiating a religious Reformation.

The Middle Ages were a time of monks and mystics, from St. Hildegard von Bingen, with her visionary medicine relating diseases to disharmony of the soul in 1100 CE, to St. Francis of Assisi in 1200 CE, to the heretical Benedictine monk Meister Eckhart in 1300 CE. The Roman Church dominated life, from the Crusades to the Inquisition to the medieval universities founded by monks. For example, Oxford and Cambridge Universities were founded by monks in 1200 CE.

Religious intolerance had led not only to the Crusades, but also to Jews emigrating throughout the world, in the Western hemisphere to Mexico and later to New Mexico. Religious corruption, the selling of indulgences, and Pope Alexander VI's installing his mistress and children in the Vatican, set the stage for Martin Luther's Reformation and the Protestantism that followed.

8.2 Avicenna's *Canon*

The *Canon* and other works of Avicenna provided the primary source of teaching for medieval medical schools. Prior to the reintroduction of Greek medicine through Avicenna's works, the medicine of the Middle Ages had been only to provide succor to patients and to care for their souls. Generally, these "hospitals" were associated with monasteries, and the monks did provide some herbal remedies in some cases. An important class of remedies, not infrequently used, was that of purges, cathartics, or "physiks." Physiks acted to oppose symptoms, i.e., according to the Law of Contraries, therefore that use was following Galen's approach to curing patients. The term came to be used for all medicines, then to mean "to cure," and so those who cured with medicines became known as "physicians."

Although Avicenna's *Canon* encompassed all of Greek medicine, together with a reflection of medical influences from the Middle East and India, the primary thrust of the translated *Canon,* and of medieval medicine, was to adhere to the concepts of Galen, including the Law of Contraries. Thus, the medieval physician was in general one who followed Galen's approach to curing: he was a Rationalist who treated "diseases" rather than patients, and was trained in medieval universities with a heavy Church influence, (most universities were founded by monastic orders).

It should be noted that Hildegard's medicine—although to us considered a major advance over the medicine taught in the universities of her time—was ignored by her contemporaries and forgotten after her death. It was hundreds of years before the value of her work was recognized. Hildegard medicine was *not* taught in medieval universities.

8.3 Women Healers

One of the consequences of this university orientation of medicine, (particularly when combined with the views of the Inquisition,) was the suppression of women as healers. Women were not admitted to the men-only universities, and therefore women were not admitted to the medical profession.

In contrast, for many centuries there has been, a tradition of women healers in many cultures and traditional medicines. For example, *Kahunas La'au Lapa'au* are traditionally women, and this status of women as healers was also true in Europe.

The women healers were very knowledgeable regarding herbal medicine and healing, and they were often far more effective healers than were the university-trained physicians, The rivalry that developed between them was not surprising. The male physicians were very effective in suppressing their rivals by the simple method of declaring them to be witches. The women's success as healers was taken to be proof of their being in league with the Devil, and they were burned at the stake. Thousands of women were killed in this fashion, and much of their knowledge of herbal medicine was lost.

8.4 The Alchemists

The Middle Ages were a time of religious ferment that eventually led to the Reformation. Natural science was heavily influenced by religious concepts, and it was the time of the medieval alchemist. The alchemist was searching for connections between man, spirit and nature, often heeding the Hermetic view, "As above, so below."

This teaching was attributed to Thoth (Hermes Trismagistus—"Thrice Great Hermes"), the Atlantean spiritual leader who had foreseen the destruction of Atlantis and had led his disciples to Egypt. Thoth was the founder of Egyptian religion, medicine, science, and language. It is no coincidence that alchemy is named after the ancient name of Egypt, "Al Chem." The science and medicine that followed (in Egypt) was influenced in a profound way by the spiritual concepts and writings attributed to Thoth. It had a noteworthy impact on the leading thinkers of the day, from the Middle Ages through the Renaissance, and down to the present time: Paracelsus, Copernicus, Kepler, Galileo, Leonardo da Vinci, Leibniz, and Newton, and the Rosicrucians. Mathematician and philosopher Giordano Bruno was burned at the stake by the Roman Inquisition for adhering to such heretical views. As Picknett and Prince describe in *The Forbidden Universe*, "The Hermetic philosophy and cosmology is not only mystical but emphatically magical, embracing different realms of being, from gross matter to the divine spheres, and that of supernatural beings, divine, angelic and demonic. But ultimately it is monotheistic, ascribing all creation to a single God, while also encompassing lesser gods and goddesses, a category to which even mortal humans can aspire if they become sufficiently advanced."[353]

The alchemists were heavily influenced by Gnostic and neo-Platonic mysticism, (neo-Hermetic, if these views are traced back to their source) and there was a major mystical component in alchemical writings. Indeed, much of the work of alchemists anticipated the science that followed, as represented by the scientific luminaries listed above. Paracelsus believed that all physicians should be students of alchemy as well as practicing medicine, and it is hardly surprising that the Rosicrucians that followed Paracelsus placed a major emphasis on healing.[354]

Historian Tobias Churton has written:

> [The alchemist/healer] was suspicious of treatments that did not fully involve nature, hard work, patience, and experiment. He understood that a human being was a marvelous, divine construction about which we actually knew very little. One thing Paracelsus was sure of, however, was that humans find their being encompassed at all times by nature in its full extension, from the stars to the Earth, and that it was therefore reasonable to assume—and by proof of practice—that

there was something of the stars in human beings themselves, made in the divine image.

The essence of life flowed largely unseen, but was frequently blocked. Paracelsus was therefore not surprised when a successful treatment might have very little, visibly speaking, to do with the disease. A great deal of modern visible cause-and-effect treatment eschews this insight. If things cannot be shown to be connected, then they should not work, even if they do! Examples of this phenomenon abound, from 'miraculous' healings following Near Death Experiences to healings by shamans as a result of shamanic journeying.

The essence of Paracelsus's medical theories was the idea of freeing up energy flow, putting people back in touch with vital spiritual and cosmic energies of which the natural forms we see with our eyes are expressions—all poppycock, of course, to the materialist. Paracelsus's famous tripartite division, his three principles, show the levels through which human beings should be addressed for treatment. Using the symbolic language of alchemy, Paracelsus's followers referred to mercury (spirit), sulfur (soul), and salt (matter).

In the truly sound wholeness of a spiritual body, spirit (the divine likeness), is wedded to soul (the sum of all faculties, including reason). This couple are then bound harmoniously to the carnal person, the person of matter, flesh, and blood. A fourth principle may be described as *lux*, light, or the *astrum* (star), the life-giving light that, unless obstructed, separates the pure from the impure, thus unveiling a general illumination derived from this light or inner sun.[355]

Today we think of the alchemist as searching to transmute base metals into gold, but in truth, the alchemist was searching more for spiritual transformation than for physical. Far more important to the alchemist than the physical realm was the invisible, the astral and the spiritual, so the development of modern chemistry from the material aspects of alchemy reflected only the least important of the alchemist's concerns.

In time, the study of nature became "natural magic" ("magic" signifying wisdom), the study, by experimental or observational approaches, of nature and all of man's environment. The study of Nature was the study of God's Creation, so there were close ties between science and spiritual understanding. This included everything from astronomy to metals to plants. Out of the alchemist's experimental studies today's chemistry developed, and nature was considered to be ruled by divine law. Knowledge was considered a divine favor whether gained by direct mystical experience or by experimentation in nature. Science and research were considered divine service, the connecting link with divinity.

8.5 Paracelsus

Theophrastis Paracelsus (1493-1541CE) was without doubt the outstanding medical figure in Reformation-era Europe, and he has been referred to as the "Luther of Medicine."[356] Columbus had just discovered the West Indies when Paracelsus was born, and Martin Luther was ten years Paracelsus' senior. Paracelsus has been described as "a blunt man, crude and opinionated," yet at the same time he was the most revolutionary in spirit of all the great leaders of the Scientific Revolution. He was a mystic; he enjoyed fighting orthodoxy, and he was not one to call a 'spade' a 'garden implement.'

Paracelsus was the son of a peasant woman and a physician who was the illegitimate son of a Swiss nobleman. The stigma of the latter circumstance, plus his affection for his very devout and caring mother, made Paracelsus sympathetic to the plight of the peasants throughout his life.

Trained in medicine by his father, Paracelsus entered the University of Basel at 16, which he left after about a year to study with a Benedictine scholar at the Monastery of Sponheim. There he learned much of alchemy, astrology and natural magic (wisdom).

However, this too proved short-lived, and he left to work with miners in lead mines, learning about minerals and observing and treating the miners' illnesses. He concluded that he could learn far more from the direct observation of nature than he ever could from books. From that time on, he spent most of his life wandering across Europe, learning from his observations and from those he conversed with, from the wise women of the countryside, to gypsies, to those physicians whom he found to have useful experience.

He also traveled in India, and many of his philosophical concepts relate closely to those of the East. Paracelsus considered himself an alchemist as well as a physician, and he felt an understanding of alchemy, including its mystical aspects, was important to the practice of a physician. In short, he was a mystic and theologian as well as a physician, and we have noted that much of Rosicrucian philosophy is tied to Paracelsian thinking.[357]

Paracelsus, as noted above, was a theologian and mystic as well as a physician. Dr. Carlos Gilly has written, in his paper that Paracelsus had written a series of theological works (not published until after Paracelsus's death) that provided a basis for the development of Rosicrucianism in the 17th century.[358] After ten years of such wandering, Paracelsus returned to Basel in 1525, and in 1527, at age 34, he was appointed Basel's city physician and also professor of physic, medicine, and surgery at the University of Basel. He proceeded to give a series of lectures at the university that made him highly unpopular with the traditionalists. First of all, he committed the academic sin of lecturing in German rather than in Latin. Further, he insisted on lecturing about the diseases of the day rather than about the matters discussed in the classic texts of Galen and Avicenna. In this, he was flying in the face of academic medical tradition, and he made many enemies by so doing. Paracelsus also incurred the wrath of the university-trained physicians by burning their medical texts, declaring everything written since Hippocrates useless (see below).

Paracelsus nevertheless attracted many young physicians to his point of view for a simple reason: his medicine healed, and that of the university-trained physicians, based on Galen's teachings, did not. One of the reasons for his leaving the university himself was when he recognized that what he was being taught was quite useless. His success as a physician was phenomenal, for he was succeeding in healing many illnesses that the university-trained physicians had considered incurable.

Note the similarity with our situation today, where healing by non-MDs, (e.g., by Frank Fools Crow, John of God, or Papa Henry Auwae,) is generally problematical for Western scientific medicine. Only recently have acupuncturists, herbal healers, naturopaths, and chiropractors been recognized as legitimate health care givers.

However, fighting the system proved dangerous, and even Paracelsus' success led to trouble. After a nobleman had been healed by Paracelsus (having promised a handsome sum for a cure, as the other physicians had given up on the patient), the nobleman reneged, and Paracelsus took him to court. The judge found for the nobleman, and Paracelsus delivered such a blistering attack upon the court that he was advised by his friends to leave town *immediately*. Paracelsus wisely did as his friends urged.

Paracelsus had also incited the wrath of Basel's pharmacists for attacking their practice of selling long, complicated, expensive and useless prescriptions to the poor.

Paracelsus spent the remainder of his life wandering, but also teaching his students. He died at age 48, most probably after being set upon by thugs in the employ of rival physicians, thugs who fractured his skull with a rock.

Paracelsus' works were mostly dictated to his students and published after his death. His reputation as a healer was such that these works attracted great attention, and centuries of Paracelsian physicians followed his lead. His views of health, disease, and healing were a great step forward from the medicine of the universities, who followed Galen, and his influence was profound. He had a major influence on the Rosicrucians, with their concern for healing and their own mystical views.[359]

Where the Hippocratic tradition considered that there was no such thing as a disease—only diseased individuals, and that the issue for health was the balance of the humors, Paracelsus held the view that disease is a "thing" and that disease has its own *specific seed.*

That *seed* was not a physical entity, and Paracelsus referred to the importance of a vital force, which he termed *Archeus,* in all living creatures. Thus, Paracelsus considered disease to be heavily influenced by invisible and metaphysical entities rather than by imbalances within the person. An important concept of Paracelsus was that the physiology of the body is ruled over by *archei* acting more or less like internal alchemists in the different organs of the body. The most important of these is the *archeus* of the stomach, which separates the pure from the impure parts of the food, distributes the valuable portions to those parts of the body where they are needed, and discards the poisons. If the *archei* fail to act properly, poisons can accumulate within the body instead of being eliminated, and when this happens disease can result.

Historian Tobias Churton adds that Paracelsus felt that "the spirit and soul needed willfully to wed in order to harmonize and spiritualize the body."[360] The founding document of the Rosicrucians, the *Fama Fraterutatis,* has been described as the "gospel according to Paracelsus;" furthermore, the Rosicrucian movement, following Paracelsus' lead, was focused on medicine. Paracelsus was considered the leader; he had written in his book, *De secretis secretorum theologia,* that a true church would be built of spirit, not of stone, and he labeled the Pope, together with Luther, Zwingli, and other reformers, as born liars. He wanted all to be subject only to God and to nature; truth would be found within the human being. Churton points out that this powerful idea resonated with the philosophies of 18th century Freemasonry and may account for much of its success.[361]

8.6 Law of Similars

Albeit Paracelsus departed from Hippocrates regarding the existence of disease, his views were Hippocratic in most respects. He was outspoken in his attacks on the Galenists in the university medical schools, and he differed sharply with them in his approach to therapeutics. Whereas Galen had relied on the Law of Contraries, Paracelsus followed the Law of Similars.

Paracelsus accepted the principle that like cures like, and that principle became the hallmark of Paracelsian physicians. This concept was associated with the herbal healers of the day, and Paracelsus not only rejected most of the medical books of his time, in particular those of Galen and Avicenna, but he learned from the herbal healers of the countryside. He wrote, *"A Physician ought not to rest only in that bare knowledge which their Schools teach, but to learn of old Women, Egyptians [gypsies], and such-like persons; for they have greater experience in such things than all the Academians."*[362]

Paracelsus was an admirer of Hippocrates (the *Corpus Hippocraticum* had been translated from Greek to Latin by refugees following the fall of Constantinople in 1453, i.e., around 50 years earlier), and he considered all medical writings since Hippocrates to be useless. He incited the wrath of his university colleagues by publicly expressing his contempt by burning all the post-Hippocratic medical texts. He had found the university-trained physicians, who followed Galen's precepts, to be far less effective than the wise-women healers, and he said so without hesitation.

Perhaps equally important with Paracelsus approach to therapeutics was his call for a new medicine based on fresh observations rather than reliance upon ancient authority. The Galenists, still entrenched in the medical schools, wrote diatribes attacking Paracelsus, and the result was to publicize Paracelsian theories. In consequence, within thirty years of Paracelsus' death in 1541, there had sprung up a group of Paracelsian physicians with a perspective quite different from that of the university-trained physicians of preceding centuries.

All Paracelsians insisted that the study of medicine and nature should be based on fresh observations and experiments rather than the outdated writings of an Aristotle or a Galen—and they called for a revision of the university curricula on this basis.

To Paracelsus, every object in nature, by virtue of its life, was a *"spiritual being,* an invisible and incomprehensible *real thing* and a *spirit* and a *spiritual thing."* To Paracelsus, the spiritual force in the organism was primary healthy or sick. Life in all its forms, including disease, was derived from spiritual forces, including the relationships between different people. We note that this perspective is that often found in traditional medicines, e.g., *Ho'oponopono* (in Hawai'i).

We also note that basic to Paracelsian thought was the conviction that chemistry or alchemy should serve as the key to the secrets of the universe. To them, chemistry could do two things:

Chemistry formed the basis for an understanding of the macrocosm as a whole (ergo, understanding Creation).

Chemistry was believed to hold the key to understanding the human body. Bodily functions were chemical functions, and diseases were pictured as chemical malfunctions which chemically prepared medicines would cure.

The chemical philosophy of the Renaissance Paracelsians was characterized by:

1. Rejection of ancient tradition and authority
2. Search for physical truth through chemistry
3. Use of a philosophical basis in Pythagorean, neo-Platonic and Hermetic thought. *"As above, so below"* implies a relationship between microcosm and macrocosm; *that there was a natural healing power, and that both disease and its cure have a spiritual nature. This was a fundamental tenet of Paracelsus' thought, his alchemy, and his medicine.*[363]

With Paracelsus' use of similars in treatment, one of the challenges of his chemical approach was to find a way to take chemicals that were poisonous in themselves and make them effective in healing. He recognized that the size of the dose was the critical factor here, but this problem was only finally resolved by the work of Hahnemann centuries later, and that became the foundation of modern homeopathic medicine. There is thus a direct lineage from Hippocrates to Paracelsus to Hahnemann and homeopathy, just as there is from Hippocrates to Paracelsus to present-day holistic medical practitioners.

In Elizabethan England, there was acceptance of the new chemical medicines associated with the Paracelsians, but in general physicians stuck with Galen in their use of these medicines. Both Paracelsians and Galenists considered chemistry to be the tool of the physician. The English physicians were not interested in the (alchemical) mystical aspects of chemistry of the Paracelsians; they merely wanted to use chemical medicines. In the end there was a major split between the Paracelsians and the Royal College of Physicians.[364]

In general, the Galenists prevailed, and chemistry was shorn of its alchemical and metaphysical aspects, laying the groundwork for chemists such as Robert Boyle to expand the field of chemistry beyond pharmacy into general chemistry. This movement was also philosophically in tune with the materialist teachings of Descartes, whose influence was becoming stronger at that time.

8.7 Paracelsus and the Power of the Imagination

Paracelsus should be remembered not only for his mystical views, for his role in the advancement of medicine and chemistry, his espousal of similars and his views of the role of spirit in disease, but also for his recognition of *the power of the imagination.* Paracelsus was an eloquent advocate for recognizing the power of imagination in life, healthy and sick. In his opinion imagination was instantly convertible into corporeal effects, and he considered *imagination second to none in causing disease.* This perspective is reflected today in our recognition of many psychosomatic causes of illness.

Paracelsus often used the example of the imagination of the pregnant women that impresses its corporeal seal on the body of the fetus. [Note the relationship to the Child's Song of expectant African mothers, where the expectant mother sings the song describing the child she wants to bear.]³⁶⁵ Today we are learning how the emotions of the mother can affect the developing fetus. This influence has been emphasized by Bruce Lipton in his work presented in the *Biology of Belief*.³⁶⁶

The author experienced this effect personally. He has a stepson whose biological mother hated being pregnant. That circumstance had a malignant effect on her fetus, and the child was born severely autistic. Fortunately, the child's adoptive mother (the author's wife) followed Paracelsus' prescription cited below, providing love for her adopted son that overcame his autism. The "autistic" child ultimately graduated from college.

Paracelsus held that, "The ultimate cause of illness is a weakness of the Spirit," very much in keeping with other traditional healers. Above all, Paracelsus' creed was one of compassion for his patients, writing, *"Compassion is the physician's schoolmaster."*³⁶⁷

8.8 Paracelsus and Love

Paracelsus considered *love* as a *key aspect of medical treatment*. He wrote, "This is my vow...to love the sick, each and all of them, more than if my own body were at stake ...not to trust any apothecary, nor to do violence to any child." And again, "The difference between a physician and the rest of men is this, that the others need think only of themselves, while the physician must care not only for himself but also for others. *His office consists of nothing but compassion for others."*³⁶⁸

Note the contrast with the present-day practice of instructing medical students *not* to become emotionally involved with their patients. Current research suggests Paracelsus was correct, as love for the patient does much to speed up the healing process. [See *Consciousness & Healing: Integral Approaches to Mind-Body Medicine.*]³⁶⁹

Compare Paracelsus's approach with Stephen Levine's admonition in Susan Trout's *To See Differently*: *"Love is the optimum condition for healing.* The healer uses whatever he intuits will be of the greatest aid, but his energy cannot come from the mind. *His power comes from the openness of his heart."*³⁷⁰

See also Paul Pearsall's *The Heart's Code*,[371] and Leonard Laskow's *Healing With Love*[372], for it has been demonstrated experimentally that a loving intent can change even DNA configuration.

8.9 Van Helmont

Among the physicians following Paracelsus, probably the most important was Van Helmont. Jean Baptiste Van Helmont (1597-1644) was the other major figure in the Paracelsian revolution. Van Helmont considered disease an affair of the *Archeus*. To Van Helmont, disease is generated by it, takes place in it, and its outcome depends upon it. To him, nothing can happen in the organism—healthy or sick—without the *Archeus*.[373]

By *Archeus* Van Helmont meant the "vital principle." To Van Helmont, the *Archeus* governs the whole of the organism. It has its seat in the stomach and spleen. Each organ also possesses its own *Archeus insitus*. The *Archeus* is a vital and spiritual force, though it is not the "soul." It is the psychic aspect of an individual.

Van Helmont was the discoverer of what he termed, as does chemistry today, "gas," a smoke with properties specific to the material studied. By "gas" Van Helmont meant the *Archeus* that vitalized all objects, a *spiritual gas.*

In the view of Van Helmont, nothing can happen without the *Archeus*. Corporeal agents cannot attack the body directly, for *the living substance is essentially spiritual. Any bodily defect is of necessity subordinated to spiritual stimulation.* Further, since all objects possess spiritual, vital power, it is thought that that power can interact with the *Archeus* of man. The real cause of disease is an *Idea* generated by the *Archeus*. When the *Idea*, or seed, takes hold, as in fear of the plague, then the disease symptoms become manifest. Outside agents are not responsible for disease, though they can spur the generation of an *Idea* that can cause disease. Disease is basically and essentially a distinct *Idea* or *Image*. This concept we know today as the psychosomatic causes of illness, and we saw previously the impact that belief systems can have on illness.

Van Helmont rejected the Aristotelian/Galenic idea of contraries, but he also rejected Paracelsus's mystical views, as in the analogy between macrocosm and microcosm. He further rejected Paracelsus' astrological concepts, but he remains an important successor to Paracelsus in the years following Paracelsus' death.

8.10 The Renaissance[374]

The Renaissance was a time of great ferment, intellectually as well as religiously. It is conventionally considered to have occurred during the period from the 14th to the 16th centuries. However, due to the important roles played by Bruno, Galileo, and Sir Isaac Newton, we will consider the Renaissance to have extended into the 17th century. If we define the Renaissance as that period between the medieval and modern periods, then Newton's role cannot be omitted.

The Renaissance incorporated three great steps in science:
1. The publication of Copernicus's heliocentric theory in 1547.
2. The trial of Galileo by the Roman Inquisition in 1633, and his being sentenced to house arrest for the remainder of his life.
3. The publication of Newton's *Principia Mathematica* in 1687.

A major influence on all three of these events, and on Leonardo da Vinci as well, was Masileo Ficino's translation, under the sponsorship of Cosimo de' Medici, of the *Corpus Hermeticum* in 1473. The *Corpus Hermeticum* contained the ancient wisdom of Egypt, originally provided by the spiritual teacher Thoth, or Hermes Trismegistus,

Fourteen years later, Giovanni Pico della Mirandola published his *Oration on the dignity of man*, stressing the brilliance of humankind and its privileged place in creation. That book's insight was based on Hermetic principles. Pico stressed man's intellect, his search for knowledge, citing Hermes Trismegistus among other non-Christian authorities. Pico's work, defining humankind as brilliant and possessed of wondrous abilities rather than weighed down by original sin, was anathema to the Vatican. His book was quickly banned by the Roman Church.

Shortly prior to his death in 1543, the Polish canon Nicolaus Copernicus published his *On the Revolutions of the Celestial Spheres*, in which he adduced, from his lifelong studies of astronomy, his hypothesis about heliocentricity. This hypothesis included three concepts that were contrary to Ptolemaic cosmology, Church dogma and accepted academic tradition, and were therefore both controversial and heretical:
1. That the earth moves in space.
2. That the earth revolves on its own axis, producing night and day.
3. That the earth and the other planets circle the sun.

Copernicus' hypothesis was of course in conflict with Aristotle's concept of a fixed universe and with the Ptolemaic model adopted by the Church, a model that held that the Earth was the center of the universe. Ptolemy used a complex system of cycles and epicycles to account for the movement of the planets.

Worse, from the standpoint of the Vatican, was that Copernicus stated the following, "Accordingly [considering the sun's central position], it is not foolish that it has been called the lamp of the universe, or its mind, or its ruler. [It is] Hermes Trismegistus' visible God..." This description of the universe referred to the *Corpus Hermeticum*, and that was deeply heretical to the Vatican.

Thoth, or Hermes Trismegistus, produced his *Emerald Tablet* and *Asclepius*, presenting his philosophical, theological, and spiritual concepts, closely related to those presented in the *Corpus Hermeticum*. The Hermetic works were believed to come from Thoth, "God's chosen teacher of humankind, 'the all-knowing revealer'." Thoth's philosophy and cosmology were both mystical and embracing different realms of being, from matter to the divine spheres, including supernatural beings. They too advanced the concept adduced by Pico: "For the human is a godlike living thing, not comparable to the other living things of the earth but to those in heavens above, who are called gods. Or better—if one dare tell the truth—the one who is really human is above these gods as well, or at least they are wholly equal in power to one another."

Ficino's study of the *Corpus Hermeticum* led him to state, "The whole world, it seemed, had always followed a single faith whose ancient priests included Zoroaster, Hermes Trismegistus, Orpheus, Pythagoras, Plato, St Paul, and St Augustine." Ficino wrote *Three books on Life*, published in 1489, expressing his deep convictions regarding Hermeticism. Many considered Egypt as the origin of the spiritual wisdom inherited by the Jews and then by the Christians.[375]

8.11 Giordano Bruno

Giordano Bruno (1548-1600) was known as one of the greatest intellects and philosophers of his time, particularly in the realms of science and mathematics. In 1584 Bruno published both *The Ash Wednesday Supper* and also his *Expulsion of the Triumphant Beast*, both relating to Copernicus and heliocentricity and both from the perspective of Hermeticism. He also published, in the same year, *On the Infinite Universe and Worlds*. He wrote:

"For there is a single general space, a single vast immensity which we may freely call *Void*; in it are innumerable and infinite globes like this on which we live and grow. This space we declare to be infinite, since neither reason, convenience, possibility, sense-perception or nature assign to it a limit. In it are an infinity of worlds of the same kind as our own.... Beyond the imaginary convex circumference of the universe is Time."

Clearly Bruno was centuries ahead of his time, with the last sentence, above, even anticipating Einstein. His concepts were not only ahead of their time but were antithetical to those of Aristotle and therefore to Church dogma. He looked upon the *Corpus Hermeticum* as the guide to a utopian state, a Hermetic utopia. He was attempting either to replace the Church or to reform it from within. Neither alternative was welcomed by the Vatican, and so the Roman Inquisition came into the picture. Bruno was arrested in 1592, and he was burned at the stake in 1600, for he refused to disavow his beliefs in heliocentricity and the *Hermetica*. Bruno was condemned for holding opinions contrary to the teachings of the Catholic Church, including denying the Trinity, Jesus' divinity, and asserting that Jesus was a magus. Hungarian biographer Ksenija Atanasijevic's *The Metaphysical and Geometrical Doctrine of Bruno* (1923) described Bruno as "certainly the greatest philosopher of the XVIth century" and wrote concerning Bruno: "If the Inquisition had not managed to put its jackal's claws upon him when he was forty-four and if he had not been burned alive at the age of fifty-two, Bruno would have left to humanity some more of his inspired and farsighted conceptions."[376]

Bruno was a martyr for Hermeticism and the symbolism of heliocentricity that he felt would bring about a Hermetic society.

8.12 Galileo Galilei

Galileo Galilei (1564-1642), Professor of Mathematics at the University of Padua, Italy, in many respects initiated the beginning of modern science. Indeed, both Albert Einstein and Stephen Hawking have considered Galileo as the father of modern science. He made great contributions in optics—inventing the first telescope, and using it for astronomical observations as well as for military purposes—and in acoustics and mechanics. He established a mathematical description of the motion of a falling body, and establishing the principle that bodies fall at a rate determined by the square of the time they have fallen (Galileo's Law). This and his other achievements were major contributions to science.

His telescope provided new evidence showing that Copernicus' heliocentric theory was correct. He described those results in his *Dialogue Concerning the Two Chief Systems* (1632) showing close parallels to Bruno's *The Ash Wednesday Supper*, written forty years earlier. It was the *Dialogue* that was used as evidence of his heresy in his trial before the Roman Inquisition. It may be noted that Galileo considered the movement of the tides as providing proof of heliocentricity. In this, Galileo was mistaken, and the final proof that Copernicus' theory was correct had to wait for the publication of Newton's Laws of Motion, demonstrating that Kepler's laws, which were derived from Copernicus' theory, were correct.

Galileo was certainly familiar with Bruno's work, and he owed an intellectual debt to Bruno. One of his lifelong friends was Tommasio Campanella (1568-1639), who wrote a defense of Galileo when the latter was on trial before the Inquisition. Campanella was a disciple of Bruno, and he continued Bruno's work after the latter's execution. There is little doubt that Galileo was well acquainted with the Hermetic works of the time. Campanella, author of *City of the Sun* (1623), believed, with Bruno, that heliocentricity was key to a Hermetic vision. That vision was of a "new city-state, led by a philosopher-priest-king, and guided by Hermetic magical principles." as one authority described *City of the Sun.*

The thought that Galileo might provide proof of Copernicus' heliocentric theory caused great anxiety in the Vatican, and Galileo was called before the Inquisition. Before leaving for his trial, Galileo wrote to a friend, "I hear from a good source that the Jesuit Fathers have impressed the most important person 'in Rome' with the idea that my book 'the Dialogo' is execrable and more dangerous to the Holy Church than the writings of Luther and Calvin."

Galileo was duly tried by the Roman Inquisition. He pointed out that in *Diologue* he had presented both Ptolemaic and Copernican theories, and he disavowed believing in Copernicus' theory of heliocentricity. He was nevertheless convicted of being "Vehemently suspected of heresy" and was condemned to house arrest for the remainder of his life. He continued his experiments with the laws of motion, and he continued to make major discoveries before his death a few years later.

His friend Campanella had urged him to stand firm *because of the spiritual [Hermetic] importance of his work*, the return to ancient truth that heliocentricity represented. However, Galileo, well aware of Bruno's fate, recanted and therefore was able to live out his life in relative comfort.[377]

8.13 The Rosicrucians

In 1614 a book appeared that caused a great stir in German philosophical circles, the *Fama Frateritatis*, or, *Discovery of the Order of the Rosicrucians*. The following year the book *Confession of the Fraternity R.C. to the Learned of Europe* appeared. The two constituted the 'Rosicrucian manifestos', announcing the existence of a secret order, the Fraternity of the Rose Cross, a fraternity of scholars that would bring about a major reform in the arts, sciences, and religion. The fraternity felt that the Reformation had failed, and they intended to fix all the 'faults of the Church'. As a consequence, the Rosicrucians were held to be a major threat to the Vatican. Neverthe less, two years later another book appeared: *The Chemical Wedding of Christian Rosenkreuz in the Year 1459*, authored by a Lutheran cleric, Johann Andreae, that continued the theme of the earlier manifestos.

The Rosicrucian brotherhood considered itself Christian, though of a reformed kind. It followed an alchemical philosophy, aiming to transform 'base souls into divine gold.' They considered the Pope to be the Antichrist, thus earning the enmity of the Vatican. They also were influenced by Campanella, whose *City of the Sun* was reflected in Andreae's *Christianopolis*.

The final blow to the Rosicrucian influence (though Rosicrucian groups continued, but their influence was muted), was delivered by the Jesuit educated René Descartes, whose separation of the physical from the invisible led to a mechanistic view of the universe. The Church strongly supported Descartes' writings as providing an anti-Hermetic and anti-Rosicrucian influence.[378]

8.14 The Late Renaissance

The late Renaissance proved to be a time of great Hermetic influence. John Dee, author of *The Hieroglyphic Monad* an astrologer and advisor to Queen Elizabeth I, was a champion of Copernicus' theory and a devotee of the Hermetic tradition. Giordano Bruno was also well known to the Queen and was not only an admirer but a frequent visitor to her court. While in

London, Bruno published two works, the *Explanation of the Thirty Seals*, and in 1584, *The Ash Wednesday Supper*, in which Bruno lauds Copernicus and his theory. He also published *Expulsion of the Triumphant Beast*, a "glorification of the magical religion of the Egyptians."

Sir Francis Bacon, editor of the King James translation of the Bible, was another Hermeticist prominent in the queen's court. He was a man of many talents, prominent in the court and enjoying the patronage of the queen. Ernest Tuveson noted that Bacon's "conception of natural processes owes much to hermeticism and other traditional (i.e., esoteric) sources," and he shared the philosophy of Dee and Paracelsus. Bacon's political progress culminated in his being appointed as Lord Chancellor in 1618, a position through which he was able to put many of his goals into practice.[379]

8.15 Leibniz and Kircher

Gottfried Wilhelm Leibniz (1646-1716) was another Renaissance notable who was influenced in a major way by the Rosicrucians. He is known today as being the co-discoverer (with Isaac Newton) of the differential calculus, and he also invented the binary system on which all modern computers are based. Leibniz was an alchemist, and his works reveal a deep familiarity with the Rosicrucian manifestos. His calculating machine earned him a Fellowship in London's Royal Society. The metaphysical influence on Leibniz was revealed when he wrote, "But when I looked for the ultimate reasons for mechanism, and even for the laws of motion, I was greatly surprised to see that they could not be found in mathematics but that I should have to return to metaphysics."[380]

Another Renaissance figure whose Hermetic influence had a major impact was the Jesuit Athanasius Kircher (1601-1680). Kircher has been described as "the most famous Jesuit scholar of his time." He was a mathematician, an Egyptologist, and writer of the four volume *Oedipus Aegyptiacus*. His understandings were close to those of Bruno, believing the ancient Egyptian civilization provided a model in both politics and religion.

As Picknett and Price write, "Kircher showed that Bruno's intellectual legacy was not only still alive but also still shaping the development of science."[381]

Ingrid Rowland, art historian and Fellow of the American Academy in Rome, wrote:

> Kircher's cosmology and its attendant concept of a universal *panspermia* . . . show that, however dramatically the eight-year trial and gruesome public execution of Giordano Bruno had been designed to prove that the heretic philosopher was a lone and terrible fanatic, the performance had failed. Bruno's books had been read by Kepler, Galileo and Athanasius Kircher, and they were enough to change the course of natural philosophy. For both Bruno and Kircher argued with passionate eloquence that nothing but an infinite universe did justice to an omnipotent God, and once the idea of that vastness immeasurable had been conceived, it really did burst the crystalline spheres of Aristotelian physics.[382]

8.16 The Royal Society

In England the Royal Society was the outcome of a group of scholars who had met in John Wilkins' rooms at Wadham College, Oxford. This group included the chemist Robert Boyle, who had significant Rosicrucian ties, John Wilkins, inventor of the metric system who referenced the Rosicrucian *Fama* in his *Mathematicall Magick*, architect Christopher Wren, and others from 1548 to 1600. In 1600 they joined with a group of natural philosophers to establish a society to use the experimental method to investigate natural phenomena. There were other Rosicrucian and Masonic ties, and they received the approval of Charles II and so became the Royal Society. There ensued a struggle between the Hermetically-inclined Oxford group and those natural philosophers that had a more materialistic approach. The materialists won out, and so the Hermetic roots of John Wilkins' group were set aside. Isaac Newton was elected a Fellow of the Royal Society in 1671 and the President of the

Royal Society in 1703. He held that position until his death in 1727. The story of Isaac Newton will be told in the following chapter.[383]

Timeline

100 CE	Galen
400 CE	Rome fell
	— Dark Ages —
1000 CE	Crusades, European recognition of Arabic medicine, Avicenna
1100 CE	Translation of Avicenna's *Canon,* Galen, Aristotle, into Latin.
	St. Hildegard von Bingen
1200 CE	Founding of Oxford and Cambridge by monks
	St. Francis of Assisi
1300 CE	Meister Eckhart
1400 CE	Inquisition begins; Church corruption (selling indulgences)
1453 CE	Constantinople fell; Hippocratic Corpus translated
1471 CE	Ficino's translation of *Corpus Hermeticum*
1492 CE	Columbus to West Indies
	Jews in Mexico/New Mexico
1493 CE	Theophrastus Paracelsus born
	Pope Alexander VI, mistress and children in Vatican
1500 CE	Religious Reformation (Martin Luther/Protestantism)
	Medical Reformation (Paracelsus; the Paracelsian physicians, forerunners of Homeopathy)
1543 CE	Copernicus publishes his heliocentric theory in *On the Revolutions of the Celestial Spheres*
1600 CE	Giordino Bruno burned at the stake by Roman Inquisition for promoting Copernicus' theory
1633 CE	Galileo convicted by Roman Inquisition for promoting Copernicus' theory, sentenced to lifelong house arrest
1687 CE	Newton publishes *Principia Mathematica*

Notes

352 Coulter, Harris *Divided Legacy: A History of the Schism in Medical Thought*, Vols. I & II, Wehawken Book Co. 1975.
353 Picknett, Lynn and Clive Prince, *The Forbidden Universe: The Occult Origins of Science and the Search for the Mind of God*, New York, Skyhorse Publishing, 2011.
354 Churton, Tobias *The Invisible History of the Rosicrucians's: The World's Most Mysterious Secret Society*, 2009.
355 Ibid.
356 Hartmann, Franz *Paracelsus: Life and Prophecies*, Steiner Books, 1973.
357 Churton, Tobias *The Invisible History of the Rosicrucians's: The World's Most Mysterious Secret Society*, 2009.
358 Gilly, Dr. Carlos "Theophrastia sancta, Paracelsianism as a Religion in Conflict with the Established Churches", *Transformation of Paracelsism 1500-1800: Alchemy, Chemistry and Medicine* (Glasgow-Symposium 15-19 September 1993), Leiden, Brill, 1998, pp. 151-185.
359 Churton, Tobias *The Invisible History of the Rosicrucians's: The World's Most Mysterious Secret Society*, 2009.
360 Ibid.
361 Ibid.
362 Ibid.
363 Ibid.
364 DeBus, Allen G. *The English Paracelsians*, Franklin Watts, New York,
365 Traditional African proverb.
366 Lipton, Bruce *The Biology of Belief*, Mountain of Love/Elite Books, 2005.
367 Churton, Tobias *The Invisible History of the Rosicrucians's: The World's Most Mysterious Secret Society*, 2009.
368 Ibid.
369 Schlitz, Marilyn and Tina Amorok, *Consciousness & Healing: Integral Approaches to Mind-Body Medicine*, Churchill Livingstone, 2004.
370 Trout, Ph.D. Susan S. *To See Differently* Three Roses Press, Wahington D.C., 1990.
371 Pearsall, Paul *The Heart's Code: Tapping the Wisdom and Power of Our Heart Energy*, New York, Doubleday Dell, 1998.
372 Laskow, M.D., Leonard *Healing With Love: A Breakthrough Mind/Body Medical Program for Healing Yourself and Others*, San Francisco, Harper Collins,1992.
373 Pagel, Walter "Van Helmont's Concept of Disease—To Be Or Not To Be? The Influence of Paracelsus" in *Bulletin of the History of Medicine*, Johns Hopkins University Press, No. 46, Sept-Oct 1972.
374 Picknett, Lynn and Clive Prince, *The Forbidden Universe: The Occult Origins of Science and the Search for the Mind of God*, New York, Skyhorse Publishing, 2011. Author's note: The section is based on this book, and the

author wishes to express his indebtedness to those authors for this material.
375 Ibid.
376 Atanasijevic, Ksenija *The Metaphysical and Geometrical Doctrine of Bruno*, 1923.
377 Picknett, Lynn and Clive Prince, *The Forbidden Universe: The Occult Origins of Science and the Search for the Mind of God*, New York, Skyhorse Publishing, 2011.
378 Ibid.
379 Ibid.
380 Letter written by Gottfried Leibniz to Nicolas Remond in 1714, reprinted in the *Stanford Encyclopedia of Philosophy*, 2013.
381 Picknett, Lynn and Clive Prince, *The Forbidden Universe: The Occult Origins of Science and the Search for the Mind of God*, New York, Skyhorse Publishing, 2011.
382 Rowland, Ingrid "Chapter 8: Athanasius Kircher, Giordano Bruno, and the Panspermia of the Infinite Universe," *Athanasius Kircher: The Last Man Who Knew Everything*, Paula Findlen editor, 2004.
383 Picknett, Lynn and Clive Prince, *The Forbidden Universe: The Occult Origins of Science and the Search for the Mind of God*, New York, Skyhorse Publishing, 2011.

Chapter 9
Descartes, the Cartesian Dichotomy, Newton, and Mathematical Models

9.1 René Descartes

René Descartes has been aptly termed the father of modern philosophy, and his materialistic philosophy pervades our culture today.[384] He was a leading mathematician of his day, and he developed his philosophy based on mathematical logic. As described later in this chapter, in mathematics one proceeds from an axiom (an assumption) and develops a mathematical structure from that axiom. This, Descartes felt, would provide a certainty missing from the Aristotelian philosophy taught in the universities of his time. The axiom from which Descartes developed his philosophy was *Cogito, ergo sum* ("I think, therefore I am"; originally, "Je pense, donc je suis"). Although René Descartes is often referred to as the founder of modern philosophy, he is best known to science for three major contributions:

(1) He was the originator of the discipline in mathematics known as Analytic Geometry, and his Cartesian Coordinates are constantly used today to express mathematical relationships.

(2) He was the first philosopher (to the author's knowledge) to espouse the view that to solve a complex problem, the most effective approach is to break it into smaller and smaller pieces. This approach has become known as *reductionism* in science, and that approach led in turn to a materialist science.

(3) Most important from the perspective of medicine, he is the person who, more than any other, represents the 17th century separation in medical science of the physical body from the mind and spirit of man, often referred to as the Cartesian Dichotomy. This separation fit well with the temper of his time—in particular the influence of the Vatican and the Roman Inquisition—and the work being

done in other areas of science. The Cartesian Dichotomy ushered in a new era of expanded medical experimental science. It has had a profound impact on the way Western scientific medicine is practiced, so it bears careful scrutiny.[385]

René Descartes (1596-1650) was a contemporary of Van Helmont, living 100 years after Paracelsus. However, Descartes took a very different viewpoint from that of Paracelsus or Van Helmont.

9.2 Descartes' Background

Descartes was the son of a wealthy professional family, his father a very successful attorney, giving Descartes the financial resources to live his life as he wished, which was to study philosophy. He was sickly as a youth, and as a consequence he developed a strong interest in medicine. He became a student at the Jesuit College at La Fleche, which Descartes described as "one of the most renowned schools in Europe." There, Descartes studied Latin, Greek, mathematics, science, the classics, and scholastic philosophy. At La Fleche Descartes, flourished, becoming strong, healthy, and developing an interest both in the outer world and in knowledge, with a particular interest in medicine. He then took a degree in law at the University of Poitiers. Despite his Jesuit training and studies of the classics, together with his studies of law, Descartes came away convinced he had really learned nothing. Like Paracelsus, he believed he could learn more—through travel, independent study of problems in science and philosophy that interested him, and his own contemplation—than he could from books. This he proceeded to do, working often in solitude but corresponding with stimulating colleagues and writing of the issues he examined.

As a young man, Descartes has been described as a "Papist swashbuckler." He fought as a soldier in the Thirty Years War in the Netherlands, Bohemia, and Hungary. At age twenty-four he was fighting with the Catholic forces at the Battle of the White Mountain (1620) in the army of the Prince of Orange. He then wintered in Prague, which gave him the leisure to develop his ideas. In Descartes' words, "The arrival of winter delayed me in quarters where, finding no company to distract me and, luckily, having no cares or passions to trouble me, I used to spend the whole day alone in a room that was heated by a stove, where I had plenty of time to concentrate on my own thoughts."[386]

While in Prague, Descartes learned of the Rosicrucians and found their principles appealing. The Rosicrucians kept their membership secret, and as a result were termed 'the Invisibles,' being suspected by many of sorcery and of being part of a devilish plot. Upon his return to Paris in 1623, Descartes found himself endangered by his known interest in the Rosicrucians. He found it expedient to distance himself from the Rosicrucians, and he made a point of denouncing the Rosicrucian 'calumny.'

Descartes' negative perspective on the Rosicrucians was reinforced by his fellow student and close friend, the monk Marin Mersenne. Mersenne was the mathematician who developed prime number theory, and was a scientist as well as a theologian and devout Catholic. He was an influential friend of Descartes and was openly opposed to the Rosicrucians in Paris.

Following his time in the army, Descartes traveled extensively in Europe. He pursued his scientific and philosophical interests, and at the age of 33 he moved to the Netherlands. He spent 21 years there, and it was during that time that he published most of his works. He moved to Stockholm in 1649 at the invitation of Queen Christina, and he died there of pneumonia the following winter.

Descartes was 32 years younger than Galileo (1564-1642) and 25 years younger than Kepler (1571-1630), and he was clearly influenced by their work in astronomy and physics. Descartes found their mathematical approach, and mathematics itself, much more satisfying than the Scholastic philosophy (that of Aristote and Thomas Aquinas') taught in the universities. Descartes' views of Aristotle were provided by his observation, "The best way of proving the falsity of Aristotle's principles is to point out that they have not enabled any progress to be made in all the many centuries in which they have been followed."[387]

He set out to develop a philosophy in the likeness of mathematics, rather than relying on the Bible and on ancient authority as did the Scholastics, developing all knowledge from a set of ultimate principles (axioms – ergo, assumptions). The use of mathematical logic would give this new philosophy a certitude that he found missing in Aristotle. Aristotle had lived 2,000 years earlier but, through the influence of Saint Thomas Aquinas, Aristotle's philosophy and science were still accepted as dogma by the Church. As a consequence, it was Aristotle's philosophy that was taught in the universities. Descartes hoped to become Aristotle's successor as the ultimate philosophical authority.

9.3 Analytic Geometry

Descartes had the ability to contemplate concepts in juxtaposition, and he joined together algebra and geometry to form a new branch of mathematics, analytic geometry. Analytic geometry gives us an extremely valuable tool for looking at mathematical relationships, and most of the relationships studied in science and mathematics today are expressed graphically in Cartesian coordinates. Descartes' development of analytic geometry gave him a well-deserved reputation as a leading mathematician of his day, and it also confirmed for him the value of expressing physical relationships in mathematical terms. That is, Descartes found it valuable to use mathematical models to describe nature, just as had Galileo and Kepler, and anticipated Isaac Newton's view as well as much of the science that followed.

However, Descartes' Jesuit teachers and his profound Catholic beliefs had a major influence on him, causing him to reject the Hermetic writings that influenced Copernicus, Kepler, Galileo, Newton, and Leibniz.

9.4 The World

Descartes was not timid! He set out to understand all of physical and spiritual reality, describing his conclusions in a compendium he referred to as *The World*. This book was to be in two parts: the first devoted to physical theory and entitled *A*

Treatise on Light, the second part devoted to anatomy as the basis of medicine.

Unfortunately, before *The World* was published, Galileo was condemned to life-long house arrest by the Roman Inquisition for his allegedly "heretical" ideas. He was suspected of agreeing with Copernicus that the earth revolves around the sun. (Galileo was convicted of having been "vehemently suspected of heresy," so he recanted and disavowed any agreement with Copernicus, thus avoiding Bruno's fate).

Descartes had written material in *The World* that agreed with Galileo, so he decided perhaps it would be wise not to publish that work. [Note that the Inquisition was still active in Descartes' time, and, via the Cartesian Dichotomy, Descartes influences Western scientific medicine to this day.] However, many of the ideas in *The World*, were later included in his *Discourse on Method*, probably Descartes' most important work, and *The World* was published in two parts following Descartes' death, in 1662 and 1664.[388]

9.5 Descartes' Discourse on Method

In *Discourse*, Descartes set down the logic he used to develop his philosophy as having four key rules. He described those rules as follows:

> The first was never to accept anything as true if I did not know clearly that it was so, that is, carefully to avoid prejudice and jumping to conclusions, and to include nothing in my judgments apart from whatever appeared so clearly and distinctly to my mind that I had no opportunity to cast doubt on it.
>
> The second was to subdivide each of the problems that I was about to examine into as many parts as would be possible and necessary to resolve them better.
>
> The third was to guide my thoughts in an orderly way by beginning with the objects that are the simplest and easiest to know and to rise gradually, as if by steps, to knowledge of the most complex, and even by

assuming an order among objects in cases where there is no natural order among them.

And the final rule was: in all cases, to make such comprehensive connections and such general reviews that I was certain not to omit anything.[389]

To us today, perhaps the most important of these rules is the second, *"To subdivide each of the problems that I was about to examine into as many parts as would be possible and necessary to resolve them better."*

This process is that of *reductionism*, an important principle followed by many scientists, and it is one that has important implications for medical science and research. This principle *assumes* that the whole is *not* greater than the sum of its parts, and in practice, it sets aside any consideration of invisible factors.

Descartes' axiom, *Cogito, ergo sum*, became the foundation of Cartesian philosophy. His goal was to exhibit all varieties of knowledge as the consequence of ultimate principles that could be universally accepted as axioms. *Cogito, ergo sum* was his fundamental axiom, and from this, Descartes went on to prove the existence of God and to develop a new physics based on this metaphysical principle.

Cartesian physics has been described in modern times, by Coulter, as follows: "The most basic assumption of the entire Cartesian physics project in physics is that all natural phenomena may be explained in terms of the motions and interactions of small parts of matter." And, "Descartes was extremely reductionist; for example, there was no room in his physics for electrical or optical properties, or for any attractive forces between particles, that are not reducible to the mechanical interactions of parts of matter."[390]

Cartesian physics provided a materialistic view of the universe, a clockwork universe, and it was the vogue among intellectuals for more than a generation after Descartes' death.[391]

However, when Isaac Newton published his *Mathematical Principles of Natural Philosophy*, the *Principia*, in 1687, Newtonian physics soon replaced Cartesian. Even so other ideas of Descartes', most importantly the Cartesian Dichotomy as well as reductionism, and so materialism, together with the mathematical approach of Analytic Geometry, remained a permanent influence on Western thought.[392]

9.6 The Cartesian Dichotomy

The most crucial of Descartes' conclusions for Western medicine was the Cartesian Dichotomy, the separation of matter (body) from mind and soul/spirit. In Descartes' view, the soul and spirit are essentially thought, and Descartes posited that there is no connection between the idea of body and the idea of thought. Therefore, in Descartes' view, as the idea of soul or mind contains nothing pertaining to a body, the soul itself is radically separate from the body, on the principle that distinct ideas are representative of distinct existences.

Historian of science Desmond Clarke (the translator of Descartes' *Discourse*) has written, "This initiative in physical theory presuppose, for Descartes, a fundamental distinction between the physical world and the spiritual world. The human soul, angels and God were classified as spiritual or non-material substances; apart from them, all other realities were classified as physical, and the kind of explanation that is appropriate for physical phenomena is a scientific one. This metaphysical distinction between two radically different types of reality was a question that Descartes had begun to work on soon after his arrival in the Netherlands, and it was summarized in another unpublished draft essay at that time."[393]

Clearly Descartes' separation of the physical and visible from the invisible placed him in sharp contrast to the hermetically influenced scientists of his time (Copernicus, Bruno, Galileo, Newton, and Leibniz), to say nothing of the shamans of the indigenous peoples, as well as the mystics and the mystery schools. Descartes' separation of the material from the spiritual gave birth to a separation between body and mind that pervades medical science to this day.

Descartes' philosophical conclusion fit in well with the sentiment of the time. Galileo's work had been condemned by the Church. Further, both Rosicruianism and Hermeticism were considered threats to the Church, and so Descartes' views, which were considered not to be Rosicrucian or Hermetic, were welcomed by the Church.[394]

Descartes' separation of body from soul made possible the removal of medicine from the Church's jurisdiction. So long as medicine concerned itself with a body that did not involve the soul, leaving the mind and soul to be the province of the Church, there was no conflict of interest, a solution that freed medicine to go its scientific materialistic way.[395]

However, in devising a solution that enabled medical science to proceed without interference from the Church and the Inquisition, Descartes enabled the Inquisition to have a profound influence on Western medicine even to this day. Clearly, Descartes' separation of body from mind and soul initiated a major break from the concepts of Pythagoras, Socrates, Plato, and Hippocrates, to say nothing of the respect for the invisible that was the hallmark of shamanism and of the mystery schools and traditional medicines.[396]

9.7 The Body as a Machine

The Cartesian Dichotomy led, in turn, to the concept of the *body as a machine* and was in stark contrast with the views of Hippocrates, Socrates, and Plato, as well those of shamans and mystery schools regarding the importance of the invisible world. Descartes wrote, in his *Discourse,* "Just as a clock composed of wheels and counterweights is as obedient to the laws of nature when it is badly made, and does not mark the hours properly, as when it fully satisfies the desire of its maker, so too, if I consider the human body to be so constructed and composed of bones, nerves, muscles, veins, blood, and flesh, that even if it were mindless, it would still move in the same way as it does now, when it moves involuntarily, without, that is to say, the help of the mind, and only through the disposition of the bodily organs, I recognize easily that it would be as natural for this body, if it were suffering, for example, from the dropsy, to suffer from dryness of the throat (which usually signifies to the mind a sensation of thirst), and to be disposed by this dryness to make those nervous and muscular movements that are required for drinking, and so increase its sickness and do itself harm, as it would be natural for this same body, when it is well, to be induced to drink for its own good by a similar dryness of the throat."[397]

Later he wrote to a friend, "Now I am dissecting the heads of different animals in order to explain what imagination, memory etc., consist of."[398]

Descartes extended these views to his concept of a clockwork universe. This view paved the way, a generation after Descartes' death, for the Newtonian physics and the concept of separate and interacting bodies that followed.

Note the contrast between Descartes' and Newton's concepts of separateness and that of indigenous peoples' recognition of the unity of all nature. This contrast, and Descartes' influence, has carried on into the present time with an important (and negative) impact on medical science.

Descartes also wrote in *Discourse* about the circulation of the blood, adding his interpretation to that of his older contemporary, Harvey (1578-1657), the first Western physician to describe the role of the heart and the circulatory system. Again, physical laws were the key to Descartes' view of the circulation, albeit his views were slightly different from Harvey's.

9.8 Descartes and Rationalism, Materialism

Descartes became known as representing a 'shift from magic to mechanism.' He argued that all physical phenomena could be explained in purely mechanical terms. He led the way for the 17th century Rationalists, holding that sense-perception and experience were far less reliable than was reasoning power, and that medicine should be based on a comprehensive theory of physical and physiological causes of disease. *This materialistic approach pervades medical research to this day.* That perspective is well reflected in the title of Carlson and Johnson's physiology textbook, *The Machinery of the Body*.[399]

With his allegiance to mathematics and physical laws and his denigration of observation, Descartes became the founder of a whole school of Rationalist, Cartesian physicians. He also could be considered a major spur in the development of modern scientific medicine for, although scientific medicine may have begun with Hippocrates, the Cartesian Dichotomy gave medical exper-imentation an impetus that continues to this day. Since animals were held by Descartes to have no souls [Descartes had referred to animals as 'brute animals'] and therefore cries of pain could be ignored as mere reflex responses to the (painful) stimulus, there were unfortunate implications for the animal experimentation that followed. Fortunately, we have moved beyond Descartes' views of animal experimentation, and practice a more humane approach to animals in recent years.

9.9 The Cartesian Physicians

A series of European physicians followed Descartes' lead in the 17th Century, including several whose names are enshrined in medical terminology today: Sylvius, Willis, Cheyne, and Hoffman. Typical was Hermann Boerhaave, Professor of Medicine at Leiden University, who taught and wrote that the body was a collection of mechanical elements obeying mechanical laws.[400]

The Cartesian physicians felt, for example, that the laws of hydraulics were the key to understanding the circulatory system. This perspective provided an approach that is still in use today—the "Principles of plumbing," as one of the author's professors put it—the engineering of the body, a view that permeates the physiology currently taught to medical students.

These Rationalist physicians followed the *Law of Contraries* as their guiding principle in therapeutics, just as had their Rationalist predecessors, albeit the Cartesian physicians tended to analyze the actions of drugs as being dependent on their physical properties. Thus, as mercury was heavy, so it was thought that this property would effectively remove obstructions to circulation. This was, of course, in contrast to the emphasis on chemistry of their predecessors, and it proved to be a malignant influence on therapeutics.

9.10 Sir Isaac Newton

Sir Isaac Newton (1642-1727) was a child when Descartes died. Although from an impoverished family, his uncle recognized his scientific curiosity and arranged for him to attend a school at Grantham, where he supported himself working as a servant for wealthier students. Newton later won a scholarship to Trinity College, Cambridge. He graduated from Cambridge in 1665; however, upon graduation he was forced by a plague epidemic to return to his family farm, where he remained for two years. During that time, he experimented with a prism and studied the properties of light, and he also began to think about gravity (the apple tree story), recognizing that the same gravitational force that caused an apple to fall to the ground also governed the motion of the heavenly bodies.

Following the plague's subsidence, Newton returned to Cambridge, where he was named a Fellow of Trinity College, becoming a professor of mathematics in 1660, at the age of twenty-seven. He continued his studies of light and of motion, and in 1687 his Laws of Motion were published in *Philosophia naturalis principia mathematica (Mathematical Principles of Natural Philosophy)*, often referred to as, simply, the *Principia*. Most scholars recognized the *Principia* for the major contribution it made to our understanding of the forces governing our universe. However, in describing the mathematics of the interactions of separate bodies, his work led to the concept of a "billiard ball" universe, a universe consisting of separate bodies and their interactions. Nevertheless, there were those who objected to its Hermetic origins. Historian Richard Westfall has written,

"The cry of occult qualities greeted the publication of the *Principia*. In more than one sense, the mechanists who raised the cry were justified. Not only did the concept of attraction violate their sense of philosophic propriety, but the origin of the concept was the very Hermetic tradition they suspected...The [Cartesian] champions of mechanical orthodoxy failed to realize what benefit the Hermetic idea would bestow on the mechanical philosophy of nature."[401]

This view of Newton has not abated to this day. Christopher Hitchens, writing in *God is Not Great*, described Newton as "a spiritualist and alchemist of a particularly laughable kind."[402]

As a consequence of his development of the first reflecting telescope, Newton was elected a Fellow of the Royal Society in 1671, and, thirty-two years later, he was elected President of the Society.

One consequence of the publication of the *Principia* was that his Laws of Motion provided the final proof of Copernicus' heliocentric theory.

Newton was also the co-inventor (with Leibniz) of the *differential calculus*, an extremely valuable mathematical tool for the analysis of physical systems.

Newton received many honors: he was named Warden of the Mint in 1696, then Master of the Bank of England, and, of course, President of the Royal Society in 1703, a position he held until his death. He was knighted by Queen Anne in 1705, and upon his death he was buried in Westminster Abbey.

In recent years it has become known that Newton's foremost interest was not on optics or mechanics but on alchemy. Fully one-third of his personal library were books on alchemy, and he had a significant esoteric interest. Economist John Maynard Keynes, a collector of Newton's alchemical writings, described Newton in a paper presented to the Royal Society, as follows: "Newton was not the first of the age of reason. He was the last of the magicians...Why do I call him a magician? Because he looked on the whole universe and all that is in it *as a riddle* [Keynes' emphasis], as a secret which could be read by applying pure thought to certain evidence, certain mystic clues which God had laid about the world to allow a sort of philosopher's treasure hunt to the esoteric brotherhood."[403]

There is also evidence that Newton was keenly interested in the Rosicrucian documents. Newton's copies of the Rosicrucian manifestos, now held in the Yale University library, contain significant annotations by Newton.[404]

Newton was influenced by his association with the Cambridge Platonists. They were a misnamed part of a spiritual brotherhood stretching back to the *Corpus Hermeticum* and its translation by Ficino in 1473.[405]

Modern historians have recognized Newton's esoteric interests. Picknett and Prince comment in *The Forbidden Universe,* "But the reality is simple: if Newton had never become privy to the Hermetic philosophy, he would never have achieved his work and the world would be—literally—much the poorer for it. It is universally acknowledged that if the *Principia* had never been written, our modern technological world would not exist. But without the Hermetica, Newton would never have written the *Principia.* Emphatically Newton did not make his great scientific discoveries *despite* his esoteric beliefs, but *because* of them." They later add, "He *applied* those [Hermetic] principles to physical systems. Like many esotericists before and after him, Newton was a great believer that the earliest civilizations, such as Egypt, knew more than people in his own day—that they possessed the *prisca sapientia,* or 'ancient wisdom'."[406]

The impact of Newton's discoveries provided further impetus to scientific experimentation, including experiments in medical science. Despite Newton's own views on the invisible source of reality, (a perspective that stemmed from his esoteric beliefs), the scientists of the 17th and 18th centuries, in accomplishing the advances in physics and chemistry of those centuries, built upon the Cartesian dichotomy and reductionism, together with Newton's Laws, to produce a 'billiard ball' universe, a mechanical, *materialistic* science and—importantly to us—scientific medicine, one in which all bodies are separate and interacting. This interaction of separate bodies provides a sharp contrast to the intermingling world of the shamans and the mystery schools, in which the visible and the invisible importantly affect each other.

Newton's Laws of Motion proved to be invaluable to science and are still routinely used today. However, they also led to what physician Deepak Chopra has described as, "Scientists are superstitious, and their superstition is called materialism."[407]

9.11 Mathematics and Mathematical Models

This brings us to mathematical models and the Trap of Mathematics: that mathematical modeling is a *game*. [This section is based upon a seminar on "How to do Research," given by Professor Allendoerfer, Chairman of the Department of Mathematics at the University of Washington, to physiology graduate students in the 1950s.] In his discussion of mathematics, Professor Allendoerfer made the point that *mathematics is a game!* That game follows the logic of *Axiom, Theorem, Prediction*, and that game may or may not have any relationship to nature.[408]

Thus, mathematics is *not* a science, the study of nature, even though it is sometimes called the "Queen of Sciences." Science studies nature; mathematics plays logical games, each game based on a set of axioms (rules, assumptions). The impact of these assumptions is well illustrated by geometries. We are taught and are familiar with Euclidian geometry, which is based on the axiom that parallel lines neither converge nor diverge as they go to infinity. However, one can postulate different axioms, assuming that parallel lines do diverge (or converge) as they go to infinity. These non-Euclidian geometries have proven valuable both in engineering applications (e.g., the design of suspension bridges) and physical theory (Einstein's relativity theory which utilizes a non-Euclidian geometry).

It becomes apparent that Descartes' philosophy, based on the axiom, *Cogito, ergo sum,* is only the result of a mathematical game. Thus, the materialist conclusions derived by Descartes are only as valid as is his axiom. There are other axioms that can be postulated, such as those of Hermeticists and the mystery schools, the shamans, and many Renaissance scientists, who postulate the presence of an invisible world fully as much of a reality as the physical world we can see and/or measure.

The issue of mathematical models needs also to be addressed. Isaac Newton commented, "Nature can be described as a second-order differential equation." Why a second order system? Because most physical systems contain the elements of mass, viscous resistance, and elasticity. Those elements can be described mathematically by a second-order differential equation. To a first approximation, Newton's assertion is often true. However, Newton's statement only works within the limits in which the system's behavior is *linear*, and then only to a first approximation. Nevertheless, Newton's statement is still a useful approximate statement. Further, just as Newtonian mechanics don't hold under quantum mechanical conditions, so also can such approximations prove misleading.

This situation can be illustrated with the behavior of a spring. Hooke's Law, L = kF, (Length is proportional to Force) describes this elastic behavior. However, Hooke's Law holds true in linear regions only (this will be discussed in a later chapter) and under certain conditions.

In fact, recent research suggests that nature is much better described by the tools of non-linear mechanics and chaos theory than by linear equations. This is the opposite of the linear, reductionist approach espoused by Descartes and illustrated by Newton's Laws of Motion, an approach still preferred by many research scientists.[409]

The most serious danger for medical science is in the assumption that such a linear model or description has biological meaning. This ignores the invisible that lies behind the visible universe (Plato's Cave), and that the whole is often greater than the sum of its parts. It also ignores the question of how diagnostic information can be obtained at a distance by sensitive individuals, including many shamans.

Additionally, we are rapidly gaining a better understanding of the holographic nature of the universe, which provides an understanding of how ear or hand acupuncture can be effective, and how the ear points can provide an accurate representation of the body's organs, or how iridology can be a useful diagnostic tool. As we understand our holographic universe, we also gain a much greater recognition of the interdependence of mind/body/spirit than could have been conceived by the Cartesians or by Newtonian science.[410]

The map is not the territory! Models can be useful, for they provide great assistance by predicting experimental outcomes if the model is an accurate representation of the system under study, but *models must be used with great caution*. The author finds, for example, the models of negative feedback systems, developed by engineers, to be useful in understanding the general nature of biological control systems. An example is provided by the body's ability to maintain itself at a quasi-steady temperature despite changes in environmental temperature. However, that usefulness does not contradict the caution stated above, that while using these models one must always be aware of their limitations, and often, inapplicability.

If one is to use a model, one *must* understand the limitations of that model, especially the *assumptions* that were made in constructing the model, or one can be seriously misled. *This was the basic flaw in Cartesian reasoning, yet it reverberates, still, in much of today's medical research.*

Timeline: 15th – 17th Century Europe

Copernicus	1473-1543
Paracelsus	1493-1541
Bruno	1548-1600
Galileo	1564-1642
Kepler	1571-1630
Harvey	1578-1657
Van Helmont	1597-1644
Descartes	1596-1650
Newton	1642-1727

Notes

384 Shorto, Russell, *Descartes' Bones: A Skeletal History of the Conflict Between Faith and Reason*, Doubleday, 2008.
385 Descartes, René, *Discourse on Method (including Meditations, and the Letter-Preface to the Principles of Philosophy)*, Penguin Books, London, 1960.
386 Ibid.
387 Descartes, Reneé, *The Philosophical Writings of Descartes*, Vol. 1, Cambridge University Press, 1985.
388 *The World* (Descartes) https://en.wikipedia.org/wiki/The_World_(Descartes).
389 Descartes, René, *Discourse on Method (including Meditations, and the Letter-Preface to the Principles of Philosophy)*, from the Introduction by translator Desmond Clarke Penguin Books, London, 1960.
390 Coulter, Harris, *Divided Legacy: A History of the Schism in Medical Thought, Vols. I & II*, Wehawken Book Co., 1975.
391 Ibid.
392 Ibid.
393 Descartes, René, *Discourse on Method (including Meditations, and the Letter-Preface to the Principles of Philosophy)*, from the Introduction by translator Desmond Clarke, Penguin Books, London, 1960.
394 Ibid.
395 Ibid.
396 Ibid.
397 Descartes, René, *Discourse on Method (including Meditations, and the Letter-Preface to the Principles of Philosophy)*, Penguin Books, London, 1960.
398 Ibid.
399 Carlson, Anton and Victor Johnson, *The Machinery of the Body*, Chicago, University of Chicago Press, 1942.
400 *Herman Boerhaave, Medical contributions*, https://en.wikipedia.org/wiki/Herman_Boerhaave.
401 Picknett, Lynn and Clive Prince, *The Forbidden Universe: The Occult Origins of Science and the Search for the Mind of God*, Skyhorse, 2011.
402 Hitchens, Christopher, *God is Not Great*, Twelve Books, 2007.
403 Picknett, Lynn and Clive Prince, *The Forbidden Universe: The Occult Origins of Science and the Search for the Mind of God*, Skyhorse, 2011.
404 Dobbs, B.J.T., *The Foundations of Newton's Alchemy*, Cambridge University Press, 1975.
405 Quinn, Arthur, *The Confidence of British Philosophers: An Essay in Historical Narrative*, E.J. Brill, Leiden, 1977.
406 Ibid.
407 Chopra, Deepak personal communication, 2003.
408 Allendorfer, Prof., Professor of Mathematics, University of Washington,

personal communication 1958.
409 Gleick, James, *Chaos: Making a New Science*, Penguin Books, 1987.
410 See, for example:
Goswami, Amit, *The Quantum Doctor: A Physicist's Guide To Health and Healing*, 2004. Also, Goswami, Amit and Richard Reed and Maggie Goswami, *The Self-Aware Universe: How Consciousness Creates the Material World*; Hunt, Valerie, *Infinite Mind: Science of the Human Vibrations of Consciousness*; Laskow, Leonard, Personal communication, 1989.

Chapter 10
Methodism: Hahnemann & Homeopathic Medicine

10.1 Rationalism after Descartes

In the century following the death of Descartes, and following the influence of Descartes and the Rationalist Cartesian physicians, the emphasis came more and more to be on a Rationalist approach to medicine. Theory was emphasized, together with the application of the developments in chemistry, physics and mathematics. Material medical science became the order of the day, a perspective that remains with us to this day. This trend culminated in Methodism, which took Rationalism—together with Reductionism and the consequent reduction of the value of experience, to a limited number of hypothesized "causes"—to an extreme limit. Methodism reduced the number of "causes" to a mere two or three, advocated by such adherents as William Cullen and John Brown in Scotland.[411]

10.2 Brown and Brownism

John Brown (1735-1788) was the pupil of Edinburgh professor of medicine William Cullen. Cullen was an advocate of Methodism, but Brown went even beyond Cullen. Brown so greatly simplified diagnosis and therapeutics that Brownism became very popular in the early 19th century. One historian writes, "Of all medical systems known to history this most peculiarly bore the personal imprint of its inventor: Brown suffered from gout and, finding that whiskey and opium relieved his pain—most effectively when consumed at the same time—he spun a whole theory of health and disease from this single observation. He lectured with a glass of whiskey and opium on the lectern; red meat and "diffusible stimulants" had a prominent role in his therapeutics; and the drug-addiction and drunkenness which his system promoted contributed greatly to its roaring popularity."[412]

Both Cullen and Brown defined "disease" as a deviation from normal physiology, and therapeutics as restoring the physiology to normality. Cullen divided diseases into four classes as a function of the flux of nervous energy through the organism. Brown went further, managing to reduce all diseases into two categories. He simplified his classification of diseases along a spectrum representing the balance of a body's "excitability" and external or internal "exciting powers." When "excitability" is not adequately aroused, the body suffers from "direct debility." When the "excitability" is too high, the body suffers from collapse and diseases of "indirect debility." *Brown urged the physician to ignore most symptoms*, and, essentially, all diseases ended up being classified as one or the other form of "debility." Brown ended up treating all diseases either with stimulants or with debilitating remedies.[413]

Needless to say, Brownism greatly simplified the practice of medicine. A German professor reduced the entire system to 30 propositions which could be mastered in a few weeks. In the United States the Methodism of Brown and Cullen was espoused by Benjamin Rush (1745-1813) and taught for decades by him as professor of medicine at the University of Pennsylvania. Opium, alcohol, and other stimulants became standard treatments of these physicians. Mercury was also a favorite treatment, to the great detriment of the patients.[414]

The extremes of Rationalism represented by Methodism, and their failures therapeutically, led to a swing back to Empiricism, a move most effectively promulgated by Samuel Hahnemann, founder of homeopathy.

10.3 Hahnemann and Homeopathy

Homeopathy was described by Hahnemann as the *Hippocratic method combined with a new interpretation of pharmacology*.[415] It provided a response to Rationalism, Reductionism, and Methodism that proved to be a highly effective method of therapeutics.

Samuel Hahnemann (a generation younger than Brown, 1755-1843) was the only son of a poor family, his father a painter of porcelain. Although Hahnemann was a very bright student, poverty led to his education being interrupted many times. As a result, Hahnemann became very much the individualist and independent thinker. He also espoused the importance of "utility," and his homeopathy was intended to make all pharmacological knowledge immediately useful to the medical practitioner. He was not interested in theory, and his exclusive stress was on symptoms as the source of medical knowledge.

Hahnemann began the study of medicine at Leipzig at age 20, supporting himself by tutoring other students in languages and translating English documents. He later studied in Vienna and Erlangen, finally obtaining his medical degree at age 24. As he began the practice of medicine, he gradually became disillusioned with the medicine he had been taught. He struggled to support a family with a medical system in which he had lost faith. He wrote, "To become in this way a murderer or aggravator of the sufferings of my brethren of mankind was to me a fearful thought—so fearful and distressing was it that shortly after my marriage I completely abandoned practice and scarcely treated any one for fear of doing him harm, and—as you know—occupied myself solely with chemistry and literary labors."[416]

10.4 Provings

Hahnemann retired from medical practice to think out a new approach. In 1796, at age 41, seventeen years after receiving his medical degree, he published his idea of "provings," his method for determining the curative powers of remedies. Medicines were to be administered to healthy individuals and a record made of the symptoms that they produced. A given substance was then used to treat the patient whose symptoms were identical to the symptom-pattern developed in the "proving" of the substance. This interpretation of the Empirical *"cure through similars"* was called by Hahnemann the *"Law of Similars,"* and it became the basis of homeopathic practice.[417] This approach to healing made use of the Hippocratic interpretation of symptoms—that they represented the body's self-healing mechanism, and that the job of the physician was to assist the body in that endeavor.

Hahnemann then returned to medical practice and spent the rest of his life developing his ideas and attempting to convert other physicians to his views, a rather hopeless task given the irreconcilability of homeopathic doctrines and Rationalist and Methodist thinking. He did teach for a time at the University of Leipzig, but he was not an effective lecturer and was not well received by most students. Nevertheless, the influence of homeopathy was spreading, particularly after its success in treating a typhus epidemic in 1813, endemic scarlet fever, and an epidemic of cholera in 1831-32.[418]

Hahnemann's success was bitterly opposed by his allopathic colleagues, especially inasmuch as he was quite vocal in attacking their practices, in particular that of blood-letting. The pharmacists were also vehemently opposed to his insistence that physicians prepare their own medicines, not trusting the pharmacists to prepare his medicines properly.

Hahnemann's wife died in 1830, and in 1835, at age 80, he married a 35-year old French woman who was "well-born, beautiful, and capable, and had apparently journeyed to Koethen, dressed as a young man, with the express purpose of marrying him." [419] She moved him to Paris, and his last years were very happily spent with her in the thick of Parisian society, welcomed by the French homeopaths and with a fashionable and flourishing medical practice. This move gave Hahnemann an excellent position from which to expound his homeopathy, and it gave his system of medicine a stage and world attention that contributed significantly to its success.

Hahnemann was highly critical of the medical profession, feeling that they wasted their time on their medical theories and were so focused on treating many patients (as many as sixty per day) and writing prescriptions that caused their patients to suffer greatly. Allopathic physicians achieved great social standing and were prosperous, but they were quite ineffective in benefiting the health of their patients. Worst of all, the treatments of the Rationalists often caused great harm to their patients, the final straw, from Hahnemann's perspective.[420]

To Hahnemann, the reductionist thrust of Rationalism was designed (1) to limit the variety of recognized diseases by ignoring many of their symptoms, and (2) to limit the variety of remedies by assuming a limited number of medicinal "powers" of value in therapeutics. Instead of accepting the variety of diseases and remedies that exist in nature, Rationalism found lowest common denominators in each and based its thought on these.[421] *The Rationalist physician also prescribed multiple drugs, since he didn't really understand their effects and hoped one might be effective.*[422]

As a medical professional, beware of this trap! In the classic Chinese herbal text, the *Shang Han Lun*, herbal prescriptions are very simple—the mean number of herbs in all the book's prescriptions is 4.5 herbs.[423] This is good medical practice. It implies you must know your herbs!

To Hahnemann, as with shamans, *the true cause of disease was spiritual*, because it was a derangement of the vital force of the body, the *physis* of Hippocrates, that which acts to maintain health and to cure it when sick. We note that in Tibetan Medicine all disease ultimately comes from a false sense of self.

Hahnemann also recognized that this protective force (*physis, die Natur*) often takes the form of a patient's instinctive knowledge of what is needed for health, for example, a particular diet, as in the instance of an animal will ingesting a medicinal herb. He wrote, "*The patient's own feelings are a much surer guide than all the maxims of the schools.*"[424] Hahnemann also felt that to understand a person's health needs required far more than knowledge of chemistry and physics, i.e., that *we are far more than machines*. He wrote, "*Human life is in no respect regulated by purely physical laws, which only obtain among inorganic substances.*"[425] He was looking for the cause of an illness. His therapeutics were, of course, quite contrary to allopathic medicine as taught today. Hahnemann was *not* a materialist![426]

Hahnemann was as emphatic as Hippocrates on the importance of observation of the patient's symptoms. He felt there was no substitute for experience in learning how to treat disease. To him, this was the physician's duty, to learn how to restore the sick to health, to cure and, if possible, to heal.

Eliminating the theories of disease of the Rationalists, Hahnemann developed the concept of *Provings* as being both more efficient and effective than trial-and-error in determining effective remedies. He had adopted Paracelsus' doctrine of similars, recognizing, with Hippocrates, that symptoms were representative of the body's way of healing itself.

Hahnemann recognized that some useful remedies had been discovered by trial-and-error, but he felt that this method was far too inefficient for use in developing new therapeutic remedies. So, he developed a *method* of discovering the curative powers of medicines, which filled the gap in Empirical therapies. By testing the effects of medicines on healthy individuals (himself, his family, etc.), in moderate doses, he determined the effects of those medicines on the health of the body and the mind.

This method of testing medicines led to a major discovery— *the biphasic action of drugs.* Hahnemann found that *"most medicines have more than one action: the first a direct action which gradually changes into the second, which I call the indirect (or secondary) action. The latter is generally a state exactly the opposite of the former... It may be almost considered an axiom that the symptoms of the secondary action are the exact opposite of those of the direct action."* [427]

Hahnemann's theory was that *disease* symptoms reflect, in part the impact of the morbific cause, and in part reflect the organism's healing response. As an example, a cut produces pain, which is an immediate response to the injury, and that pain calls attention to the injury and thus provides protection from further injury; in contrast, the bleeding and swelling that follow are parts of the healing response. This is a theme which reappears periodically in medical thought, but it had never been dealt with methodically and never extended to cover the action of drugs. Hahnemann found that if the *primary* actions and the symptoms produced by the drug were similar to the patient's symptoms, then the *secondary* actions of the drug would remove the disease.

He coined the term *'homeopathy'* to indicate that *cure results from similarity between the symptoms of the patient and the primary symptoms produced by the drug.*[428] Therefore, he would select that drug whose primary symptoms most closely resembled the symptoms of the patient. This drug would slightly aggravate the patient's symptoms. This response was considered as proof that the correct drug had been chosen, and as the patient's curative processes were then stimulated by the secondary action of the drug, the cure would be hastened.[429]

This drug action was, of course, just the opposite of that of allopathic drugs, chosen to *oppose* the patient's symptoms. Hahnemann wrote how the allopathic treatments, whose primary action was to suppress the patient's symptoms, only led to more serious illness as a consequence of the secondary action of the allopathic drug.[430]

Hahnemann commented, "How often, in one word, the disease is aggravated, or something even worse is effected by the secondary action of such antagonistic remedies, the 'harmful side effects,' the Old School with its false theories does not perceive, but experience teaches it in a terrible manner."[431] That is, the primary action of allopathic drugs suppresses symptoms; the secondary action exacerbates the problem. This is *iatrogenic* disease (*Arzneikrankheit*), often far worse than the original complaint, and a far too common occurrence today. This is illustrated by a statement in the *Annals of Internal Medicine,* 1978: "Iatrogenic disease in the U.S. has become a serious public health problem. This includes an estimated two million hospital-related infections and many thousands of deaths per year." As a result, iatrogenic disease is now the third leading cause of hospital deaths in the United States, per a Johns Hopkins University study published in the *British Medical Journal* in 2016.[432]

Hahnemann wrote, "The physician is proud of his power of palliating, and of being able to allay pains for a few hours, but the after-effects—they do not trouble him." He pointed out, "Do not the poor, who use no medicine at all, often recover much sooner from the same kind of disease than the well-to-do patient who has his shelves filled with large bottles of medicine?"[433] We note that a study in Atlanta, published in the *New England Journal of Medicine*, showed that children from affluent families, frequently treated with antibiotics for minor ailments, were less able to cope with drug-resistant pneumonia than their "less fortunate" counterparts from the slums.[434]

The first controlled clinical study in the United States of particular diseases, performed in the 1830s and described by Lewis Thomas in *The Fragile Species*,[435] demonstrated that supportive diet and bed rest were superior to the allopathic medicine of the day. The results of that study reinforced Hahnemann's viewpoint with its finding that the self-healing properties of the patient resulted in a far superior outcome than did the administration of the allopathic medicine.

Since Hahnemann found that the only useful knowledge of remedies was that obtained from provings, and the provings yielded only symptoms, it followed that the only useful way to describe diseases was in terms of their symptoms. Thus, he felt that knowledge of internal pathology was useless, even misleading, since the prover was a live person, not a cadaver under autopsy. Only symptomatic descriptions were useful to Hahnemann, but this required a *careful and detailed study of the patient and the patient's history*, even to using the same expressions used by the patient to describe his or her symptoms.[436] Thus, Hahnemann followed the Empiricist position that observation was the key to understanding a patient's illness, and he railed against his Rationalist colleagues for their cursory examination of their patients.

Hahnemann also stressed the importance of looking for the particular symptoms that a particular patient might exhibit, in contrast to noting merely the symptoms that most patients with a similar malady might exhibit, for *it was* those particular symptoms that would provide the clue to the most effective treatment of that patient's illness.[437]

Hahnemann also placed great importance on emotional symptoms, as those often gave important clues in addition to the physical symptoms. As Hahnemann put it, "One of the chief symptoms in diseases...is the 'state of the disposition,' "[438] and he would use a remedy that had a similar effect on the disposition as well as producing similar physical symptoms. In this way, Hahnemann was addressing emotional cause, not merely managing symptoms.

By focusing on the *propria,* (the particular) as opposed to the *communia* (the symptoms common to all similar patients), Hahnemann was again going contrary to his Rationalist colleagues, for he was destroying all their disease categories, the latter being based on common symptoms held to define diseases. He was back to the Empiricist position that diseases are infinite in number, and that the physician must focus on the individual patient.

Since he felt that the only way to define a disease was by the symptoms produced in a remedy's proving, he urged his colleagues to stop using conventional disease names. Hahnemann wrote, "*All diseases are, in fact, diseases of the whole organism.*" Thus, the physician must treat the *entire* patient, not merely respond to a few prominent symptoms as defining a particular disease. He continued, "The local affection depends solely on a disease of the rest of the body and should only be regarded as an inseparable part of the whole, as one of the most considerable and striking symptoms of the whole disease."[439]

In modern times, cardiologist Dr. Bernard Lown, whose clinic *treats patients, not diseases*, discusses the dangers of attending merely to the patient's "chief complaint," in his book *The Lost Art of Healing*.[440] Far more than merely the obvious symptoms are required to provide an adequate diagnosis for a patient. [It should be noted that it was Dr. Lown's clinic that advised David Rodman regarding his atrial fibrillation, and the prayerful sweat lodge resolution of that illness, described in Chapter One.]

Hahnemann emphasized that all diseases have both a physical and a mental/emotional aspect, both somatic and mental symptoms. The latter are as diverse as the former, and his *provings* yielded a wealth of information on their variety. In treating patients, Hahnemann followed the Empiricist principle that *treatment points to cause*, that theory arises out of practice, that by healing his patients the physician comes to know them.

The physician understands a patient's needs *through his knowledge of remedies*, i.e., from *provings*. Since the particular cause of disease is healed when the physician administers the single remedy whose symptomatology most closely matches that of the patient, that remedy heals the entirety of the patient's illness.

Hahnemann thus insisted that patients be given only one remedy at a time, attacking his allopathic colleagues for their multi-ingredient prescriptions. Even in epidemics, Hahnemann insisted on treating individual patients.[441] Each patient would manifest the epidemic disease in different ways and so require different treatments. This approach by Hahnemann is similar to that of Oriental medicine, where the treatment addresses the *root* of the problem, not only the symptoms, and so is specific to the individual patient.

The author recommends Harvard Medical School faculty member Dr. David Eisenberg's *EncountersWith Qi: Exploring Chinese Medicine*, in which Dr. Eisenberg describes the treatment given a group of patients exhibiting symptoms of pneumonia. Western physicians prescribe an antibiotic; traditional Chinese physicians will look for the *root* of their patient's illness and will prescribe different herbs depending on the particular patient's history.[442] The Chinese physician is using the same logic as did Hahnemann.

10.5 Preparation of Homeopathic Remedies

As Hahnemann's experience grew, he reduced the size of his doses. He had noted that large doses of medicines, given according to the law of similars, caused severe aggravation of the symptoms, so he began reducing his doses. His experiments led him to the conclusion that it was the *essence* of the remedy that was key, and that that essence was retained no matter how small the dose. This view was reinforced by his clinical experience, and he gave instructions for preparing medicines with doses as small as a decillionth (0.0000001) of a grain.[443]

Hahnemann would mix one part of the medicine with 99 parts of milk sugar if a dry medicine, or 99 parts of alcohol if a liquid medicine, then triturate it (grind to a powder) if dry, or shake it if liquid, until it was thoroughly mixed. This he called the "first centesimal dilution." He would then take one part of that dilution, mix it with 99 parts of milk sugar or alcohol, and obtain the "second centesimal dilution." He would repeat this even down to the 30th centesimal dilution, well beyond Avogadro's limit, the dilution at which no molecule of the original medicinal substance can statistically be expected to be present in the dilution.[444]

Even more fantastic to his allopathic colleagues, Hahnemann found that successive stages of dilution, trituration, and succussion actually *enhanced* the power of the remedy.[445] Thus the more dilute preparations were more powerful in healing the illness than were the less dilute ones. The theory underlying this finding presented an important question. Hahnemann wrote that trituration and succussion released the "spirit-like power" of the medicine, consistent with his view that medicines act through their spiritual impact upon the organism.[446] Today homeopaths would suggest that the reason for the enhanced potency is related to a transmission of electromagnetic energy of the medicine's molecules into the energy of the solvent, but the question is still unresolved. The answer appears to relate to the bioelectric energy fields, which is discussed below.

The use of high dilutions enabled Hahnemann to use, as medicines, materials that would, in large doses, be quite poisonous, and a number of his remedies did fall into this category. It may be noted that *any* substance, in large enough quantity (even water), can be poisonous, so Hahnemann's approach does follow pharmacological logic. Hahnemann's key contribution here was to discover a method of producing doses that retained the healing power of the remedy while eliminating its toxic effects.

Empirical tradition viewed *physis* as the self-healing capacity of the body, and it viewed symptoms as representing the efforts of the *physis* to overcome the disease. As Hippocrates put it, "Through vomiting, nausea is cured." Symptoms were thus beneficial, and treatment aimed to intensify and further their development. *Hahnemann interpreted symptoms in part as the onslaught of the disease and in part the curative effect of the vital force.* He felt that if the curative force needed assistance, that was the role of homeopathic remedies. His logic was that if the *physis* had been strong enough, the patient would not have become sick, and that the "disease" was an impairment of the vital force itself. Thus, the job of the physician was to assist the body to heal itself rather than to assume that the *physis* would do the job unaided. He wrote, "By giving a remedy which resembles the disease [symptoms] the instinctive vital force is compelled to increase its vital energy until it becomes stronger than the disease which, in turn is vanquished. Then, by interruption of the medication, health follows... "*All* the symptoms of a disease are therefore the reaction of the vital force, the *physis*." [447]

Thus, homeopathy was a new variant of Hippocrates' and the traditional Empirical reliance on the *physis* as the principal instrument of cure. Instead of permitting the *physis* to cope with disease unaided, the homeopathic physician reinforced and guided it by using the secondary actions of his remedies.

Hahnemann recognized that persons varied in their susceptibility to disease-producing influences. He also found that the diseased organism is more susceptible to the action of the medicine than is the healthy one. The opposite of susceptibility is of course immunity, which he noticed particularly in epidemics, concluding that the gradual introduction of an individual to the disease enabled the individual to develop an immunity to the disease. He also noted that the appropriate homeopathic remedy for the disease could have a prophylactic effect when administered to a healthy individual, since that remedy would arouse the body's defenses against the disease just as it would in the sick. This concept was the basis for later immunization procedures.

10.6 Isopathy

Isopathy was the concept that infectious diseases contained in their infectious material the means of their cure. Several homeopathic physicians and scientists pursued this idea, and *nosodes* (substances derived from animals that had diseases similar to those of humans) were gradually developed. The principal use of the nosode was to stimulate a suppressed disease to manifest all its symptoms. The use of nosodes became a common homeopathic addition to their stock of remedies, and this use was the forerunner of the development of immunizations and antitoxins later in the 19th century.

10.7 Prayer, Ceremony, and Healing

A theme found repeatedly in traditional medicines is that of invoking the divine, usually through prayer and/or ceremony. The author discovered this personally through studying Hawaiian medicine, as prayer is used in the preparation of tinctures of the herb *olena* to treat *otitis media* or sinus infections. This is not unique: shamans, including *kahunas,* invoke the divine; Tibetan monks' prayers are part of the preparation of "Precious Pills." The importance of prayer in David Rodman's sweat lodge ceremony in his healing of atrial fibrillation was described in Chapter One. Homeopaths have used prayers as they prepared homeopathic remedies. Homeopathy by *not* separating the body from mind and soul is akin to traditional medicine.

10.8 Modern Homeopathy

Homeopathy today, in contrast to allopathic medicine, has changed only in detail from the homeopathy of the early 19th century. We now have more information available about bioelectric fields, and with it more refined hypotheses about how the individual becomes ill and how homeopathic remedies can cure that illness. These theories have been well expressed by one of the leading contemporary homeopathic physicians, George Vithoulkas, in his *Homeopathy: Medicine of the New Man.* Vithoulkas suspects that the electromagnetic field of the body is the vital force to which Hahnemann referred. Vithoulkas writes, "The function of homeopathy is to powerfully strengthen the organism's natural defense mechanism by adding to it resources and energy. It works in the same direction as the vital force and

Methodism: Hahnemann & Homeopathic Medicine 235

not against it. This direction, this natural intelligence of the vital defense, is precisely that set of symptoms that allopathy would so diligently suppress."[448]

The modern homeopathic concept is that all substances have a natural electromagnetic field, a particular vibration rate. *The vibration rate of a remedy, if matched to the vibration rate of the patient during illness, will, by a resonance phenomenon, reinforce the patient's electromagnetic field at precisely the frequency needed to bring about a cure.* The task of the homeopathic physician is,—by studying the totality of the patient's symptoms, which are the outward manifestation of the patient's electromagnetic field—to select a remedy that exactly matches the patient's needs and so produce a cure. It is for this reason also that multiple remedies do not work together—either a remedy's frequency matches that of the patient, or it does not. Two remedies that almost match will produce dissonance rather than resonance, and no cure will be produced—any more than two Beethoven sonatas, played simultaneously, will produce a harmonious result.

Modern homeopathy has an excellent track record, albeit it was quite effectively suppressed in the U.S. by the Flexner Report (to be discussed in a later chapter). It is now enjoying a resurgence due to its effectiveness, but it is still used far less extensively in the United States than in Europe (e.g., Queen Elizabeth and the British Royal Family have used homeopathy exclusively for their health care for many years).[449] Homeopathic practice—with the necessity of detailed case histories and a broad knowledge of the symptoms produced by the provings of many remedies—not only requires extensive training and experience on the part of the homeopathic physician, but it is *not* readily adapted to the demand for rapid turnover of patients, especially in HMOs.[450] It may be noted that the effectiveness of homeopathic medicine has repeatedly been proven in veterinary practice (e.g., with chickens in Germany).[451]

To a not inconsiderable degree, the conflict between allopathic medicine and homeopathic medicine has not changed significantly in two hundred years. The homeopaths are aghast at the harm they see being done by allopaths, and the allopaths mount their scientific forces against the perceived absurdity that remedies which are so extraordinarily dilute could have any effect on the patient. Consider the *assumption* that drug actions must obey chemical laws, and that chemistry's Law of Mass Action therefore applies to those actions on patients.

This clearly reflects the sharp contrast between two distinct philosophies of medicine. The allopaths follow a materialistic creed and so imbed in their medical practice and in modern medical science what Dr. Deepak Chopra described as a materialistic superstition.[452] The homeopaths, in contrast, hark back to the recognition of the invisible shared by Pythagoras, Socrates, Plato, and Hippocrates, as well as by shamans both ancient and modern, and by mystery school healers.

Nevertheless, double-blind studies of homeopathic treatments published in prestigious scientific journals[453] have been conducted, generally in Britain and in Europe, and modern scientific evidence is confirming the efficacy of homeopathic remedies—to the outrage of allopaths!

Notes

411 Coulter, Harris, *Divided Legacy: A History of the Schism in Medical Thought*, Vol. II, Wehawken Book Co., 1975.
412 Ibid.
413 Ibid.
414 Runes, Dagobert D., *The Selected Writings of Benjamin Rush*, Read Books Ltd, 2013.
415 Coulter, Harris, *Divided Legacy: A History of the Schism in Medical Thought*, Vol. II, Wehawken Book Co., 1975.
416 Ibid.
417 Rogers, Naomi, *An Alternative Path: The Making and Remaking of Hahnemann Medical College and Hospital of Philadelphia*, Rutgers University Press, 1998.
418 Hahnemann, Samuel, *The Chronic Diseases: Their Specific Nature and Homeopathic Treatment*, Advance Publishing Company, 1889.
419 Haehl, Richard, *Samuel Hahnemann: His Life and Work*, B. Jain Publishers, 2003.
420 Coulter, Harris, *Divided Legacy: A History of the Schism in Medical Thought*, Vol. II, Wehawken Book Co., 1975.
421 Ibid.
422 Ibid.
423 Zhang, Zhongjing et al., *Shang Han Lun: The Great Classic of Chinese Medicine*, Oriental Healing Arts Institute, 1981.
424 Hahnemann, Samuel, *Lesser Writings*, Dudgeon R.E., editor, New Delhi: B Jain; 1994.
425 Ibid.
426 Ibid.
427 Ibid.
428 Coulter, Harris, *Divided Legacy: A History of the Schism in Medical Thought*, Vol. II, Wehawken Book Co., 1975.
429 Ibid.
430 Ibid.
431 Hahnemann, Samuel, *Lesser Writings*, Dudgeon R.E., editor, New Delhi: B Jain; 1994.
432 Makary, Martin A; Daniel, Michael "Medical Error—The Third Leading Cause of Death in the US", *British Medical Journal*; London 353, 2016.
433 Hahnemann, Samuel, *Lesser Writings*, Dudgeon R.E., editor, New Delhi: B Jain; 1994.
434 Hofmann, Jo, MD et al., "The Prevalence of Drug-Resistant Streptococcus pneumoniae In Atlanta" *New England Journal of Medicine*, 1995.
435 Thomas, Lewis, *The Fragile Species*, New York, MacMillan Publ. Co., 1992.
436 Demarque, Denis, "The development of proving methods since

Hahnemann," *British Homeopathic Journal*, April 1987.
437 Ibid.
438 Demarque, Denis, *Medicine and Specificity*, CEDH, 2009.
439 Hahnemann, Samuel, *Organon of Medicine*, London, W. Davey & Son, 1849.
440 Lown, Bernard, MD, *The Lost Art of Healing*, Ballantine Books, 1999.
441 Hahnemann, Samuel, *The Chronic Diseases: Their Specific Nature and Homeopathic Treatment*, Advance Publishing Company, 1889.
442 Eisenberg, David, *Encounters with Qi*, New York, Penguin Books, 1985.
443 Davenas, E. et al., "Human basophil degranulation triggered by very dilute antiserum against *IgE*," Nature, 333: 816-818, 1988.
444 Coulter, Harris, *Divided Legacy: A History of the Schism in Medical Thought*, Vol. II, Wehawken Book Co., 1975.
445 McCabe, Vinton, *Homeopathy, Healing, and You*, St. Martin's Press, 1999.
446 Hahnemann, Samuel, *Organon of Medicine*, London, W. Davey & Son, 1849.
447 Vithoulkas, George, *Homeopathy: Medicine of the New Man*, New York, Arco Publishing, 1979.
448 Ibid.
449 Ullman, Dana, *The Homeopathic Revolution: Why Famous People and Cultural Heroes Choose Homeopathy*, North Atlantic Books, 2007.
450 At the Vivekananda Polyclinic and Institute of Medical Sciences Centre, in Lucknow India, a very modern hospital, patients are allowed to choose between allopathic and seven other forms of medical approaches, including homeopathic, Ayurvedic and naturopathic medicines. http://www.ramakrishnalucknow.org/hospital.php
451 Madrewar, B.P., *Veterinary Homeopathy: A Scientific Clinical Research*, B. Jain Publishers, 2007.
452 Chopra, Deepak, *Science and the Superstition of Materialism*, beliefnet.com, 2009.
453 Torkos, Sherry, *The Canadian Encyclopedia of Natural Medicine*, John Wiley & Sons, 2012.

Chapter 11
European Medicine in the 19th and 20th Centuries

11.1 Introduction

At the same time that Hahnemann was developing homeopathy in Germany, there were also significant developments in the struggle between Empiricism and Rationalism elsewhere in Europe, with France an area of particular ferment. One of the two major centers of French medical education, the Medical College at Montpellier, was firmly in the Empiricist camp, albeit with a rather complex form of Empiricism (see Béchamp, below), and some of its faculty espoused homeopathy. Many of the Montpellier graduates went to Paris and influenced thought in the capital, but most of the Parisian medical academy faculty were in the Rationalist camp. A hot controversy persisted throughout the 19th century, with the Paris Academy of Medicine coming down firmly opposed to homeopathy, albeit individual members of the Academy were more willing to consider alternative approaches in their medical practices, and some ended up adopting portions of homeopathic principles.

11.2 Pathology vs. Symptoms

One of the major issues of the day was the argument over the relative importance of pathology and symptoms. Rationalists believed pathology was the key to understanding disease, while Empiricists looked to symptoms. In Germany, Rudolph Virchow (1821-1902) had pioneered the new field of pathology, using microscopes to study cellular changes in disease. Virchow believed that understanding a disease required understanding its effects on body cells. One problem for Virchow and for the Rationalists was that some diseases could be identified at autopsy by pathological changes, but others could not. Further, some diseases showing similar pathological changes would manifest differing symptoms in different patients. So the struggle continued.[454]

11.3 Infectious Diseases

Infectious diseases were a particular health concern in the 19th century, and there was much controversy over the causes of contagion. Europe had been plagued by epidemics for centuries, with an outbreak of the Black Death (plague) killing about one-fourth of the population of Europe 500 years earlier (mid-1300s). Poor nutrition and sanitation had provided a fertile ground for infectious disease to spread. Hahnemann had shown that immunity was important in resisting disease, but contagion itself long remained a mystery. A case in point was the tragedy of Semmelweis, now recognized as a pioneer who solved a deadly contagion with simple hygiene but was reviled in his day. Semmelweis had gone against the assumptions and dogma (the belief systems) of his medical colleagues, and he was castigated rather than honored for his discovery.

11.4 Semmelweis

Ignaz Philipp Semmelweis (1818-1865) was a Hungarian physician who became very concerned about the fact that many women who delivered children in his hospital succumbed to a deadly fever following childbirth, a situation so serious that many women recognized the danger of going to the hospital and wisely chose to have their children at home. Semmelweis observed that some physicians would go directly from the autopsy laboratory in the hospital's morgue to the obstetrics ward, and that they never concerned themselves with cleanliness as they examined their patients and went from one patient to another. What is now known as puerperal fever would often follow, many times causing the death of the mother and/or the baby.

Semmelweis concluded that hygiene was the problem and, against the objections of his colleagues, he insisted that physicians on his ward wash their hands before entering the obstetrics ward to examine their patients and between patients. The mortality rate dropped rapidly, and his obstetrics ward became safe for mothers. In 1847 Semmelweis announced his discovery to the medical world, but he was roundly denounced for the absurdity of his conclusions [*Assumptions* had led to *Dogma*]. It was only very belatedly, well after his death, that the importance of Semmelweis' discovery was appreciated. There is now, in Hungary, a medical school named in his honor.[455]

11.5 Leeuwenhoek's Microscope

An amateur Dutch scientist, Anton van Leeuwenhoek (1632-1723) had invented the microscope in the 17th century and had observed tiny objects invisible to the naked eye. In time, Leeuwenhoek's microscope made an important contribution to medicine's views of the cause of infectious disease, the microscope proving to be a useful tool for the developing science of bacteriology as well as microscopic anatomy.[456]

11.6 Smallpox and Jenner

One of the contagious diseases that caused many deaths for centuries was smallpox. Edward Jenner (1749-1823) had shown that cowpox could provide immunity to smallpox, a discovery that paved the way for the development of immunization procedures in the 19th century.

11.7 Robert Koch

Robert Koch (1843-1910) played an important role in the late 19th century with his development of ways of staining and culturing bacteria, together with his association of specific bacteria with particular diseases. Koch's four postulates became the standard for associating bacteria with diseases. His procedure and postulates were as follows:

1. Pathogenic bacteria were taken from diseased animals or patients,

2. The pathogenic bacteria would be isolated and grown in a laboratory,

3. The laboratory-grown bacteria would be injected into experimental animals, and

4. Bacteria isolated from the diseased experimental animals would be shown to be of the same kind as the original bacteria.[457]

If all of Koch's postulates were satisfied, then a direct connection between bacteria and disease would be inferred. Koch worked particularly with anthrax, tuberculosis, cholera, rinderpest, and sleeping sickness.[458]

It should be noted that satisfying Koch's postulates does *not* say the bacteria *caused* the disease (experimental results relevant to this issue will be discussed below), though in an animal with a weak immune system the presence of the pathogenic bacteria would produce the *symptoms* of the disease.

This issue is an important one: *Association does* not *imply causality*. Buicks do not *cause* doctors in the Midwest, even though most midwestern physicians drive Buicks. The Northeast power blackout of circa 60 years ago did not *cause* the many babies born nine months later.

Koch's work was greatly lauded. He founded and was director of the Institute for Infectious Diseases in Berlin in 1891, and he received the Nobel Prize for his work on tuberculosis in 1905.[459]

The issue of the cause of infectious diseases was an important one in 19th century European medicine. Bernard, Pasteur, and Béchamp all contributed their respective views, and the controversy has yet to be resolved.

11.8 Francois Magendie

Francois Magendie played an important role in early 19th century European medicine. Magendie (1783-1855), who came to Paris in 1835, was a contemporary, but a generation younger than Hahnemann. Magendie was a physician and physiologist, and was the Chairman of Physiology at the Collège de France. He was firmly of a Rationalist perspective, but he adopted Hahnemann's principle of proving drugs by testing them on healthy animals to observe the drug's effect. This was later extended to human trials, and Magendie became known as the father of experimental pharmacology. He is often given credit for a method that had been previously developed by Hahnemann. However, Magendie_remained a convinced allopath (really a Methodist) despite his adoption of Hahnemann's method of testing medicines.[460]

Magendie's work was followed by many others, and by the end of the 19th century Hahnemann's principle of testing medicines on healthy individuals had become accepted medical practice among allopaths as well as homeopaths. It became a major influence on both forms of medical practice, and Hahnemann's procedure continues to be followed in today's clinical trials of new drugs. Many homeopathic remedies were adopted by allopaths, and homeopathic medicine gradually became better accepted in Europe (including England, where homeopathy has long been the medicine of choice of the royal family) despite official allopathic opposition. Allopathic *materia medica* texts included homeopathic remedies, and Empirical medicine made major inroads.[461]

11.9 Claude Bernard

Claude Bernard (1813-1878) was a peasant's son who studied medicine in Paris and became a student in Magendie's physiology laboratory. Bernard succeeded Magendie in his Chair of Physiology at the Collège de France in the mid-19th century (1855), and he became highly influential in the history of both medicine and physiology. His *Introduction a l'Etude de la Medecine Experimentale* (1865)[462] is often considered the founding work of experimental physiology, and Bernard is frequently referred to as the father of modern physiology.

A confirmed Methodist, Bernard was firmly opposed to homeopathy, and in particular the principle of vitalism. Following Descartes, *Bernard considered the body to be a machine*, and his physiological research was a study of that machine's characteristics. He considered the body to be a self-regulating device that worked to maintain a constant *milieu interieur* (internal terrain), a concept that proved to be not only a major contribution to physiology (the origin of our understanding of physiological homeostasis) but an important contribution to medicine as well. To Bernard, the internal *terrain* was all, and the body functioned to maintain the constancy of that *terrain*.[463]

Le terrain included all aspects of the body's functions, including the immune system, and Bernard believed that if *le terrain* were healthy, then the body was capable of defending itself against external attack. In this he broke sharply with his student, Louis Pasteur, and Bernard demonstrated his belief in *le terrain* with a dramatic demonstration to the Collège de France. Cholera was a dread disease that had caused great suffering in Paris as elsewhere in Europe, and Bernard shocked his medical colleagues by drinking a glass of cholera-contaminated water before a medical assembly. As he had predicted, his digestive, immune, and endocrine systems (his *terrain*) were sufficiently robust that he suffered no ill-effects (an experiment later repeated by German colleagues), thus demonstrating that Pasteur's *microbes* were not the whole story.[464]

Given his stature as a highly regarded professor of physiology, Bernard's attack on the vitalism of Hahnemann and homeopathy was telling. The concept of an *archeus*, an *elan vital*, in short, *vitalism*, came to be rejected by all physiologists even into the 20th century. They found no necessity to include vitalism in their studies of the body's physiology, and the concept came to be considered a relic of primitive and unscientific thought. That view still holds today, with vitalism routinely labeled as "unscientific," a reflection that *the materialistic views of Descartes and Bernard still hold full sway*.

A parallel might be made with other areas in which experiments suggesting a different point of view from that accepted by the scientific community are routinely rejected as unscientific. A comparison may be made with the response to Joseph Rhine's Duke experiments on Extra Sensory Perception, the disbelieving letters he received in response to a paper he published in *Science*.[465] We might also note the experiments of Davenas, et al.,[466] that provided support for homeopathy, and the attack on Davenas by allopaths that followed, sending a committee—including a stage magician, Randi—to debunk Davenas' work. This incident occurred in the 1980s, and the fight between allopaths and homeopaths continues to this day.[467]

Bernard's rejection of vitalism was abetted by the earlier work of Luigi Galvani (1737-1798), who had shown that a frog's muscle twitched when stimulated by an electric current. Galvani's work is considered the foundation of neurophysiology, for his demonstration of the relationship between electricity and muscle contraction laid the groundwork for later work on the electrical nature of the nerve impulse.[468]

Charles Darwin's monumental work on evolution fit well with Bernard's views. Darwin (1809-1882) had shown that species could evolve rather than each being separately created, a view that again suggested no need for a vital force in species or individuals, thus a materialistic perspective.[469] We should note that recent research suggests that, contrary to Darwin's views, nature is far more cooperative than competitive, and "survival of the fittest" is probably a misinterpretation of the historical data. Further, our makeup is *not* determined solely by the DNA we inherit from our parents, as many recent studies in epigenetics have shown. Environment, diet, and emotions matter—all affect our health and the persons we are, modifying our physiology and that of our offspring as well. (See Lynne McTaggart's *The Bond* for an in-depth discussion of epigenetics and its implications).[470]

A pioneer in physiological research, Bernard was not a practicing physician. However, regarding therapeutics, he was a staunch adherent of the Doctrine of Contraries. To Bernard, if *le terrain* was sufficiently unhealthy that disease needed to be combated, one should look upon disease symptoms as something to be opposed, thus use contrary medications. He did not approve of Hippocratic medicine, for the Hippocratic physicians regarded disease symptoms as something to be respected. This, Bernard felt, was all wrong.[471]

Bernard was clearly a Rationalist, despite the apparent similarity of his view of *le terrain* and Hippocratic views of the body's *physis* and its self-healing capacity.

11.10 Louis Pasteur

Louis Pasteur (1822-1895) was originally a chemist, but he went on to make major contributions to medicine and bacteriology as well as to chemistry. A student of Bernard, Pasteur's studies of bacteriology led him to the view that diseases are caused by external bacteria—though see below regarding his deathbed recantation. Pasteur's development of vaccines was successful in combating anthrax, chicken cholera, rabies, and other diseases. His demonstration that heat can kill bacteria led to the process of pasteurization, still the standard method of ensuring that milk is not contaminated by pathogenic bacteria.

By the end of his life, Pasteur recognized that his view had been too narrow. On his deathbed, Pasteur confessed to one of his colleagues that his own focus on external germs as the cause of disease had been an error. In Pasteur's words, *"Bernard a raison, le terrain est tout! Le microbe n'est rien!"* (Bernard is right, the terrain is all! the microbe is nothing!).[472]

Despite his deathbed recantation, Pasteur's view that external bacteria are the cause of infectious disease became accepted by the medical community, and Pasteur has been honored in book and film. Allopathic infectious disease treatment, to this day, follows the perspective adduced by Pasteur, that disease is caused generally by external agents, and that the challenge of medicine is to find means of counteracting those agents. Thus, e.g., if a modern allopath finds *pneumococci* in a pneumonia patient, he/she administers an antibiotic to destroy the *pneumococci*. This of course *assumes* that the *pneumococci cause* the pneumonia, an assumption not shared by a traditional Chinese physician, who will look for the *root* of the problem rather than suppressing the pneumonia's symptoms.

This perspective is described by Harvard Medical School professor Dr. David Eisenberg in his *Encounters with Qi: Exploring Chinese Medicine*,[473] where Eisenberg describes the situation where a group of patients exhibiting the symptoms of pneumonia go to a medical clinic and are given a choice of being treated by either a Western or a traditional Chinese physician.

The Western physician, finding *pneumococci* present in the patient's sputum, administers an antibiotic to all, on the assumption that the *pneumococcus* is the source of the patient's problem. The Chinese physician, in contrast, treats each patient differently, for the Chinese physician is looking for the *cause (root)* of the patient's weakness (that which is reducing the effectiveness of the immune system, thus *le terrain*), rather than assuming the *pneumococcus* is the source of the patient's illness.

We note the parallel between the practitioner of Traditional Chinese Medicine and Bernard's views of *le terrain*. Albeit we now understand more and more the role of the immune system, together with the role of emotions, mind, and spirit in influencing the immune system, and the appropriateness of Pasteur's recantation, his earlier views regarding the external cause of disease are still widely held.

11.11 Antoine Béchamp

Antoine Béchamp (1816-1908), Professor of Medicine at the University of Montpellier, was Pasteur's opponent in the debate about the issue of external versus internal cause of disease. Béchamp's research was elegant and his findings profound. It has been suggested that some of his bacteriological research was stolen by Pasteur; however, the important issue is that Béchamp's data indicated a very different view of disease than did those of Pasteur.[474]

Béchamp, Pasteur and other 19th century scientists had studied the process of fermentation, important to the wine and beer-producing industries of France. In the course of his research, Béchamp discovered the existence of the fundamental living particle that he named *microzymes*. Béchamp found the microzymes to be the building blocks of microbes as well as cells.[475]

Béchamp found this microorganism in all living cells, and he found further that microzymes lived on after the death of their host, being found even in ancient chalk deposits. He found that microzymes were an essential element in the process of nutrition, that they are found in all living and dead tissues, and that they can change into forms that are destructive to tissues and cells. He demonstrated that under toxic conditions the microzymes change into pathogenic forms that then bring about pathological changes in the host organs. Béchamp's conclusion: "The microzymes, living agents of all organization, are also the agents of disease and death." When the body becomes toxic, the microzymes adapt by changing into pathogenic microbes.[476]

Béchamp's studies of the microzymes had answered the fundamental question of the day: "Does the germ cause the disease, or does the disease cause the germ?" He was able to show that under toxic conditions the microzymes are changed into pathogenic forms that produce disease.[477] This conclusion was of course in direct conflict with Pasteur's concept that infectious disease can be caused only by external microbes. It was consistent, however, with Bernard's views of *le terrain*.

Béchamp showed microbes to be a secondary manifestation of the disease, a symptom rather than a cause.[478] The microbes play a role in manifesting the symptoms of the disease, so when a diseased immune system is producing pathogenic microbes, and those microbes are augmented by other microbes from external sources, serious symptoms can develop. The appearance of microbes themselves, however, are caused *by* the disease, and *not* the other way around. A healthy immune system kills external bacteria and no disease symptoms will appear, as illustrated by Bernard's cholera demonstration.

Béchamp's work laid the foundation for what has come to be known as the Pleomorphic theory of disease—the concept that his microzymes change into pathogenic forms in the face of environmental, dietary, emotional, and other stresses. As Béchamp put it, the answer to maintaining health is "hygiene," a healthy lifestyle that includes all aspects of body, mind, and spirit and that maintains Bernard's *terrain*, the strength of the body's systems, including the immune system. Thus, there is ultimately no disagreement between Bernard and Béchamp.

11.12 Günther Enderlein

Günther Enderlein (1872-1968) was the successor to Béchamp in developing our understanding of the Pleomorphic

Cycle. Enderlein was a German physician and bacteriologist who spent nearly sixty years studying fresh unstained blood using darkfield and phase-contrast microscopes. Enderlein was posted to a hospital in Berlin during World War I, where he was able to spend much of his time on microbiological research. His initial discoveries of the cycles of bacteria were made in 1916. In 1925, Enderlein published *Bakterian Cyclogenie*,[479] describing the life cycles of bacteria and showing how healthy particles in the blood, which Enderlein called *protits*, can develop into pathogenic forms in an unhealthy bodily environment. That work continued throughout the first half (plus) of the 20th century, providing much of the documentation of the Pleomorphic Cycle as we know it today.

Enderlein found that, when the body is healthy, these *protits* work symbiotically with other cells and assist the immune system in its function. However, when there is a deterioration in the body's internal environment, with a change in the pH of the blood, tissues, and fluids for extended periods—due to poor nutrition, emotional stress, smoking, synthetic drugs, radiation, or carcinogenic substances in the environment—the beneficial microorganisms change to pathogenic forms which have been identified as *causing* disease. (Note that Chinese medicine has long recognized that emotional stress alters the pH of the blood. Thus, the emotions that alter pH are identified as *causing* disease).

This was fundamentally important in showing that an unhealthy body produced the disease, with the associated microorganisms being produced *inside* the body by the *unhealthy conditions, including unhealthy emotions, that were the true cause of the disease*. Enderlein went on to develop therapeutic measures to reverse the deterioration of the blood's immune system elements via the Pleomorphic Cycle—the Enderlein therapy used effectively today in North America as well as in Europe.

We might note the implication that an unhealthy body would affect not only the production of pathological *protits*, but would also, per recent studies in epigenetics, affect offspring yet unborn.[480]

11.13 Gaston Naessens

The work of Béchamp and Enderlein has been extended in the 20th century by the French (now Canadian) scientist Gaston Naessens and others. Naessens has also studied the Pleomorphic Cycle, again finding minute particles in the blood that are pleomorphic and in their pathological forms are associated with a variety of degenerative diseases.

For a detailed discussion of Béchamp, Enderlein and the Pleomorphic Cycle, including the work of Virginia Livingston-Wheeler, Royal Rife, and Gaston Naessens, see Smith, et al., *Your Cure for Cancer*, 1998.[481]

Note that the work of Bernard, Béchamp, Enderlein, and Naessens, et al., provides a scientific understanding of the cellular mechanism responsible for the success of traditional medicines. This understanding, combined with the invisible, has been successful for millennia, from shamans to mystery school healers to Hippocrates to Hildegard von Bingen to Tibetan Medicine to Ayurvedic Medicine to Classical (Taoist) Chinese Medicine. In short: *Restore the patient's system to balance, and you reverse the Pleomorphic Cycle. You assist the patient to heal him/herself, and you prevent degenerative disease.*

European Medicine in the 19th and 20th Centuries 251

Pleomorphic Cycle

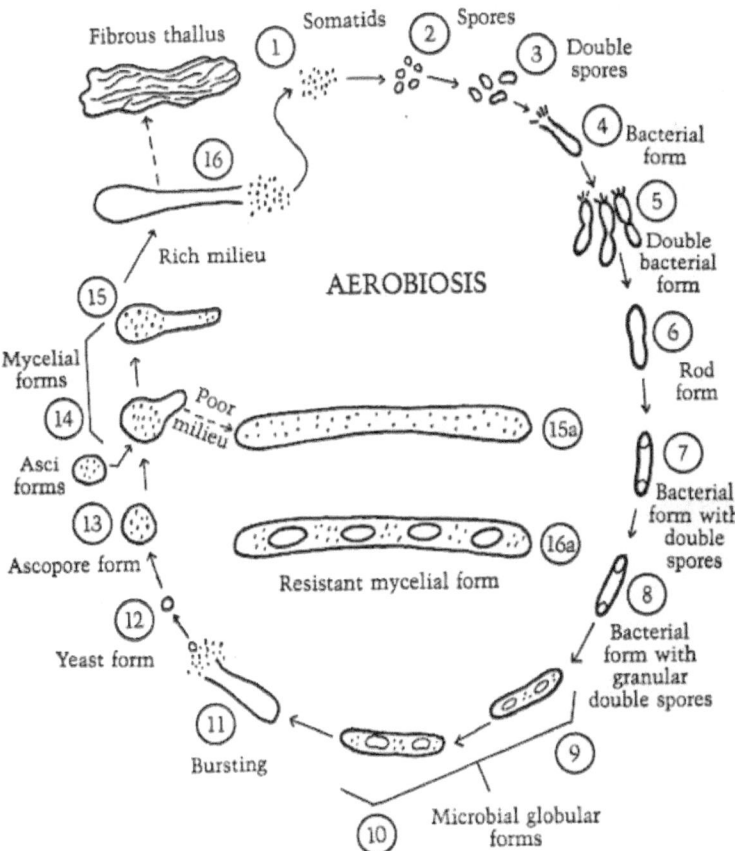

Timeline: 17th, 18th, 19th and 20th Centuries

Anton van Leeuwenhoek	Microscopist	1632-1723
Edward Jenner	English physician	1749-1823
Samuel Hahnemann	Homeopathic physician	1755-1843, Paris 1835
Francois Magendie	Physiologist/pharmacologist	1783-1855
Charles Darwin	Biologist	1809-1882
Claude Bernard	Physiologist	1813-1878
Antoine Béchamp	Microbiologist	1816-1908
Ignaz Semmelweis	Obstetrician	1818-1865
Rudolph Virchow	Pathologist	1821-1902
Louis Pasteur	Chemist/bacteriologist	1822-1895
Robert Koch	Bacteriologist	1843-1910
Günther Enderlein	Microbiologist	1872-1968
Gaston Naessens	Microbiologist	20th century

Notes

454 Coulter, Harris, *Divided Legacy: A History of the Schism in Medical Thought,* Vols. II, Wehawken Book Co., 1975.
455 http://semmelweis.hu/english/
456 Zuylen, J. van, "The Microscopes of Antoni van Leeuwenhoek", *Journal of Microscopy,* Vol. 121, Issue 3, March 1981.
457 Brock, Thomas D., *Robert Koch: A Life in Medicine and Bacteriology,* Berlin, Springer, 1988.
458 Ibid.
459 Ibid.
460 Coulter, Harris, *Divided Legacy: A History of the Schism in Medical Thought,* Vols. II, Wehawken Book Co., 1975.
461 Ibid.
462 Bernard, Claude, *Introduction a l'Etude de la Medecine Experimentale* 1865
463 Winters, Eric R., *Personal Terrain: Living the Vigorous Life,* Lulu.com, 2007.
464 Ibid.
465 https://en.wikipedia.org/wiki/Joseph_Banks_Rhine
466 Davenas, e. et al., "Human basophil degranulation triggered by very dilute antiserum against *IgE*", Nature, 333: 816-818, 1988.
467 Ullman, Dana, "Luc Montagnier, Nobel Prize Winner, Takes Homeopathy Seriously," *HuffPost,* January 2011
468 Cajavilca, Christian et al., "Luigi Galvani and the Foundations of Electrophysiology," *Resuscitation,* Vol. 80, Issue 2, February 2009.
469 Darwin, Charles, *The Origin of Species,* Wordsworth Editions, 1998.
470 McTaggart, Lynne, *The Bond: How to Fix Your Falling-Down World,* Simon & Schuster, 2011.
471 Coulter, Harris, *Divided Legacy: A History of the Schism in Medical Thought,* Vols. II, Wehawken Book Co., 1975.
472 DuBos, René, *Louis Pasteur: Freelance of Science,* Charles Scribner's Sons, 1976.
473 Eisenberg, David, *Encounters with Qi,* 1985.
474 Hume, Ethel Douglas, *Béchamp or Pasteur? A Lost Chapter in the History of Biology,* Bechamp.org, 2006.
475 Béchamp, Antoine, *The Blood and its Third Anatomical Element,* Boerick & Tafel, 1911.
476 Ibid.
477 Ibid.
478 Ibid.
479 Enderlein, Günther, *Bakterien Cyclogenie,* W. de Gruyter & Co., 1925.
480 Lipton, Bruce, *The Biology of Belief,* Mountain of Love/Elite Books, 2005.
481 Smith, R.E., P.K. Smith and H. Bigelsen, *Your Cure for Cancer,* Promotion Publishing, 1998.

Chapter 12
American Medicine in the 19th and 20th Centuries

12.1 Assumptions

Before proceeding with the history of American medicine in the 19th and 20th centuries, the issue of assumptions needs to be addressed. This issue has been mentioned in preceding chapters, but it has not been addressed explicitly.

The dangers of assumptions were made clear when an undergraduate engineering student encountered a structures professor who commented to his students that no structure that they designed would ever fail because they misread the third decimal place on their slide rule. It might well fail, however, because of a factor they had forgotten to include in their calculations, an assumption that they had made.

This danger had been illustrated in Southern California when freeways were designed on the *assumption* that there was an infinite supply of air and that therefore exhaust fumes would be no problem. As anyone who has flown into Los Angeles International Airport can attest, that assumption was wrong, and a blanket of smog has been the consequence.

Now to continue with the history of American medicine.

12.2 Homeopathy vs. Allopathy

The history of medicine in America during the 19th century is one of a struggle between competing medical systems, with particular emphasis on the competition between allopathic (Rational) and homeopathic (Empirical) medicine.[482] Benjamin Rush, signer of the Declaration of Independence and for many years Professor of Medicine at the University of Pennsylvania, was a staunch Rationalist, and he had an important influence on medical practice in the early part of the nineteenth century. However, allopathic medicine was in competition with frontier doctors, who had learned their medicine from Native American medicine men and women (shamans), and later, from homeopathic physicians. The struggle between homeopathic and allopathic medicine led in time to the formation of the American Medical Association, with allopathic medicine finally winning the upper hand early in the twentieth century with the implementation of the Flexner Report.[483] Thus, the struggle between Empirical and Rational medicine had become the battle between homeopathy and allopathic medicine.

12.3 Benjamin Rush

Benjamin Rush (1745-1813) was a student of William Cullen and John Brown in Scotland, and he brought their Methodism (also known as the Solidist tradition) to America. Although there were, at that time, four medical schools in the United States: Harvard University, Dartmouth University, New York College of Physicians and Surgeons, and the University of Pennsylvania; it was from the last that about three-fourths of U.S. physicians graduated. Rush was Professor of Medicine at Pennsylvania for 44 years, so in that time he had a tremendous influence on the education of American physicians.

Rush's influence on medicine was not benign. Without going into the details of Rush's theoretical views of disease, suffice it to say that his treatments were "heroic," and their effect on patients was often devastating. As might be expected from a student of Brown, Rush simplified therapeutics into a relatively few agents, but they were not harmless. He used large doses of calomel (mercury), quinine, opium, and other, mostly mineral drugs, together with a generous use of the lancet. His prescription for the treatment of pneumonia, for example, was *"Copious bleeding ... up to 140 ounces" (almost 9 pints); the bleeding should be continued until the fifth, seventh, or even the fourteenth day.* His favorite medicine was mercury, about which he stated, *hence its usefulness and fame in all general and chronic diseases."* [emphasis added]

A note regarding bloodletting: The use of bloodletting originated with Galen two thousand years earlier. I have emphasized Galen's role in developing Rationalist medical theories ("identify a disease; find the antidote"), but Galen also based treatments on Greek medicine's four humors. Galen's approach to restoring balance among the humors was not, however, a harmless one. His treatment was to "relieve the patient's congestion" by bleeding the patient, often copiously. Lewis Thomas, in *The Fragile Species*, described this therapy as follows:

> Congestion of the various organs was the trouble to be treated, according to Galen, and by the eighteenth century the notion had been elevated to a routine cure-all, or anyway treat-all: remove the excess fluid, one way or another. The ways were direct and forthright: open a vein and take away a pint or more of blood at a sitting, enough to produce faintness and a bluish pallor, place suction cups on the skin to draw out lymph, administer large doses of mercury or various plant extracts to cause purging, and if all else failed induce vomiting.
>
> George Washington perhaps died of this therapy at the age of sixty-six. Hale and hearty, he had gone for a horseback ride in the snow; unfortunately, later in the day he developed a fever and a severe sore throat. He then took to his bed and called in his doctors. His throat was wrapped in poultices, he was given warm vinegar and honey to gargle, and over the next two days he was bled from a vein for about five pints of blood. His last words to his physician were, "Pray take no more trouble about me. Let me go quietly."[484]

Rush was opposed to the use of botanical remedies, the favorite of the Indian-influenced doctors, preferring mercury and other mineral medicines. Not only did he use powerful mineral medicines, but in large doses. This practice of "heroic medicine" continued for the first half of the nineteenth century, the allopath being confident in his medical theory and distrustful of the recuperative power of the patient. Rush wrote, "Physicians are in practice the masters of nature. Instead of waiting for the slow operations of nature, to eliminate a supposed morbid matter from the body, art should take the business out of her hands."[485] Rush was *not* a Hippocratic physician!

The consequence of this kind of treatment was a serious deterioration in the health of many Americans. Calomel (mercury) was known to cause severe deterioration to the teeth, and one commentator noted, "*Perhaps the most universal symptom of the physical decay was the condition of America's teeth; one seldom talked to a dentist, it was affirmed, who did not despair of the republic.*"[486]

In 1845, citizens of one Pennsylvania county petitioned the state legislature to pass a law prohibiting the use of mercury in medicine. The legislative committee examining the matter concluded that mercurial medicines are indeed capable of damage to the patient, but it added that *if physicians were to be deprived of all agents capable of doing harm, they would have no medicines left*. The petition was denied.

Rush had his detractors. One Philadelphian described Rush's therapeutics as, "one of those great discoveries which are made from time to time for the depopulation of the earth." Somewhat more scientific, a hospital study (1830s) of the relative therapeutic values of allopathic medicine and of no treatment at all for two of the major diseases of the day (typhoid fever and delirium tremens) showed that *no treatment at all* was clearly more successful than was the standard medical treatment. Lewis Thomas describes this clinical research in *The Fragile Species*: "*One (group of patients) was treated by bleeding, cupping, purging, and the other athletic feats of therapy, while the other group received nothing more than bed rest, nutrition and observation. The results were unequivocal and appalling.*"[487] Nevertheless, Rush's many graduates continued to influence American medicine for much of the nineteenth century.

12.4 Indian Doctors and Eclectics

Many early American settlers had been treated by Native American healers, and from those healers they had learned of herbal and other treatments. These treatments worked, and in time there developed a body of American physicians who learned their mentors' lore and came to be known as Indian Doctors. They were, of course, looked down upon by the university-trained physicians, albeit the success of the Indian Doctors often exceeded that of their allopathic competitors. There were also a few university-trained physicians who recognized the effectiveness of the Indians' methods, and the latter became known as "botanical practitioners."

Though the Indian Doctors were primarily a frontier phenomenon, they eventually joined with a related group (Thompsonians, who used steam baths and other Indian medical remedies) and became known in the 1840s as the Eclectic medical school.[488] They had learned the physical and spiritual benefit of sweat lodges and herbs from Native American healers.

12.5 Homeopathy and Constantine Hering

Homeopathy came to the U.S. in 1825, and by the 1840s it was providing serious competition to allopathic medicine. The first American homeopath was a Danish_Bostonian (Dr. Gram) who had gone to Copenhagen for his medical education. He had discovered homeopathy while in Denmark, and he practiced it exclusively upon his return. The second was a Swiss physician who immigrated to Pennsylvania, read of homeopathy, and adopted it in the late 1820s.

In 1830, Constantine Hering (1800-1880) came to Pennsylvania, and he came to be known as the father of American homeopathy. The German influence was strong in Pennsylvania, and the first homeopathic academy in Pennsylvania (Nordamerikanische Academy der Homoeopathischen Heilkunst) was established in 1835 with all instruction in German. It was succeeded in 1841 by the Homoeopathic Medical College of Pennsylvania, established in Philadelphia by Hering. It became the international center of homoeopathic education in the 19th century.

Hering was both an educator and a medical scientist, and one of his principles came to be known as *Hering's Law*, that "As diseases go from acute to chronic phases, symptoms move from the surface to the interior, from the lower part of the body to the upper, and from the less vital organs to the more vital."[489] This perspective of course further emphasized, to the homeopathic physician, the *importance of addressing cause rather than suppressing symptoms.*

German immigrant physicians and graduates of Hering's Academy carried the doctrine of homeopathy to the West, and in Ohio, the homeopaths and the Eclectics established a friendly relationship, with the result that Cincinnati became a center of homeopathy west of the Alleghenies (even today the term Eclectic is known in Cincinnati). The German physicians spread around the country and maintained close relations with the German-American population of the country.

Homeopathy also spread from its Boston origin (Dr. Gram's colleagues) to other areas of New England and New York. Many allopaths were converted to homeopathy, and the new system's influence spread.

The American Institute of Homeopathy was founded in 1844, with Constantine Hering the first president. The purposes of the Institute were:

(1) The reformation and augmentation of the *materia medica*

(2) The restraining of physicians from pretending to be competent to practice homoeopathy who have not studied it in a careful and skillful manner [490]

Thus, the American Institute of Homeopathy was a self-regulating body.

The popularity of homeopathy led to a severe conflict with allopathic medicine. Homeopathy was well accepted by the intellectuals and professionals of the country. This caused great despair among the allopaths, especially when many graduates of allopathic medical schools became convinced of homeopathy's superiority. Repeated attempts by allopaths to achieve legislation restricting licensing to allopaths failed—if such laws were passed, they were almost inevitably repealed at the next legislative session due to voter pressure. Finally despairing that the American voters lacked the intelligence to see the superiority of their cause, and suffering economically because of the public's acceptance of homeopathy (homeopathic practitioners were practicing medicine with much more success and better remuneration than were the allopaths), leading allopathic medical societies to join forces to found the American Medical Association (AMA).

12.6 The American Medical Association

The American Medical Association was founded in 1846, primarily due to the influence and efforts of Dr. Nathan Smith Davis, of New York, who was described as *"a bitter foe of homoeopathy and scornful of those who would treat it as simply another theory of etiology; he was too thoroughly imbued with the positivism of nineteenth century clinical medicine to accept such reasoning."*[491] Immediately after graduating from medical school, Davis joined his county medical society's anti-quackery committee, and he fought what he considered quackery throughout his life. As the leader of the AMA for half a century, Davis was the single man most responsible for the extreme anti-homeopathic orientation of American medicine.

The AMA formally endorsed Galen's concepts upon its founding, and its stated purpose was to accomplish (allegedly) three goals:

(1) To improve medical education, (this was a code phrase meaning to improve the economic status of allopathic physicians—this was a BOGUS goal.)

(2) To educate the public as to the superiority of allopathic medicine. (This was also BOGUS, as previous attempts to "educate the public" had failed, and homeopathy had a better record than had allopathic medicine.)

(3) *To eliminate the competition from homeopaths.*

Homeopaths, being organized, were considered a far more serious threat than were the Eclectics, and the vituperation heaped upon the homeopaths by the allopaths was extreme. They were labeled as uneducated quacks, even though many were graduates of allopathic medical schools.

The AMA did essentially nothing about medical education, possibly because academic medicine was well-represented in the Association, and these universities liked the *status quo.*

Education of the public was considered to be a lost cause, inasmuch as the public had already formed a low opinion of allopathic medicine, and nothing much had changed there.

The real focus of the AMA's efforts was its attack on homeopathy, albeit at the same time American allopaths did gradually adopt many homeopathic tools. Significant amounts of the homeopathic remedies were absorbed into allopathic use, and allopaths moved away from the use of multiple drugs. They also moved to smaller doses of medicines instead of using the "heroic" dosages of Rush.

The AMA attacked homeopaths on many fronts. It threw them out of county and state medical societies, even though they might have MD degrees from highly regarded medical schools. They banned consultation with homeopaths, which led to such extremes as a physician's being expelled from a Connecticut medical society for consulting with a homeopath—his wife. Allopathic medicine's principle bastion was the allopathic medical schools, and students could be discharged for professing an interest in homeopathy. Nevertheless, many prominent Americans remained convinced of homeopathy's superiority, and it was not until the twentieth century that the AMA finally won its fight.

As indicated above, homeopathy became the treatment of choice for many Americans during the nineteenth century, with perhaps the best-known adherent to homeopathy being Lincoln's Secretary of State, William Seward. Seward was joined in his confidence in homeopathy by many prominent figures, particularly in the Boston area, including such notables as Harvard physiology professor William James, authors Mark Twain, Henry Wadsworth Longfellow, Nathaniel Hawthorne, Louisa May Alcott, Henry James, and Daniel Webster, together with journalists Horace Greeley and William Cullen Bryant, and industrialist John D. Rockefeller. This popularity reached its peak when homeopathic physicians proved far more effective than their allopathic competitors in treating the Yellow Fever epidemic in Louisiana and the Mississippi Valley in 1878. The homeopathically-treated patients had a mortality rate less than half that of those treated allopathically (around 7%, versus at least 16% for those treated with allopathic medicine).[492]

The 1870s and 1880s proved to be a peak for homeopathy. Several factors were responsible. The first was a division within its own ranks between those such as Hering, who adhered to Hahnemann's teaching, including the use of high dilution remedies, and other homeopathic physicians who found the Hahnemann methods too demanding, preferring low potencies and gradually shifting to the use of multiple drugs and a less rigorous examination of patients' symptoms than the older homeopaths demanded.

This split between the "highs" and the "lows" led to a relaxing of homeopathic standards at the same time that allopathic medicine was adopting many homeopathic remedies (e.g., nitroglycerine for angina). Thus, the "lows" and the allopaths became less separated in their practices, even though the AMA was still calling the homeopaths "quacks."

Another important factor was that the homeopaths were conducting highly successful medical practices. They prospered, in contrast to allopaths, who left medical practice in droves when they found themselves unable to make a satisfactory living practicing allopathic medicine. One result of the homeopathic complacency was their lack of interest in joining homeopathic medical societies, in sharp contrast to the dedication of the allopaths, who used the AMA as a weapon to destroy homeopathy.

The internal division among homeopaths set the stage for the decline of homeopathy, but the active opposition of the AMA proved to be the death knell. The AMA was guided, between 1899 and 1910, by a very capable and dedicated anti-homeopathy physician, Dr. George Simmons. The AMA's efforts were aided financially by the pharmaceutical companies, whose advertising revenues in the Journal of the American Medical Association (JAMA) provided a war chest in the AMA's fight against homeopathy. Much of that advertising raised serious ethical questions, but Dr. Simmons guided the AMA through compromises that maintained the appearance of ethical standards without decreasing the revenues from the pharmaceutical companies.[493]

Another of Simmons' maneuvers was to reverse the AMA's previous combativeness against homeopathy and to encourage homeopaths to join the AMA ranks. This was done by inviting homeopaths to join county medical societies, where the national Ethical Code regarding consultations with homeopaths was held not to apply. The gist of it was: "If you don't call yourselves homeopaths, and if you don't try to recruit homeopaths, then you can join our society; we won't call you 'quacks' anymore, you can practice any way you wish, and we'll refer patients to you."

The implication was that there would be open discussion in the medical societies of therapeutic approaches. The homeopaths soon learned that this was not the case, but many still were absorbed into the allopathic medical societies. Since the "lows" were practicing medicine in a manner not very different from that of allopaths, the shift to collaboration with their allopathic colleagues became more and more palatable. A similar situation occurred in California in the 1950s, when Doctors of Osteopathy were designated as equivalent to MDs, and the Southern California School of Osteopathy was converted into an allopathic medical school.

The final blow against homeopathy struck by the AMA was against homeopathic medical schools. There were too many homeopathic medical schools (22 in 1900) just as there were too many allopathic schools for the patient population, and the AMA intended to reduce the number of both. Further, many of the homeopathic schools had abandoned Hahnemann and were teaching "low" homeopathy, really a mix of homeopathic and allopathic medicine.[494]

12.7 The Flexner Report

In 1904 the AMA proposed new standards for medical education, following the pattern of European allopathic schools. After the proposed standards met with resistance, from both homeopathic and allopathic medical schools, the AMA in 1909 asked the Carnegie Endowment for the Advancement of Teaching to join the effort. Abraham Flexner, for the Carnegie Endowment, and Nathan Colwell, for the AMA, surveyed American medical education and issued the Flexner Report in 1910.

The Flexner Report established the pattern for medical education in the United States for the rest of the twentieth century. It used the educational model of German allopathic medical schools, instituting medical science as the sole basis for American medicine and medical education. After the Report was issued, financial incentives were provided by the Carnegie and Rockefeller Foundations to medical schools that adopted the Report's recommendations. It should be noted that there is great irony in the Rockefeller Foundation's support of the Flexner Report's recommendations. John D. Rockefeller had been a lifelong advocate of homeopathic medicine, but he had an assistant who was equally devoted to allopathic medicine.[495] It was the assistant who arranged to support the recommendations of the Flexner Report. With the offer of financial support, many medical schools were persuaded to convert to systems of training that conformed to the Report's recommendations.

The Report was systematically opposed to homeopathic principles, and it specifically recommended that no financial support be given to homeopathic medical schools, deeming them unscientific. Many of the changes proposed in the Report were beneficial in ensuring good science training for future physicians. However, this major shift in American medical education also ensured that the *chemico-mechanical (materialist) assumptions and disease-oriented dogma of the Rationalist and allopathic viewpoint became thoroughly entrenched in American medicine.*

As mentioned, the Report sounded the death knell of homeopathic education, and it also essentially eliminated women's and minority medical colleges. The mechanism for doing so was to state that these colleges didn't meet the AMA standards, so would not receive financial support. Finally, state examining boards accepted only graduates of AMA-approved schools, which was the final blow. Even Hahnemann Medical School in Philadelphia became an allopathic school, though its charter requires it to teach homeopathic medicine, a requirement that was met by one seminar course describing homeopathic principles.[496]

12.8 The AMA and the Pharmaceutical Industry

The ties between the AMA and the pharmaceutical industry continued to grow, particularly during the years (1924-1949) when Dr. Morris Fishbein was Executive Secretary of the AMA. Dr. Fishbein assumed his position with the AMA immediately following his graduation from medical school. He was *not* a practicing physician. Pharmaceutical advertising was bolstered by Dr. Fishbein's innovation of providing the AMA's "seal of approval" to drugs it deemed worthwhile, usually, of course, the same drugs that were advertised in the Journal of the AMA (JAMA). Inevitably the close ties between the pharmaceutical industry and the AMA influenced the direction of American medical research as well as American clinical medicine. Physicians came more and more to rely on drug companies' "detail men" for their information about new drugs, and American medicine became more and more influenced by the pharmaceutical companies' new products. Pharmaceutical companies even secured legislation allowing drug advertising in television ads, ensuring that the TV-viewing public viewed pharmaceutical products as the only cure for various disorders.

The Federal Food and Drug Administration (FDA) did require those ads to include the drug's side effects, but there is ample evidence of close ties between the FDA and the AMA. The most recent example of collaboration between pharmaceutical companies and the AMA was the AMA's decision to label obesity as a disease, *coincidentally* at the same time that pharmaceutical companies introduced anti-obesity drugs.

Many medical successes were achieved under this system. Many of the new drugs were successful at combating the symptoms of serious and life-threatening illnesses. *If the role of the physician is to keep the patient happy while nature does the healing, then the relief of symptoms may be all that is required for a successful recovery from disease.* So, this treatment of acute disease symptoms, especially coming at the same time that major advances were made in sanitation, refrigeration, and economic progress, was associated with a significant improvement in the nation's health.

Unfortunately, this reliance on the pharmaceutical companies' products also has had its problems. Many drugs proved to have undesirable side effects; thus a continuous stream of new drugs was produced throughout the century. We are currently seeing microbes rapidly modifying their genes and so rendering them invulnerable to antibiotics; with impotent antibiotics, hospital infections are on the rise.

Further, Dr. Fishbein's commitment to drugs as the only acceptable therapeutic measure (with surgery and radiation) led to his inveighing against the concept that *diet* might also provide valuable therapeutic assistance. In this, Dr. Fishbein was clearly opposing Hippocrates' dictum that "food is the best medicine." A consequence of this viewpoint is that, even today, nutrition is taught in American medical schools in only a cursory manner. Oriental and naturopathic medical students receive far more training in nutrition than do most Western (allopathic) medical students.

Furthermore, the result of the allopathic drug treatment has not been that effective in far too many cases, particularly in chronic disease. Dr. Kerr White, former Deputy Director for Health Sciences at the Rockefeller Foundation, summarized the situation in 1988 when he wrote, "It is still the case that *only about 15% of all (allopathic) contemporary clinical interventions are supported by objective scientific evidence that they do more good than harm.*" White went on to say that *three to four times as important in providing therapeutic benefit is the care and concern of the patient's care-givers, the love that stimulates psychoneuroimmunologic pathways.*[497] [emphasis added]

A tragic case of economic interest's superseding patient benefits is the story of Dr. Royal Raymond Rife, a bacteriologist, microscopist and engineer. He made fundamental discoveries about the nature of cancer in the 1920s and 30s, using his own ultra-high resolution optical microscope to study live cells. Rife's secret in obtaining such ultra-high resolution was to use a single frequency light source. Dr. Rife's work was ground-breaking. It supported the earlier work of Béchamp and the contemporary work of Günther Enderlein and Gaston Naessens regarding the Pleomorphic Cycle. (See Chapter 11). It also proved highly effective in the clinical treatment of cancer.

Dr. Fishbein found out about the success of Rife's cancer treatment from a patient who had been cured of a large facial tumor. Dr. Fishbein invited the patient to lunch and interrogated him about his remarkable recovery. Dr. Fishbein, upon learning of the source of the patient's cure, then attempted to become a financial partner in a clinic using Rife's method. The clinic refused, and within days AMA attorneys descended on Rife and the clinic and closed them down. A long trial ensued. Rife finally won in court, but the process destroyed him both financially and physically. He did write up his work before he died, but the microscope that he had invented was destroyed, for he had sold parts of the microscope to meet his legal expenses. His methods were effectively lost, to the apparently great detriment of generations of cancer patients.[498]

Fishbein's excesses finally led the AMA to remove him from office in 1949, but for decades he had a major and pernicious influence on American medicine, facets of which have still not been recovered from.

American medicine today is at a crossroads. The AMA is still fighting its old battles against competition, that competition today coming in the form of various modalities of alternative or complementary medicine. The executive secretary of the AMA appeared only a few years ago on national television to debunk the non-material but highly successful Healing Touch, and it was in 1987 that a U.S. District Court found the AMA guilty of an antitrust conspiracy against chiropractic doctors.

Nevertheless, there are many encouraging signs of change. American medical schools are recognizing the need to broaden their perspectives, and many are now including one or another elective in alternative medicine for their students. At an International Conference on Science and Spiritual Healing at Keauhou (Big Island of Hawaii) several years ago, not only universities and medical schools but also the NIH were represented. Hospitals such as North Hawaii Community Hospital are including non-MDs, chiropractors and acupuncturists, as well as Healing Touch practitioners, on their staffs. As yet, these hospitals are few in number, but the trend has begun and more integrated clinics are being founded. Harvard Medical School is proving to be a pioneer in recognizing the value of other healing modalities. Harvard Medical School faculty member Herbert Benson has been a leader and has written *The Relaxation Response*,[499] and his colleague David Eisenberg has joined him with his *Encounters with Qi*.[500] Harvard is not alone.

It should be noted, however, that even Harvard is influenced by financial considerations. Dr. Robert Pumphries, a White House physician and formerly on the Board of Directors of the National Cancer Institute, was refused permission to speak at Harvard on cancer prevention. (Cancer treatment is a billion-dollar business at Harvard-affiliated hospitals.)[501]

Once again, the public is leading the way, with perhaps half of their medical dollars going to alternative medical practitioners despite the lack of insurance coverage (Eisenberg, et al, *New England Journal of Medicine,* 1993).[502]

The other side of the current picture for allopathic medicine is less encouraging. The economic pressures of high-tech medicine have led to the development of Health Maintenance Organizations (HMOs), with a resultant rise in the power of accountants in the practice of medicine. The Rationalist view of disease, of course, fits well with an accountant's perspective of the practice of medicine—identify the disease, then use a standard therapy for that disease. Reduce the amount of physician time devoted to symptom evaluation, and you have a medical system that is not only Rationalist but simplistic. Base that medicine on a reliance on laboratory experiments and technology, hold to the Cartesian dichotomy, and you face another set of problems. These will be discussed in a later chapter, but suffice it to say that the HMOs' approach reinforces the limitation of Western Scientific Medicine to symptom management, which can be highly effective in acute cases, where the patient's self-healing power is the key once the crisis is past, but symptom management is of limited value in chronic disease. The consequences of restricting medical practices to symptom management will be described in Chapter 13.

The situation is changing, as more and more MDs recognize the limitations of Western allopathic medicine. Noteworthy among these is Dr. Lissa Rankin, whose book, *Mind Over Medicine*[503] is an impressive contribution to this discussion and whose work has been frequently referred to in the present text, as well as books by Louise Hay[504], and R.E. Smith, et al[505].

Key Names and Dates—American Medicine in the 19th and 20th Centuries

Benjamin Rush	1745-1813
Constantine Hering	1800-1880
American Institute of Homeopathy	1844
American Medical Association	1846
Nathan Smith Davis, Executive Secretary	*1846-1899*
George Simmons, Executive Secretary	*1899-1910*
Morris Fishbein, Executive Secretary	*1924-1949*
Flexner Report	1910
Co-Chair, Abraham Flexner, Carnegie Endowment for the Advancement of Teaching	
Co-Chair, Nathan Colwell, American Medical Association	
Royal Raymond Rife	*1920s and 1930s*

Notes

482 Coulter, Harris, *Divided Legacy: A History of the Schism in Medical Thought*, Vol. III, Wehawken Book Co., 1975.
483 See Section 12.7.
484 Thomas, Lewis, *The Fragile Species*, Macmillan, 1992.
485 Coulter, Harris, *Divided Legacy: A History of the Schism in Medical Thought*, Vol. III, Wehawken Book Co., 1975.
486 Ibid.
487 Thomas, Lewis, *The Fragile Species*, Macmillan, 1992.
488 Felter, Harvey Wickes, *History of the Eclectic Medical Institute, Cincinatti, Ohio, 1845-1902*, Alumnal Association of the Eclectic Medical Institute, 1902.
489 Coulter, Harris, *Divided Legacy: A History of the Schism in Medical Thought*, Vol. III, Wehawken Book Co., 1975.
490 https://www.homeopathyusa.org.
491 Coulter, Harris, *Divided Legacy: A History of the Schism in Medical Thought*, Vol. III, Wehawken Book Co., 1975.
492 Goddard, Jayney, "Homeopathy in Epidemics and Pandemics", *Scientific Research in Homeopathy Conference*, 2013, http://www.holistic-iasis.com/uploads/2/3/6/5/23654344/jayney_s_20presentation-2.pdf.
493 Davidson, Jonathan, *A Century of Homeopaths: Their Influence on Medicine and Health*, Springer, NY, 2014.
494 Coulter, Harris, *Divided Legacy: A History of the Schism in Medical Thought*, Vol. III, Wehawken Book Co., 1975.
495 Brown, E. Richard, *Rockefeller's Medicine Men*, University of California Press, 1979.
496 Coulter, Harris, *Divided Legacy: A History of the Schism in Medical Thought*, Vol. III, Wehawken Book Co., 1975.
497 White, Kerr L., Foreword by Lynn Payer, *Medicine and Culture*, Henry Holt, 1988.
498 Lyns, Barry, *The Cancer Cure That Worked*, Marcus Books, 1989.
499 Benson, Herbert, *The Relaxation Response*, William Morrow, 1975.
500 Eisenberg, David, *Encounters with Qi: Exploring Chinese Medicine*, Penguin Books, 1987.
501 Pumphries, Robert, MD, personal communication,
502 Eisenberg, D.M., et al., "Unconventional Medicine in the United States—prevalence, costs, and patterns of use" *New England Journal of Medicine* 328: 246-252, 1993.
503 Rankin, Lissa, *Mind Over Medicine: Scientific Proof That You Can Heal Yourself*, Hay House, 2013.
504 Hay, Louise L., *Heal Your Body*, Hay House, 1984.
505 Smith, R.E., P.K. Smith and H. Bigelsen, *Your Cure for Cancer*, Promotion Publishing, 1998.

Chapter 13
The Impact of Western Science on Medicine: Methods and Assumptions of Western Science

13.1 Assumptions Revisited

The danger of assumption is well illustrated by an incident that happened in the U.S. Navy in November 1939 (Names have been changed, but this is an historical event). Task Force Delta was steaming off the Maine coast. The date was prior to World War II and the development of radar. It was night, there was a dense fog, and lookouts had been posted on the bow of the flagship. Admiral Jackson was in command aboard his flagship, the USS Ulysses.

One of the lookouts suddenly advised the bridge that there was a light bearing down on a collision course with the task force. The captain of the flagship ordered the radioman to send a message to the ship bearing on the collision course to alter his course to starboard. A response quickly came back, "No. You change your course to starboard."

It happened that Admiral Jackson arrived on the bridge while this interchange was going on. The Admiral was not amused! He immediately took the radio from the radioman and ordered, "This is Admiral Jackson in command of U. S. Navy Task Force Delta. You are ordered to turn to starboard!"

Back came the reply. "Admiral Jackson, this is Seaman 2nd Class Barnes. We are a lighthouse."

Moral: Never assume (make assumptions), whether in the fog, conducting a scientific experiment, in a relationship, or in any other phase of life, including when you are treating a patient.

Modern Western medicine prides itself on being scientific, and the most frequently expressed response to issues regarding non-allopathic medical modalities is, "Is it scientific?" It is thus highly important that when one refers to Western Scientific Medicine (WSM), the implications of that terminology are understood. Unfortunately, all too often the practitioners of WSM are themselves unaware of the implications of their own terminology. It therefore becomes imperative that, for a complete understanding of modern allopathic medicine, science itself be understood.

13.2 The Scientific Method

Most scientists, when they are using the word "science" in a strict interpretation (a broad definition would be the study of nature), are really talking about the Scientific Method. This Method has proven invaluable in the elucidation of the *mechanisms* underlying natural processes. The dependence of science upon the Scientific Method has led to the corollary that, unless the mechanism underlying a process is understood, then, no matter how well-documented a particular phenomenon might be, that phenomenon is not considered part of scientifically accepted reality. In a recent example of this reasoning, the frequently-reported phenomenon of "Runner's High" was considered only an old wives' tale until the mechanisms underlying the euphoria given that name had been demonstrated as being caused by endorphin release during exercise.[506] Once that mechanism was understood, then "Runner's High" became accepted as scientific fact.

The Scientific Method is a process by which the mechanisms underlying an observed natural phenomenon are examined and tested. It goes like this:

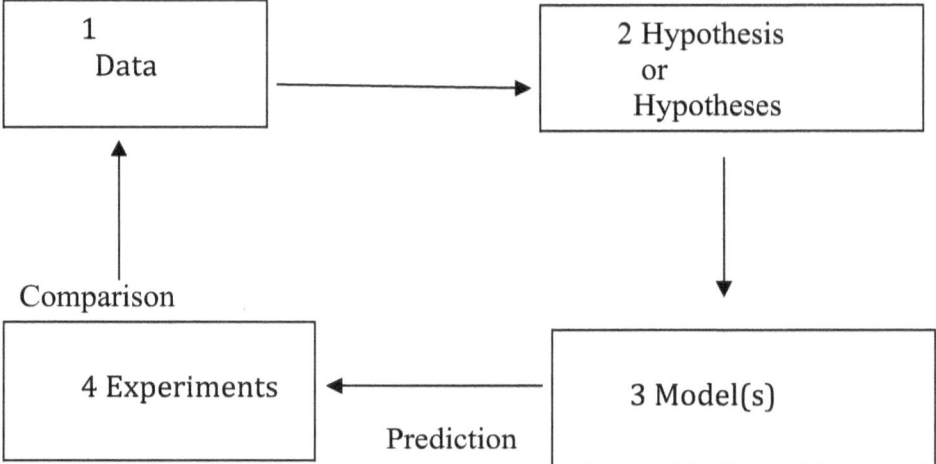

Procedure:

A. Observe the phenomenon, collecting all *data* considered useful in the understanding of the phenomenon.
B. Develop an *hypothesis* or (better) *hypotheses* regarding the mechanism believed to be responsible for the observed phenomenon.
C. Develop a *model*, capable of predicting experimental outcomes, from the hypothetical mechanism. This model is usually either physical or, preferably, mathematical.
D. Using this model, *predict* the outcome of proposed experiments with the phenomenon under study.
E. Conduct the proposed *experiments* and compare the actual experimental outcome with the outcome predicted by the model.
F. Observing any *discrepancies* between predicted and actual experimental outcomes, *modify the working hypothesis* appropriately and then repeat the process of *modeling* and *testing*.
G. When there is no longer a significant ("significance" is open to interpretation) difference between predicted and actual

experimental outcome, the hypothesis advances to the rank of theory.
H. When enough different researchers have independently confirmed the experiment and its outcome, the theory becomes accepted as scientific fact.

This process is rigorous and it has proven itself highly effective in testing proposed explanations for observed natural phenomena. It provides an intellectual feedback loop (cf. negative feedback control systems—e.g., the steersman, or anti-aircraft control) that has the highly important property of being *self-correcting.* Such a self-correcting strategy is also a crucial element of effective medical diagnostics. Unfortunately, the Scientific Method has built into it assumptions that may or may not be appropriate for the phenomenon being studied.

Some of the ASSUMPTIONS of WESTERN SCIENCE include:

Assumption 1: It is *possible* to understand nature by observation.

In fact, it appears *not* to be possible to understand observations without their being in the context of a theory. Albert Einstein has commented, "It is the theory that determines what we can observe," and "The answer you get is determined by the question you ask." For example, the supernova of 1054 was seen by Chinese astronomers but not by European astronomers, not because eyesights were different, but because European astronomers worked in the context of Aristotle's astronomical theory that held that the skies are unchanging. There are many examples of how observations are influenced by the observer's belief system.

Assumption 2: The experimenter understands all the influences that may affect the experimental outcome.

Examples of assumptions that may fail include but are not limited to the following:
- A. It doesn't matter what time of day the experiment is performed (consider Chinese medicine, or chronobiological studies). A good example of this phenomenon occurred during research determining the effect of a drug on a particular hypothalamic

response. The experimenter was cognizant of the possibility that the time of day the drug was administered might have an effect on the experimental outcome, so he performed the experiment at different times during the day and recorded the response. The results showed clearly that the drug did indeed have an impact on the hypothalamic response, a response that varied as a function of the time of day the experiment was performed. The results further showed that had the experiment been performed only at 9 am when the experimenter normally arrived at his laboratory, no drug effect on the hypothalamic response would have been found.
Note: very few Western clinicians are aware of this factor.
B. It doesn't matter what day of the month the experiment is performed (female subject).
C. An experimental animal is used, and data/theories gained from the experiment are assumed to apply to humans.
D. The experimental animal is anesthetized, and the data obtained are assumed to apply to intact animals.
Examples:
- Experiments in which different anesthetics lead to different experimental results.
- Renal autoregulation (Renal Blood Flow is not a function of Renal Arterial Pressure)—is still in physiology textbooks despite experimental data to the contrary.

E. The emotional state of the experimental subject, human or animal, is assumed not to affect the experimental outcome.
See the Rabbit experiment described below.

Assumption 3: The experimental outcome is *assumed* to be independent of the experimenter, so long as each follows the same experimental protocol (see below).

Assumption 4: The phenomenon under study can be represented by a mathematical model, usually a simple linear differential equation. This itself implies a tremendous simplification of the phenomenon (at best), as most phenomena are non-linear except within an extremely narrow range. Limiting the experimental perturbations to that range may not well represent physical reality. Assuming linearity in any case is risky, for only sometimes does it approximate reality. See discussion of mathematical models in Chapter 9 and of chaos theory in Chapter 15.

Assumption 5: The experimental testing and/or analytical procedures used are relevant to the real state of the phenomenon under study.

Convenient experimental perturbations of the system, for example, are the use of square waves or steps, pulses, or a simple change of stimulus intensity. Each of these procedures, and others, while convenient analytically, may not represent events in the real world.[507]

Examples of errors that result from making this assumption:

- Recall the situation of the drunk under the light post, searching for a coin he lost elsewhere. However, the light was better under the light post, so that was where he was searching.
- The Goldblatt Preparation has been popular as a way to study renal hypertension. This procedure *may* apply to 2-3% of cases of hypertension. This procedure is convenient experimentally, but the results do not apply to most human hypertension.
- Genetically hypertensive mice have been studied extensively and are of interest, but the experimental results so obtained do *not* extrapolate to human hypertension.

Assumption 6: It is necessary to use *accepted* scientific laws in the interpretation of experimental data.

It is precisely this issue that has led to the refusal of scientists to accept data from well-designed experiments. E.g., to most scientists it is a "given" that chemistry's Law of Mass Action applies to therapeutic drugs or other substances ingested by humans. Given that assumption, it is absurd to such scientists that homeopathic doses of medical remedies *could* work, regardless of whether laboratory or clinical data show that they *do* work. Valid experimental data is thus discarded because it does not fit the current scientifically accepted model of reality, a belief system of what is real.[508]

Note that this perspective is specifically the function of the currently accepted model of reality. If that model were to include human energy fields, for example, then the analysis of whether or not homeopathic remedies *could* work would change completely.[509]

The Scientific Method provides a valuable means for studying phenomena so long as the questions asked are appropriate for the phenomenon under study and so long as the range of the study is strictly limited. A study of the length-tension relationship of a spring, for example, is highly useful within a certain range and under certain temperature and other conditions, but outside those conditions the data collected could lead to interpretations of minimal value to the experimenter.

Example: length-tension diagram for a spring *at room temperature*:

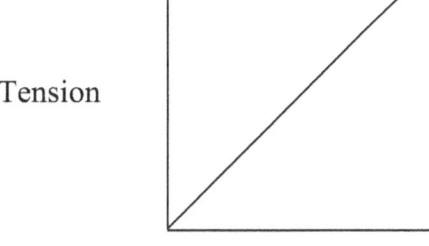

Tension

Length

The question, "What happens at –60° F?" cannot be answered without additional information.

For biological phenomena the problem becomes far more difficult, for such phenomena are subject to a vast array of influences that limit the application of the procedures of the Scientific Method.

The *assumptions* of the Scientific Method are but the beginning of the problems associated with the application of Western science to medical questions. Other important assumptions made by Western medical scientists include:

Assumption 1: In medicine, following Galen, we can define a disease, then find a treatment (antidote) to combat that disease.

Assumption 2: In medical science, following Descartes, we can consider body and mind/spirit to be separate and can study the body as a biochemical/ mechanical machine.

Assumption 3: In medical research, we can follow the principle that scientific reductionism provides an understanding of the body's function and malfunction.

Assumption 4: Scientific laboratory instruments define objective reality. Thus, if something *cannot be measured* by scientific instruments, it is *not real*. Conversely, if something *can* be measured by a scientific instrument, then it *is* real.

Assumption 5: The experimenter doesn't influence the experimental outcome. (This assumption was mentioned earlier, and it is important to understand the implications of this assumption on both medical science and medical practice. This assumption is extremely important with respect to the question of being a healer.)

Assumption 6: Each person is separate and can be considered to be an isolated entity. This is a Newtonian concept that does not conform to the findings of modern physics or to data documenting distant healing.

Each of these assumptions must be considered. Several have been previously discussed so may be addressed fairly briefly. Each assumption will also be considered from the perspective of traditional medicines, using Hawaiian medicine as an example.

13.3 Western Medical Assumption 1: The Scientific Method provides an accurate understanding of natural mechanisms and of scientific reality.

This assumption has been addressed above, as have the assumptions that come with the Method. Remember, when all else is set aside, it is the Scientific Method that is the cornerstone of modern Western science.

13.4 Western Medical Assumption 2 (Galen's Assumption): We can define a disease, then find a treatment to combat that disease.

This assumption of course derives from the Rationalist perspective generally associated with Galen and continued by medical scientists such as Claude Bernard. It is still the accepted philosophical assumption of the medicine taught in Western allopathic (and so materialistic) medical schools.[510] The theories used to define diseases have changed through the centuries, with the present theories based on our understanding of physiology and pathology. Both of these sciences are based on a biochemical/mechanical model of man, and pathology cannot escape the homeopathic criticism that pathology represents the effects of disease rather than the cause. Thus the question, does the germ cause the disease, or does the disease cause the germ? In the author's experience, Western scientific medicine is unable to define diseases unless it uses quite arbitrary methods of identifying some symptoms as useful and others as irrelevant.

Nevertheless, the current Western medical perspective is that its task is to perfect the art of differential diagnosis to identify the disease. With its focus on science, it uses laboratory research to understand the disease and to identify a treatment for that disease.

Allopathic medicine's method of combating disease uses the Law of Contraries to manage/suppress the symptoms of the identified disease. It assumes the symptoms to be the problem, and the task of the physician to be that of counteracting the symptoms (inasmuch as symptoms can sometimes kill, this assumption may well be warranted). Thus, this assumption *may* apply in some acute illness, but it does not lead to desirable results in chronic disease.

Suppressing symptoms is in total contrast to the Empiricist (Hippocratic) perspective that symptoms represent in part the body's efforts to combat disease (e.g., fever), and that the task of the physician is to assist the body in its efforts (Law of Similars) rather than to suppress symptoms. Such an approach conforms with the shamanic view that to suppress symptoms goes against nature. Symptom suppression additionally counters the homeopathic finding that symptom suppression merely drives the problem deeper, leading to more serious consequences for the patient in the future (consider Hering's Law, together with the case of the painful hemorrhoids described in Chapter One).

Hawaiian medicine, together with other holistic medicines—in contrast to Western Scientific Medicine—*treats the patient* rather than the disease. It might be noted that one of the finest of Western physicians, Sir William Osler, when Chairman of Medicine at Johns Hopkins Medical School, taught his students that, "It is far more important to know the patient who has a disease than it is to know the disease the patient has." Treating the disease rather than the patient is an unfortunate inheritance from Aristotle, and that approach merits being abandoned.

13.5 Western Medical Assumption 3: The body and mind/spirit are separate, and it is appropriate to study the body as a biochemical/mechanical machine.

This is of course the Cartesian Dichotomy, and it underlies all of modern medical science. It has led to many valuable experimental studies of human physiology, biochemistry, and more. *However*, it has within it so many limitations that it and other assumptions led to the apt comment of a colleague to a class of beginning medical students, "Half of what we will teach you (in physiology) is wrong; our problem is that we don't know which half."

Further, recent research in psychoneuroimmunology has proven the Cartesian Dichotomy to be false. It is an assumption of a materialistic medical science that can no longer be sustained.[511]

With the Cartesian assumption, there is no way that prayer could effect a healing outcome, despite evidence to the contrary.[512] Similarly, the outcome of the rabbit experiment (Nerem, et al., *Science*, 1980)[513] (discussed below) *could not* have occurred, nor *could* any of the many other well-documented examples of the effects of emotions on the body's physiology.

Hawaiian medicine, in contrast, assumes we are spiritual beings having a human experience. Therefore, Hawaiian medicine includes the impact of emotional, mental, and spiritual influences on the patient's physical health.

Hawaiian medicine was very familiar with the impact of the subconscious (*ku, unihipili*) and superconscious (*aumakua*) on health. The Hawaiian practice of *ho'oponopono* addresses the impact of emotional issues on health. The implications of this practice have been verified by scientific experiments quantifying the impact of emotions on the immune system.[514]

However, this knowledge is *not* limited to Hawaiians. It is found in a number of ancient scriptures:
1. Proverbs: As a man thinketh in his heart, so is he. (Jewish/Christian)
2. Buddha: All that we are is the result of what we have thought. (Buddhist)
3. Upanishads: Man is the creator of thought. What he thinks about in this life, that hereafter he becomes. (Hindu)
4. It is also found in contemporary literature. Harold Sherman has stated that you are today the sum total of every thought and experience you have ever had. A comment by Carolyn Myss describes the reality with the perceptive statement that your biography is your biology.

13.6 Western Medical Assumption 4: Scientific Reductionism provides an understanding of the body's function and malfunction.

Natural systems are complex, and it is most understandable that scientists have sought ways to reduce the complexities of their studies. An extremely valuable tool in prying ever deeper into the mysteries of nature has been the principle of Reductionism, that if one can gain a complete understanding of the basic element of a system, then one can understand the system itself.

The application of this principle has led to ever more focused investigations, the process of *learning more and more about less and less*. Most nuclear physics, for example, is really a study of the hydrogen atom. When physicists contemplate the helium atom, life is already too complicated, and they leave those studies to the chemists.

To biologists, the principle of Reductionism may seem simplistic, but in fact much medical research is based on this principle. We might characterize these studies as *Study the cell to understand the system*. If the system is a person, this conclusion may appear absurd, but reflect for a moment on the vast amounts of research dollars spent on research in cellular biology, on DNA research, all with the underlying theme that if we can correct the DNA problem, then we can cure the disease. Unfortunately, instead of moving towards integration, many medical physiology departments are moving more and more into cell biology under this reductionist influence.

This point was brought home forcibly to the author when he heard the author of a major textbook of neurophysiology, and a later Nobel Laureate, describe his research with a single neuron of the sea snail *aplysia*, stating confidently that from this research would come a complete understanding of the phenomenon of memory.

Reductionism appears in medical practice as specialization, with the consequence that we have large bodies of medical specialists who have little understanding of how their specialty relates to the rest of the body. A patient might be seen simultaneously by a cardiologist, an anesthesiologist and a surgeon, for example, each with only limited knowledge of the others' fields. If the same patient also has cancer, the opportunities for unfortunate treatment interactions abound.

A particular consequence of Reductionism appears in an area of potential misunderstanding between patients and specialists. An unfortunate example might be if the oncologist asserts that scientific research has shown that new super chemotherapy Drug X has an 80% record of success with the patient's particular form of cancer. The patient, and the patient's family and friends, interpret the oncologist's statement to mean that with Drug X the patient has an 80% likelihood of getting well. In fact, the oncologist was merely reporting that Drug X had an 80% record of reducing that particular tumor, and he was saying nothing about whether Drug X would increase the patient's survival odds. In fact, given Drug X's impact on the immune system, the patient's projected survival time might well decrease with the use of the drug. We read again and again of individuals who had been treated for cancer, then shortly later died of, say, pneumonia, inevitably accompanied by the statement, "He did not die of cancer."

Reductionism and the Cartesian Dichotomy of course go hand-in-hand with materialism, for without treating the body as a machine, Reductionism would be unthinkable. Thus, when a reductionist perspective is adduced, materialism goes with it as an inevitable companion.

In contrast, Hawaiian medicine and other holistic medicines are not at all reductionist, considering the patient as a whole person, not as a collection of parts. Historically, this perspective conforms well with that of Hippocrates, who was perhaps a model of the holistic physician. We know well that the whole, with all the complexity of emotional and other influences, is much greater than a sum of the parts. Epigenetics and psychoneuroimmunology have shown that emotions do affect our physiological responses and even our genetics.

For example, reductionist DNA research has proven valuable in areas of science such as anthropology and forensic pathology, but DNA is only one factor in disease. Further, the new science of epigenetics has shown that the hypothesis of genetic determinism is quite invalid.[515]

Further, genetic makeup might provide information about *where* one would most probably develop a cancer *if* one had cancer. However, a "defective breast cancer gene" would not determine *whether* the patient would have cancer at all, breast or otherwise. Should a patient found to possess such a gene have a "preventive mastectomy," then *if* a cancer did occur it would simply occur in a different organ.

In contrast, Hawaiian and other traditional medicines treat the patient as a whole, recognizing that no single part acts in isolation of the rest of body, mind and soul.

13.7 Western Medical Assumption 5: Scientific laboratory instruments provide an accurate measure of natural phenomena.

With the rapid growth of ever more sophisticated scientific instrumentation, this assumption seems naive, but it is all too real. There is no question that scientific instruments provide valuable information, but the very precision of many measurements can cause those measurements to be misinterpreted, and the assumption that our *present* instruments measure all that could be measured is unrealistic.

There is first the consequence of this assumption that says, *"If we can't measure it, it isn't real."* This is a standard scientific position, and it inevitably leads to the ignoring of information that could be extremely valuable. Measurements by humans without instruments, for example, are inevitably considered to be subjective and therefore scientifically suspect, even though the human sensory system is one of the most sensitive measuring devices known. Thus, though palpation of pulses was once part of the Western medical armamentarium, it has long been abandoned in favor of more "objective" measurements. In general, if a variable cannot be measured by a laboratory instrument, it will not be considered scientifically valid.

Even if measured by accepted scientific instruments, measurements that do not conform to the accepted scientific paradigm may also be ignored by science. Thus, although there is now ample documentation of the changes in electrical conductivity, capacitance, etc., at acupuncture points and meridians, those data have generally been ignored by Western medical science, for the concept of energy meridians does not fit into accepted Western medical theory. Science has a similar problem with homeopathic remedies—they may work, but again that effectiveness does not fit accepted (Western scientific, allopathic and rational) models of therapeutic mechanisms. As

Indigenous shamans have long known, and the sciences of epigenetics and psychoneuroimmunology are now confirming, invisible factors such as belief systems or emotional factors can have important impacts on health and upon healing.

Equally pernicious as the assumption that, if something cannot be measured it isn't real, is the assumption that if something *can* be measured, then it *is* real. This assumption can be extraordinarily dangerous. Examples: Clinical laboratory tests rarely specify the time of day that the sample is to be taken, albeit many physiological measurements vary significantly as a function of the time of day, when many physiological variables have a major circadian variation. A particular measurement made at one time of day (e.g., blood pressure in a patient with labile hypertension) may appear quite normal, yet the same measurement made at a different time of day could show significant pathology.

A particularly egregious example is one of assuming the significance of a months-old laboratory measurement. Using this outdated test result, a specialist recommended that a patient, who had formerly been paralyzed and had a tracheotomy, should never have the tracheotomy tube removed. The specialist made this recommendation based on a three-months-old laboratory test that represented the patient's clinical condition at her worst. The specialist did not consider that the patient had recovered from the paralysis (thanks to Chinese medicine, which was outside her experience and therefore not in her paradigm) in the interim. Fortunately, the attending physician questioned the specialist's conclusion and consulted another specialist, who examined the patient and, finding no reason not to remove the tube, did so with a resultant immediate improvement in the patient's vital signs.

It might be noted that had the first specialist's advice been heeded, the effect on the patient's emotional outlook, and thus on her immune system and her ability to heal, would have been profound, and very probably devastating to her health. In fact, the original specialist had already had a highly negative impact on the patient's health when by remarking, during the original "swallow" test, that the patient was "going to die with pneumonia." Fortunately, the patient was able to prevent the specialist's remark from destroying her ability to self-heal, but the remark nevertheless took a serious toll and could have been fatal.

The ultimate example of dependence on "objective" data is computer diagnosis, with all its problems. The treatment approaches of most HMOs, with their heavy reliance on laboratory tests, closely follows this reasoning.

Example within the Western context: An experienced MD, a surgeon, had a patient who had, by the surgeon's diagnosis, acute appendicitis. The hospital had a policy of not permitting surgery unless the diagnosis was confirmed by ultrasound. This acute appendix was *not* confirmed by the ultrasound scan. The (senior) surgeon overruled the hospital policy, performed the appendectomy, and saved the patient's life.

Laboratory measurements can be extremely useful, but they must be thoroughly understood, with all the implicit assumptions of the measurement, when the laboratory data are evaluated. If not, the evaluation can be greatly in error.

Holistic Hawaiian medicine recognizes that there are important aspects of reality not now measurable by scientific instruments. The effect of emotions on health provides an obvious example. This recognition is important for both diagnosis and treatment.

Hawaiian medicine also recognizes the importance of the human as a sensing device, as do other traditional medicines. Papa Auwae sensed energy with his hands. Inca shamans often sense energy disturbances in a patient's aura.

Tuning into the patient while reading pulses is an art particularly well-developed by traditional Chinese and Tibetan physicians. Recall Tibetan physician Yeshe Dhonden's diagnosis of the patient he observed at Grand Rounds at Yale Medical School.

Medical dowsing, including radionics, provides another example of the value of the healer as a sensing device. The Hippocratic healer was trained to sense his patients' needs via pulses and "tuning in," and he was tested on a related ability in his graduation examination.

13.8 Western Medical Assumption 6: The experimenter doesn't influence the experimental outcome.

This assumption is a logical consequence of Cartesian thought and the assumption that the body is a machine. *It is a fundamental assumption of Western scientists.* If research findings are not independently replicated, (i.e., by a laboratory other than the one doing the original research,) those results are not accepted as scientifically valid. That the experimenter doesn't affect the experiment's outcome is clearly disproved by the results of the rabbit experiment mentioned earlier.[516]

Unfortunately, the *assumption* that the experimenter doesn't influence the experiment's outcome severely limits the "scientific" conclusions that can be reached.

This assumption has as a corollary in medicine in the concept that the healer doesn't affect the patient's outcome, and certainly not the effectiveness of the medicine prescribed. This assumption is quite contrary to the experience of other medical traditions, particularly that of traditional medicines (which have long recognized the importance of the healer's impact on the patient), and it is an important reason for the limited effectiveness of Western scientific medicine today.[517]

The effect of the healer on the patient can readily be demonstrated by having several people successively assess the pulses of a patient. If, after several pulse takings, the first pulse taker again assesses the pulses, they will usually be found to have changed, presumably due to the effect of the energies of the intervening pulse measurers on the energy of the person whose pulse is being measured.

A dramatic example of the importance of the healer on the patient, and even of the preparer of medicine on the therapeutic effects of a medicine, is provided by the Hawaiian *lima awa* ("bitter hand") and the example of Papa Auwae's students' preparation of olena. Note that this effect was incomprehensible to a Western medical scientist, a medical school Professor of Pharmacognosy (pharmacological effects of herbs).

In short, Hawaiian and other holistic medicines recognize that the healer has a profound impact on the effectiveness of the treatment given the patient. This is a major contrast with Western medicine, where the Western physician will tell his patient the worst-case scenario (possibly in order to avoid lawsuits). His so doing instills in his patient the emotion of fear, which has a profoundly negative impact on the patient's immune system and so inhibits healing. In sharp contrast, Papa Auwae followed the policy of *always* giving *hope*, recognizing that the emotion of hope will activate self-healing in the patient.[518]

13.9 Western Medical Assumption 7: Each person is separate and can be considered to be an isolated entity.

This assumption is a logical consequence of Newtonian physics, which provides a mathematical approach to the behavior of separate objects and their interactions. It also matches the sense that each of us has that we are separate individuals. We live our lives as individuals, and we make much of our separateness, our individual choices, our individual opportunities, our individual responsibilities. Most unfortunately, when this sense of separation is applied to ethnic, religious, or national groups, conflicts and wars are the result.

However, modern science, from biological exchange to quantum physics, shows us that we are interconnected in ways we in the West have not previously recognized. Modern psychology became aware of this interconnectedness when Carl Jung spoke of the Collective Unconscious, or Teilhard de Chardin, of the Noosphere. Quantum physics now speaks of the Zero Point Field, or the Quantum Hologram, a field where information is stored holographically. Both theoretical (Bell's Theorem) and experimental results at the quantum (John Clauser and Alain Aspect) level verify that we are all profoundly interconnected, that not only our actions but our emotions affect each other. Indeed, we now know, from satellite measurements, that our emotions affect the earth's geomagnetic field, which in turn affects our weather, geologic stress (earthquakes), human behavior, and more.[519]

Traditional medicines have long been aware of these interconnections. Hawaiian medicine recognizes the *aka* threads that interconnect us all, and ancient Celtic shamans (Druids) referred in similar fashion to the *Web of Wyrd* (Being).[520] Indeed, recognition of the Web of Life is commonplace among shamans. It is precisely such interconnectedness that allows distant healing to take place, together with telepathic communication and other forms of non-physical information and energy transfer. The contemporary healer, Adam, has provided visual verification of this interconnectedness, observing how, in a group of people, changes in one person's aura (due to an emotional surge) affects the auras of the rest of the group.[521]

Notes

506 Pert, Candace, *Molecules of Emotion: The Science Behind Mind-Body Medicine,* New York: Simon & Schuster, 1997.
507 Polya, G. *How to Solve It: A New Aspect of Mathematical Method*, Garden City, NY, Doubleday Books, 1957.
508 Vithoulkas, George, *Homeopathy: Medicine of the New Man,*
509 Wallace, B. Alan, *Choosing Reality: A Buddhist View of Physics and the Mind,* Ithaca, NY, Snow Lion Publications, 2003.
510 Coulter, Harris *Divided Legacy: A History of the Schism in Medical Thought,* Vols. I, II & III, Wehawken Book Co., 1975.
511 Pert, Candace *Molecules of Emotion: The Science Behind Mind-Body Medicine*, New York, Simon & Schuster, 1997.
512 Dossey, Larry, *Healing Words: The Power of Prayer and the Practice of Medicine*, San Francisco, Harper SanFrancisco, 1993.
513 Nerem, R.M., et al., "Social environment as a factor in diet-induced atherosclerosis," *Science*, 208: 1475-1476, 1980.
514 Pert, Candace, *Molecules of Emotion: The Science Behind Mind-Body Medicine*, New York, Simon & Schuster, 1997.
515 Lipton, Bruce, *The Biology of Belief: Unleashing the Power of Consciousness, Matter & Miracles*, Santa Rosa, Mountain of Love/Elite Books, 2005.
516 Nerem, R.M., et al., "Social environment as a factor in diet-induced atherosclerosis," *Science,* 208: 1475-1476, 1980.
517 Carlson, Richard and Benjamin Shield, *Healers on Healing,* Los Angeles, Tarcher, 1989.
518 Papa Henry Auwae, personal instruction, 1990s.
519 Radin Ph.D., Dean, *Entangled Minds: Extrasensory Experiences in a Quantum Reality*, Pocket Books, 2006.
520 Bates, Brian, *The Way of Wyrd*, Hay House, 2013.
521 Adam, *DreamHealer: A True Story of Miracle Healings*, Plume, 2006.

Chapter 14
The Impact of Western Science on Medicine: Methods and Assumptions of Western Medical Science, Continued

14.1 The Present Situation of Western Scientific Medicine with Regard to its Assumptions

The assumptions of Western science, and in particular, Western medical science, that have been discussed in the previous chapter have profound implications in terms of the limitations they place upon the practice of allopathic medicine. It is *not* enough to ask, "Is it scientific?" for the question itself imposes severe limitations on what can be acceptable Western medical practice. The experiences of Hawaiian medicine described earlier have not only shown that Western medical assumptions may be incorrect, but that using those assumptions can have an important impact on the effectiveness of therapeutic procedures. Hawaiian medicine has been effective, as has Oriental medicine, in many patients whose problems have not been helped by Western scientific medicine. *It is precisely because of the assumptions of Western scientific medicine that it is often less effective than are other medical modalities that are not limited by current materialistic medical and scientific thinking.*

The assumptions cited in Chapter Thirteen are those on which Western medical science is based, and newer fields that go beyond these limitations, e.g., psychoneuroimmunology, and the healing power of prayer has not yet been generally accepted—Carl Simonton's proposed seminar was rejected due to the objection of a senior faculty member at the University of California at Davis Medical Center.[522]

However, the situation is improving: Conferences on Science and Spiritual Healing have been held, and there now exists a Center for Spirituality and Healing at the University of Minnesota School of Medicine, and the Center for Consciousness Studies is at the University of Arizona. Double blind studies of prayer's effectiveness in promoting healing have been conducted at Duke University and in San Francisco. Herbert Benson, David Eisenberg and Ted Kaptchuk are faculty members at the Harvard Medical School. Integrative Healing clinics, with East meeting West as well as integrating other medical modalities, are being established. There are, for example, now serious studies of the effects of prayer on healing, so the future does look better than the present.

14.2 Mechanisms

The *mechanism* explaining how emotions affect all our cells (ca. 30% of body mass) was described by Candace Pert, *et al*, in 1975 and subsequently.[523] That emotions affect body fluids (ca 70% of body mass) was described by Masaru Emoto in his research published in 1994.[524] The *mechanism* of such action has been described by Bruce Lipton in his *Biology of Belief*, 2005.[525]

The importance of the subconscious mind was recognized in the West in the nineteenth century. William James, the Harvard physiologist, psychologist, and philosopher, commented, "The greatest scientific discovery of the nineteenth century was the power of the subconscious mind touched by faith." James was citing a discovery in the West of an important phenomenon known in Hawaii, Greece, Tibet, and elsewhere many centuries earlier.

Healing involves all of body, mind, and soul, not just management of symptoms. Healing often involves good nutrition, healthy environment—both physical and emotional—as well as lifestyle, all contributing to the restoration of the harmony that is the key to self-healing and to good health.

For complete healing, the patient must address the often complex issue of the underlying ***cause*** of the illness—often an emotional, mental or spiritual issue. Unfortunately, although many traditional healers are fully aware of these issues, Western physicians rarely address the **cause** of the disease. Brian Weiss, M.D., is a psychiatrist who has found that the relaxation that comes when a patient is in a relaxed state under hypnosis often brings about healing (see Weiss, *Messages from The Masters* for details of his procedure).[526]

To focus on the mind, there are techniques such as visualization to stimulate action of the immune system (see Simonton, et al, *Getting Well Again*),[527] and meditation has been found to produce heart coherence and so to heal both the cardiovascular system and the immune system. Counseling as well as hypnosis or meditative techniques have proven valuable in resolving emotional problems that are often the underlying cause of the disease. All of these are useful approaches to healing both the cause and the symptoms of disease. Note that all of these methods address the subconscious mind. The scientific confirmation of the importance of these approaches has been provided by research in psychoneuroimmunology[528] and at the HeartMath Institute [529] research that has verified the impact of emotions, both positive and negative, on the immune system.

The multiple personality patient provides a remarkable example of the mind's ability to change pathologies in a seemingly miraculous fashion. When the personality changes, so do the physical symptoms. One personality may have high blood pressure; switch personality and the hypertension disappears and diabetes appears. One personality who was a child received an overdose when his adult personality was given a prescription drug. There are multiple personality patients who carry multiple pairs of glasses, for when the personality changes, so does the correction required by the patient.[530]

Healing the cause of an illness can be accomplished in many ways. Drs. Norm Shealy and Carolyn Myss had a patient who was dying of cancer and was healed by *forgiveness*. Jacqueline Aldana's husband was dying of cancer and was healed by *gratitude*. These two emotions, *forgiveness* and *gratitude*, are frequently the keys to healing the cause of an illness and so the illness itself.

Louise Hay has been a pioneer in identifying emotional *cause* of illness. Her book, *Heal Your Body*,[531] was followed by *You Can Heal Your Life,* [532] and, most recently, with Mona Lisa Schulz, M.D., Ph.D., by *All Is Well: Heal Your Body with Medicine, Affirmations, and Intuition.*[533]

Prayer has produced what we would term miracles, bringing Spirit into play. An example of prayer's effectiveness was given in Chapter One, and well designed scientific studies have confirmed prayer's effectiveness. Note that it is important to distinguish between spirituality and religion, although both can be supportive in healing illness. Prayers and spiritual healing are *not* limited to any particular religious belief.

Spectacular "miracles" have been produced by contemporary spiritual healers, as well as by many saints of history, Hawaiian *kahunas*, Tibetan lamas, Native American medicine men and women and sweat lodge ceremonies, energy balancing procedures, and many more. These "miracles" often occurred as a result of prayer and/or meditation. The Brazilian medium John of God and the 'miracles' performed through him are notable.[534] A friend of the author's was healed of pancreatic cancer at John of God's center in Abadiania and many seemingly miraculous healings have occurred there. There is a room full of crutches discarded by healed patients as the crutches were no longer needed.

A few years ago the author learned of a highly spiritual Tibetan lama who developed acute appendicitis while in a remote area in the Himalayas. He declined a helicopter ride to a hospital, and cured his appendicitis with meditation—not an approach generally recommended, for surgery might have been simpler—but it does illustrate what can be done.

The value of prayer in healing has been confirmed many times, and it is currently being studied at leading medical schools, research institutions and hospitals. Well-designed double-blind experiments have shown both that prayer works, and that it works independently of religious belief.

All of these methods are variations on the theme of activating *self-healing* via the subconscious mind.

14.3 The Problem of Statistics

Western science is well aware of the variability of both physical and biological phenomena, and its solution has been to develop quite sophisticated statistical methods to deal with random events. Unfortunately, the application of these statistical methods to medical research poses its own set of problems. This issue was recognized over a century ago by physiologist Claude Bernard, who wrote:

"Another very frequent application of mathematics to biology is the use of averages which, in medicine and physiology, leads, so to speak, necessarily, to error. There are doubtless several reasons for this: but the greatest obstacle to applying calculation to physiological phenomena is still, at bottom, the excessive complexity which prevents their being definite and comparable one with another. By destroying the biological character of phenomena, the use of *averages* in physiology and medicine usually gives only apparent accuracy to the results. . . Aside from physical and chemical, there are physiological averages, or what we might call average descriptions of phenomena, which are even more false. Let me assume that a physician collects a great many individual observations of a disease and that he makes an average description of symptoms observed in the individual cases; he will thus have a description that will never be matched in nature. So in physiology we must never make average descriptions of experiments, because the true relations of phenomena disappear in the average . . . averages must therefore be rejected, because they confuse, while aiming to unify, and distort, while aiming to simplify."[535]

Bernard's reasoning is absolutely accurate, and it addresses precisely the point made by Hahnemann and others, that we cannot generalize, that it is the *differences* between patients, often subtle physical and/or emotional symptoms, that dictate the difference in treatment required for one patient versus another, even though both may have some symptoms that might fit the same "disease's" average description. Symptoms commonly found in the "same disease" in different patients are *not* enough to establish a treatment plan, as has long been recognized by Oriental medicine. As Harvard professor Ted Kaptchuk describes in *The Web That Has No Weaver:*

"When the Chinese physician examines a patient, he or she plans to look at many, many signs and symptoms and to make of them a diagnosis, to see in them a pattern. *Each sign means nothing by itself* and acquires meaning only in its relationship to the patient's other signs. *What it means in one context is not necessarily what it means in another context.*" (author's emphasis)[536]

Follow Kaptchuk's admonition—avoid simplistic diagnostic methods!

This is not to say that statistical methods may not be useful, for they are often a necessary methodology in examining experimental data. Nevertheless, Bernard's admonition as well as Kaptchuk's must always be kept in mind, and awareness of individual differences must always be honored. Treat the patient, not the "disease"!

Averages are dangerous.

- The arrow on a clinical thermometer does *not* indicate a "normal" temperature! As time of day changes, so does body temperature.
- Not all menstrual cycles are 28 days in length.
- Is a 23-year-old female with an oral temperature of 103°F ill (feverish)? Not necessarily. She may have been running a marathon.
- Is a 30-year-old male with a blood pressure of 230/150 mm Hg ill (hypertensive)? Not necessarily. He may have just contracted his muscles isometrically.

14.4 Double Blind Experiments.

The double-blind experiment, in which neither the patient nor the administering physician, is consciously aware of whether the patient is receiving an "active" drug or a placebo, is Western scientific medicine's way of dealing with the influence of the experimenter on the experimental outcome, and in particular the emotional response of the patient to the perceived value of the drug. The data suggesting that up to 85% of the effect of drugs is due to a placebo effect is believed to be taken out of the picture by using a double-blind procedure.

Note that the concept that the double-blind experiment succeeds in eliminating the placebo effect makes *assumptions* about the transmission of information. *Someone* knows which drug is "active" and which is the placebo, and there is ample experimental data that suggest information transfer in subtle ways (not recognized by Western science), that may call into question the validity of this assumption. Note also that if one changes models of medical reality to include the body's energy fields, the assumptions of the double-blind experiment immediately collapse.

We now have solid information that the experimenter influences the experiment in ways that may have nothing to do with knowledge of the drug administered (e.g., the *lima awa* effect referred to in a previous chapter). In short, the double-blind experiment is a useful device that should without doubt be used much more often than is now the case (e.g., in testing drug interactions when newly developed drugs are marketed that will interact with other drugs being taken by the same patient). Nevertheless, the double-blind experiment has its own limitations, and it is *not* the "Gold Standard" it is often represented to be.

14.5 Western Scientific Medicine and Symptom Management

When one conducts laboratory, or clinical, experiments, one necessarily designs the experiment so that it will have a measurable experimental outcome. If the phenomenon being tested is a therapeutic procedure, drug administration or other, that experimental outcome must be a measure of the efficacy of the therapeutic procedure under study. Generally, the outcome measured is a change in the level of some symptom of the illness being treated (or physiological variable in a healthy subject), whether that symptom is a disease response or a change in one or more physiological variables.

Thus, our experimental science provides us with information about the changes in symptoms brought about by the therapeutic procedure studied. Say Drug X brings about a reduction in blood pressure, so Drug X is accepted for use in blood pressure reduction. Similar experiments have been used to assess the efficacy of the physician's entire armamentarium. *The result is a medical system that has available a wide variety of methods for managing symptoms.* This recognition provides us with the best description of modern allopathic medicine that the author has encountered. It was provided by a colleague, a Professor of Internal Medicine, who observed, "We keep the patient happy while nature cures her."

"We keep the patient happy while nature cures her" describes allopathic medicine at its best. Symptoms can kill, and "keeping the patient happy" implies managing the patient's symptoms and hopefully setting the stage so that the patient's own healing abilities can achieve the healing needed if the patient is to become healthy again. This logic proves inadequate in many chronic diseases, for managing symptoms in chronic illness is only a palliative treatment at best (often with undesirable side effects).

Symptom management may set the stage for recovery, but it does nothing to address the *cause* of an illness, especially important if that illness is chronic and symptom management disguises the *cause* of the problem. In a patient known to the author, her serum potassium was found to be low by a blood test, so her physician prescribed potassium chloride for her. This treatment was successful in restoring her blood chemistry to normal levels, but it did nothing to address the question of why her potassium level was low to begin with. Fortunately for this patient, she was also being treated by Oriental medicine, which did address the *cause* of the low potassium level. Thus, the patient was both relieved of the potassium deficiency, and the cause of that deficiency was resolved.

An important question regarding the issue of symptom management is that of the long-term effects of such procedures. There is first the issue of side effects of drugs used for symptom management, especially the long-term effects. A critical example of this is the development of antibiotic-resistant strains of bacteria and the lowered immune system strength of patients who have been given such drugs (e.g., the Atlanta study showing lowered resistance to disease in children from affluent neighborhoods—previously treated for minor ailments by antibiotics).

A further issue is the effect of bypassing the body's normal healing response. If a prescription or a surgical procedure does the body's job, the body's negative feedback system will result in reduced self-healing action.

Also of importance is the issue of the direct effects of symptom suppression. Per Hahnemman, Hering and others, the suppression of surface symptoms has the result of driving the disease process inside the body, of replacing a relatively benign condition with a more serious one. Hering's Law provides a useful guide here, and it alerts us to a potentially serious consequence of symptom alleviation without healing the cause of that symptom.

Further, if symptoms are the body's way of informing the patient that a problem exists, then one must be very careful not to miss the body's message by eliminating the symptom. We recall the patient with hemorrhoids described by John Upledger in "Self-Discovery and Self-Healing," in *Healers on Healing*, that was cited in Chapter One.[537]

Symptom management, then, can be a useful tool in acute illness, and Western scientific medicine has developed this tool with great sophistication. There will be situations where you will want to refer patients to your Western medical colleagues for precisely the symptom management at which they excel. Recognize, however, that when those symptoms have been controlled and the patient's initial condition apparently resolved, you will have to help the patient recover from the drugs or procedure that were used to manage the symptoms by the Western physician as well as to address the *cause* of the imbalance as well as the imbalance itself that led to those symptoms.

Precisely this situation not infrequently happens in the Tibetan refugee community in Dharamsala, India. Tibetan refugees in Dharamsala sometimes contract tuberculosis, a disease that traditional Tibetan medicine has no tools to treat, as tuberculosis does not exist in high altitude and cold Tibet. So, the patient is first treated with antibiotics at the Western hospital in Dharamsala. The antibiotics resolve the tuberculosis, after which the patient goes to a traditional Tibetan medical clinic to undo the damage (liver, etc.) caused by the antibiotic. The healer may very likely encounter comparable situations in his or her own medical practice.

Symptom management has been promoted by television advertisement of prescription medicines. This has had two effects, both unfortunate. First, the ads reinforce the concept that there is a way of managing symptom X. This is particularly unfortunate if that symptom is the result of a chronic illness, for then the patient will not look at the issue of what caused the symptom to start with.

The second effect, also unfortunate, is to elicit fear of the "disease" that resulted in the symptoms supposedly "cured" by the pharmaceutical being advertised. As was discussed by the shaman cited in Chapter Three, it is important *not* to give energy to what we *don't want.* Fear is an emotion that will give energy to the "disease" responsible for the symptoms that we wish to avoid.

Therefore:

Use Western medicine when that is in the patient's best interest, but be prepared to follow up on that treatment with your own restoration of the patient to internal harmony; in so doing, you assist the patient's self-healing ability to accomplish the healing.

14.6 Results of Western Scientific Medicine's Limitations

Allopathic medicine is not meeting the healthcare needs of the U.S. today, as shown in medical statistics. The first two leading causes of hospital deaths in the U.S. are chronic degenerative diseases (heart disease and cancer), and these are not well served by allopathic medicine.

The third leading cause of death is the healthcare system itself, per hospital statistics published in *Journal of the American Medical Association* in 2000 (from Johns Hopkins School of Hygiene & Public Health; see Appendix). The consequence is that although it is an international leader in medical costs, the U.S. ranks very poorly in health indicators (see Appendix).

14.7 A New Perspective

As reported in Chapter Five, German biophysicist Marco Bischof has given us an important observation of the relevance of quantum physics for today's understanding of reality with his observation, "Quantum mechanics has established the primacy of the inseparable whole. For this reason, the basis of the new biophysics must be the insight into the fundamental interconnectedness *within* the organism as well as *between* organisms, and that of the organism *with the environment.* (emphasis Bischof's).

It is the author's contention that the United States would be well served if we retained the progress of Western scientific medicine as well as returned to the perspective of the traditional medicines of the past, of Pythagoras, Socrates, Plato, and Hippocrates, who treated patients in their entirety, body, mind, and spirit. We can learn from the shamans and the mystery school healers of the past and the present. We can move into the twenty-first century with modern physics informing medical research, no longer Cartesian and Newtonian, but recognizing the implications of quantum physics and chaos theory. **We are One**, and **Gratitude**, **Compassion**, **Forgiveness**, and **Love** are keys to restoring health.[538, 539, 540]

Appendix to Chapter 14: *JAMA* paper on iatrogenic deaths

- Author: Dr. Barbara Starfield, Johns Hopkins School of Hygiene and Public Health
- Reference: *Journal of the American Medical Association, 284 (4)*, July 26, 2000: 483-485.
- 250,000 medically-caused hospital deaths per year:
    - 12,000 deaths due to unnecessary surgeries.
    - 7,000 deaths due to medication errors in hospitals.
    - 20,000 deaths due to other errors in hospitals.
    - 80,000 deaths due to infections in hospitals.
    - 106,000 deaths due to *drug side effects* (no error in prescription). [Note that this category constitutes 42% of medically-caused deaths]
- U.S. is 12th of 13 countries in 16 health indicators; Japan, Sweden, and Canada are first.

Notes

522 Simonton, O. Carl et al., *Getting Well Again*, Los Angeles, Tarcher, 1978.
523 Pert, Candace, *Molecules of Emotion: The Science Behind Mind-Body Medicine*, New York, Simon & Schuster, 1997.
524 Emoto, Masaru, *The True Power of Water*, Beyond Word Publishing, 2005.
525 Lipton, Bruce, *The Biology of Belief: Unleashing the Power of Consciousness, Matter & Miracles*, Santa Rosa, CA, 2005.
526 Weiss, M.D., Brian *Messages from The Masters: Tapping into the Power of Love*, New York, Warner Books, 2000.
527 Simonton, O. Carl, et al., *Getting Well Again*, Los Angeles, Tarcher, 1978.
528 Pert, Candace, *Molecules of Emotion: The Science Behind Mind-Body Medicine*, New York, Simon & Schuster, 1997.
529 Childre, Doc & Howard Martin, *The HeartMath Solution*, HarperCollins, 1999.
530 Talbot, Michael, *The Holographic Universe*, HarperCollins, 1991.
531 Hay, Louise L., Heal *Your Body*, Hay House, Inc., 1984.
532 Hay, Louise L., *You Can Heal Your Life*, Hay House, Inc., 1984.
533 Hay, Louise L. and Mona Lisa Schulz, MD, *All Is Well: Heal Your Body with Medicine, Affirmations and Intuition*, Hay House, 2014.
534 Wing, Josie Raven, *The Book of Miracles: The Healing Work of Joao de Deus*, 1st Books, 2002.
535 Coulter, Harris *Divided Legacy: A History of the Schism in Medical Thought*, Vols. I, II & III, Weehawken Book Co., 1975.
536 Kaptchuk, Ted, *The Web That Has No Weaver*, Congdon & Weed, New York, 1983.
537 Carlson, Richard and Benjamin Shield, *Healers on Healing*, Los Angeles, Tarcher, 1989.
538 Dossey, Larry, *Healing Words: The Power of Prayer and the Practice of Medicine*, HarperOne, 1995.
539 Adam, *Dream Healer: A True Story of Miracle Healings*, Plume, 2006.
540 Nerem, R.M., et al, "Social environment as a factor in diet-induced atherosclerosis", *Science*, 208: 1475-1476, 1980.

Chapter 15
Modern Physics and Medicine
The Modern Conflict in Western Science—The Paradigm Is Shifting

15.1 Introduction

A major paradigm shift is underway in Western science, a shift with profound implications for modern Western scientific medicine. Inasmuch as most of the assumptions of Western scientific medicine are based on the old paradigm, medicine is lagging behind most of Western science in making this transition. As Thomas Kuhn has noted in *The Structure of Scientific Revolutions*,[541] scientific ideas change only reluctantly, and too often it is the dying out of an older generation that permits new ideas truly to take hold.

Nevertheless, change does occur. The geologists of 80 years ago considered the concept of continental drift to be sheer fantasy, and the originator of that idea, Alfred Wegener, died an outcast from his scientific colleagues. Today no self-respecting geologist would dream of disputing the evidence of plate tectonics that has been repeatedly demonstrated. Similar changes have taken place in the realms of science most relevant to our understanding of human health and disease. Recall Semmelweis and puerperal fever, to say nothing of Pasteur and Béchamps.

15.2 Changes in the Physics Paradigm

Many of the most important changes in Western science have been in the domain of modern physics, in the shift from Newtonian to relativistic and quantum physics at the beginning of the 20th century (relativistic physics addressing issues of space and time, quantum physics addressing issues of matter and energy). At the end of the 19th century, physicists thought they pretty well understood the fundamental physical processes, with only one sticky problem: the nature of radiation from a black body, yet to be elaborated. Within 20 years, thanks to Planck's discovery of the quantum in 1900, followed by Einstein's theories of special and general relativity and the work in quantum physics of Bohr, Heisenberg, Dirac, Born, Schrödinger, and others, all physicists recognized that there was a new world of problems yet to be understood. The third major shift in physical thinking, Chaos Theory, came in the 1970s and will be discussed later.

Particle and quantum physics became the forerunner of a new view of the universe. None of our modern electronics, from cell phones to laptop computers, would exist today without using the equations of quantum mechanics in their design. Yet the end has certainly not been reached. The concepts of a holographic universe, mentioned below, together with the recognition that consciousness is even more fundamental than matter and energy, are having a profound impact, and one can confidently predict that there are new and yet unthought of perspectives that still lie ahead.

15.3 The Influence of the Observer and of the Question Asked

A key issue that has come to be appreciated in modern physics is that of the influence of the observer and the importance of the question asked. It is now recognized that the act of observation can influence the observed object. *In fact, it is the act of observation that brings "reality" into existence!* This led Princeton University professor of physics John Archibald Wheeler to observe, "We live in a participatory universe." The implications of quantum physics have been illustrated by the example of Schrödinger's Cat:

Imagine a box that contains a radioactive source, a detector that records the presence of radioactive particles (Geiger counter), a glass bottle containing cyanide, and a cat. The apparatus in the box is arranged so that the detector is switched on for just long enough so that there is a 50:50 chance that one of the atoms in the radioactive material will decay and that the detector will record a particle. If the detector does record such an event, then the glass container is crushed and the cat dies; if not, the cat lives. We have no way of knowing the outcome of this experiment until we open the box to look inside; radioactive decay occurs entirely by chance and is unpredictable. Per the standard interpretation of quantum mechanics (Niels Bohr's Copenhagen Interpretation), the equal probabilities of radioactive decay and no decay produce a "superposition of states," i.e., that until we look inside the box, there is a radioactive sample that has both decayed and not decayed, a glass vessel of poison that is neither broken nor unbroken, and a cat that is both dead and alive, neither alive nor dead. *Until the cat is observed both possibilities are true. It is the act of observation that changes reality from superposition to either a live or a dead cat.* Stated differently, both possibilities are not only equally real but equally unreal until we look inside the box. This sounds weird, but it is what the equations of quantum physics predict.

In the 1950s, another possibility was developed: American physicist Hugh Everett suggested that both cats are real. There is a live cat *and* a dead cat, but they are located in different worlds. It is not that the radioactive atom inside the box either did or didn't decay, but that it did both. Faced with a decision, the whole world—the universe—split into two versions of itself, identical in all respects except that in one version the atom decayed and the cat died, while in the other the atom did not decay and the cat lived. This is the "Many Worlds Hypothesis," which was derived quite rigorously from the same quantum mechanics equations that led to the Copenhagen Interpretation. The Many Worlds interpretation sounds strange, but it is coming to be accepted by more and more quantum physicists.
—Adapted from John Gribbin, *In Search of Schrödinger's Cat.* [542]

It can be noted that the Many Worlds Hypothesis provides a way of linking relativity theory—dealing with issues of time and space—with quantum physics, which deals with matter and energy. The point of intersection of parallel universes, which occurs at black holes, provides the link between relativistic and quantum physics long sought by physicists. Note: The existence of parallel universes was actually derived from the theory of general relativity before parallel universes were shown by Everett to be a mathematically correct interpretation of quantum physics addressing the issue of the observer effect.

It may further be noted that the only way the universe can have been created and obey the laws of quantum physics is for an infinite number of parallel universes to have been created at the beginning of creation. The Copenhagen Interpretation requires an observer for matter to have been defined, and only with an infinite number of parallel universes can the observer problem be avoided.[543]

It should also be noted that the Copenhagen Interpretation and the Many Worlds Hypothesis are not the only possible interpretations of Schrödinger's Equation. David Bohm has resolved the observer paradox by introducing a non-linearity into Schrödinger's Equation, the fundamental equation of quantum physics. Bohm did this by splitting the equation into two parts, one describing a quantum particle in the classical manner, the second describing a "quantum potential" in which the particle moves, a kind of infinite sensitivity possessed by the quantum particle to its surroundings. Bohm developed this interpretation as a part of his theory of the implicate order.[544]

An important result of quantum physics is the Heisenberg Uncertainty Principle, the principle that one cannot simultaneously know both the momentum and the position of a particle. This has the consequence that, as Heisenberg put it, "We *cannot* know, as a matter of principle, the present in all its details." The implications of this principle are many, one of the intriguing ones being the suggestion by Bentov that, since in an oscillating particle one knows precisely the momentum (0) at the instant that the oscillation changes direction, then one cannot know *at all* the position of the particle at that same instant. It has been suggested that there might be a connection between Bentov's observation and unexplained phenomena of apparently instantaneous information transfer at a distance. Whether or not Bentov's interpretation is correct, the Uncertainty Principle does have many profound implications. Combined with Bohm's concepts of a holographic universe (below), Bentov's and others' perspectives are enabling our understanding of the possibilities of information transfer, distant healing, and other yet inexplicable phenomena to grow rapidly.[545]

Even more fundamental is Einstein's observation that, "The answer you get is determined by the question you ask." This observation has applications in many fields, certainly including medicine. However, it is most directly exemplified by the well-demonstrated fact that one can prove experimentally that light is a wave, and exhibits all the properties of a wave, if one designs the experiment to identify the wave characteristics of light. However, if instead, one designs the experiment to demonstrate qualities of light as a particle, the photon, then one can with equal validity describe the particle's characteristics. The wave-particle duality of light has been repeatedly validated, and it is but one of many examples of the relationship between answers and questions.

It should immediately be added that the wave-particle duality applies not only to light but to all particles—electrons (it is the wave properties of electrons that make possible the electron microscope; it is the particle properties of electrons that produces an image on a television screen), protons, neutrons, all the particles that make up our bodies and our apparent realities. We tend to think of matter as made up of particles, but a more profound understanding of reality may emerge when we think in terms of waves. Pribram's studies of memory and the brain provide an example of the value of analyzing nature in terms of wave phenomena (see Section 15.14).

Examples of the importance of asking the most relevant question arises frequently in medicine. If the question asked is how to eliminate a troublesome symptom, then the answer obtained will likely be quite different from the answer appropriate to a question about how most effectively to treat the cause of the disorder that led to the symptom.

Oncologists may effectively eliminate a tumor with little effect on the life expectancy of the patient if the key question is not how to kill the tumor but rather how to bolster the immune system, whose inadequate function allowed the tumor to develop in the first place. For example, if the key issue is an unhappy family relationship, removing the tumor without resolving the unhappy relationship only sets the stage for the recurrence of the cancer with another tumor, perhaps in a different organ.

15.4 Implications of Quantum Field Physics

Quantum physics has led to totally new concepts of the nature of matter. Linear relationships are replaced with probabilistic equations. Without going into details, we must recognize that the issue is often one of scale. Newtonian equations work as an approximation of the behavior of matter on a large scale, but once we increase the magnification of our microscope sufficiently, the Newtonian relationships no longer adequately describe the behavior of the particles that make up the matter that was being observed on a macroscopic scale.

A table appears smooth and solid to us, but under a microscope we recognize that the table is really a collection of wood fibers, each individual fiber having a particular shape and texture. If we use a particularly high-powered microscope to examine the wood sample, we observe many details of those fibers. Increase the magnification further and we observe organic molecules that make up the fiber. Increase it further and the structure of the atoms becomes apparent. Study the atoms in an accelerator and the subatomic structure can be described. However, at this point in the investigation, it is apparent that there is far more space between particles than is taken up by the particles themselves (if the nucleus of an atom is visualized as a grain of sand, the orbits of electrons would take up a large concert hall). Finally, the ultimate picture is not one of particles at all, but of energy fields. These quantum fields are perhaps the basis of matter, but the energy of those fields is not matter at all. A friend of the author's who was working in a research laboratory, was invited to observe his hand under a high magnification electron microscope. When he did so, the apparent physical structure of the hand disappeared. Where the hand had been were only energy fields.

Even more fundamental than energy or matter, we are now recognizing, is consciousness. This recognition is implicit in the statement by physicist John Wheeler cited above, and is the subject of *The Self-Aware Universe: How Consciousness Creates the Material World*,[546] by University of Oregon professor of physics Amit Goswami. Wheeler's and Goswami's view has been supported by prominent physicist John Hagelin, of the international high energy physics laboratory CERN in Switzerland and SLAC at Stanford, developer of a Grand Unified Field Theory based on Superstring Theory, and a frequently cited researcher in a variety of leading areas of quantum physics. Hagelin noted that "at the foundation of the universe there is a field of pure, abstract universal existence—Universal consciousness—The unified field."

It is appropriate to quote here from Bentov's *Stalking the Wild Pendulum*:

"We human beings consider ourselves to be made up of 'solid matter.' Actually, the physical body is the end product, so to speak, of the subtle information fields, which mold our physical body as well as all physical matter. These fields are holograms which change in time [and are] outside the reach of our normal senses. This is what clairvoyants perceive as colorful egg-shaped halos or auras surrounding our physical bodies." [547]

It is at this level that we can begin to formulate hypotheses on how thought can influence matter, how, e.g., *love* might influence the fields that change the structures of the molecules. Leonard Laskow has conducted experiments in which he changed the configuration of DNA by bathing a Petri dish containing a cell culture with unconditional love.[548] Thus, the functioning of organs and individuals can be benefitted by sending those organs or individuals love. Conversely, *hate* can bring about a cancer or a heart attack. Research conducted at the Institute of Noetic Science and the Institute of HeartMath have quantified the impact of emotions on the immune system: love, compassion, and appreciation support the immune system; anger or hate depress it. We may note that in Tibetan Medicine hate/anger is one of the three fundamental causes of disease; the other causes described by Tibetan Medicine are greed/acquisitiveness and ignorance/misunderstanding. Each of these causes is related to an imbalance in one of the three primary bodily elements. All are invisible and so are not considered by materialist medical science.

15.5 Bell's Theorem and Non-Locality

In 1964, Irish physicist John Bell, investigating an apparent contradiction between conflicting theories of quantum reality, discovered an assumption made by world-class mathematician John von Neuman. Bell then developed what has become known as Bell's Theorem. Bell's Theorem states that underlying our apparent local interactions (locality is our common experience that causes and effects are directly related and due to physical connections with each other, and that the speed of light is the fastest that anything can happen) is a world behind phenomena that must be non-local. Thus, reality *must* be non-local; we are *instantaneously* interconnected. Bell's Theorem may well explain Rupert Sheldrake's morphogenetic fields, the hundredth monkey syndrome, simultaneous scientific discoveries (e.g., differential calculus, developed simultaneously by Isaac Newton in England and Gottfried Liebniz in Germany), as well as distant communication and healing. Bell's Theorem has been proven experimentally in several different laboratories (most notably in 1982 by Alain Aspect in Paris), and the result is the establishment and confirmation of the fact that *everything is interconnected*, as indigenous cultures have long known, and that the interconnection occurs at a speed faster than the speed of light. Reality really *is* non-local. Many physicists are uncomfortable with this result, but it is consistent with the insights of shamans and mystics that everything is connected to everything else: the Web of Life. We are in fact *one*!

15.6 Chaos Theory: A Major Advance

Chaos Theory is one of the three most significant advances in physics during the 20th century, with a fourth looming on the horizon as the century closed. The first was Quantum Mechanics, which dates from the discoveries of Max Planck in the year 1900. Shortly after (1905) came Albert Einstein's development of the theory of Special Relativity, followed later by General Relativity, together the second major advance of the 20th century. Both Quantum Mechanics and Relativity continued to develop and to receive experimental verification throughout the century. Chaos Theory came later, in the 1960s and '70s, and without the development of modern computers Chaos Theory would not have developed as it did.[549] The fourth major development, the study of the physics of consciousness, is still in its early stages.

15.7 Newtonian Dogma

The Newtonian dogma has been: Given an approximate knowledge of a system's starting point (initial conditions—position and velocity) and an understanding of the laws of motion, one can calculate the approximate behavior of the system. This *assumption* had become the underlying philosophy of science. It was now being overturned by the probabilistic nature of quantum mechanics.

The struggle between Newtonian Order and Quantum Mechanical Uncertainty continued throughout the 20th century. Quantum Mechanics rocked the boat by describing a probabilistic universe, and many, including Einstein (who made important contributions to Quantum Theory), felt Quantum theory to be incomplete, for Einstein couldn't believe that "God would play dice."

This concern placed Einstein in the same camp as Newton, LaPlace, and the Roman Catholic Church (and Fundamentalists of all religions). Their demand for order in the universe (after all, Bruno had been burned at the stake for asserting otherwise) had been a continuing theme in science as well as in religion. Scientists had accepted that linear differential equations provided an adequate (if approximate) description of nature, and mathematicians focused on analyzing those equations. Scientists did recognize that nonlinear equations existed, but most of those equations were unsolvable analytically, and they were generally ignored.

Science has had an orderly and a materialistic perspective since the days when the Inquisition burned Bruno at the stake for holding a belief contrary to Church dogma, and we find such scientific dogma as uniformitarianism in geology (no catastrophes allowed). More recently, Francis Crick speculated that DNA is fixed at birth (this speculation becoming scientific dogma, although it has been contradicted by the recent developments in epigenetics). Dr. Rhine had experimental results with Extra Sensory Perception. These ESP results were dismissed by one of the country's leading physicists as "impossible; therefore Dr. Rhine's results *have* to be fraudulent."

The degree to which most scientists adhered to a belief in an orderly cosmos was exhibited in an extraordinary manner when Immanuel Velikovsky suggested (1950) that there was historical evidence that extraterrestrial objects had caused ancient catastrophes on earth. Velikovsky was roundly condemned by the scientific community in a manner reminiscent of the Church's condemnation of Bruno, the attack on Velikovsky being science's equivalent of burning him at the stake (that many of Velikovsky's predictions have been verified in the years since the publication of *Worlds in Collision* has given some scientists pause—though not all).[550]

Velikovsky was not the last. In 1981 Rupert Sheldrake published *A New Science of Life: The Hypothesis of Formative Causation*, eliciting such a furor among his scientific colleagues that Britain's premier science journal, *Nature,* suggested editorially that the book should be burned.[551]

The French mathematician Poincaré had been the first to demonstrate that Newton's assurance that the solar system was orderly was not verifiable. Newton's laws do demonstrate orderly relationships between the sun and earth or the moon and earth (so-called two-body problems), but those laws had been incapable of solving the problem of the interaction of all three at the same time (the three-body problem). In short, Newton's conclusion about the orderliness of the solar system was based on faith, not facts—on a theological assumption, not mathematics. The 19th century mathematician Pierre LaPlace had supported Newton's view of an orderly solar system, but no proof was ever provided.

In 1887, Sweden's King Oscar offered Kr 2500 for a mathematical proof that the solar system is stable. Poincaré won the prize in 1889; however, what he had discovered was <u>not</u> stability, but mathematical chaos, and in developing his proof he had developed several new areas of mathematics. Poincaré discovered the predecessor of modern Chaos Theory.[552]

Note: As we will see, there is more and more evidence coming to light that the universe really is chaotic, not orderly. Bruno was right; Aristotle, the Roman Church, and the dogma of an orderly universe were demonstrably wrong.

15.8 Nonlinearities in Nature

Turning now to the issue of the nonlinearities found in nature, it turns out that the equations used by Newton and others to model nature's behavior, linear differential equations, in fact model far less than 1% of that behavior. As Enrico Fermi exclaimed, "It does not say in the Bible that all laws of nature are expressible linearly!" or, as one mathematician put it, to call the study of chaos "nonlinear science" was like calling zoology "the study of nonelephant animals."[553] Unfortunately, most nonlinear differential equations are not solvable analytically. A common approach to solving these equations is to guess at the answer, insert the assumed answer into the equation, determine how great an error you have made, then try another guess. Keep up this process for however long it takes, and hope for the best. Computers help out, but even with computers there can be serious problems—too often the results are not deterministic at all, but are chaotic.

Solving a nonlinear equation has been described as like walking through a maze whose walls rearrange themselves with each step you take. The highly respected mathematician, John

Von Neuman, commented regarding a nonlinear equation describing fluid motion (the Navier-Stokes equation), "The character of the equation ...changes simultaneously in all relevant respects: Both order and degree change. Hence, *bad* mathematical difficulties must be expected." [554]

Nature has not been kind to mathematicians. Nonlinear systems are in general far more efficient than are linear systems, and nature has designed most of the world around us as nonlinear systems. This has been fortunate for us even if not so good for mathematicians.

As example: Driving a car on a winding road. One succeeds in keeping one's car where it belongs thanks to a very efficient (negative—to minimize error) feedback system. We observe the road's bends as we approach them, and we adjust the steering wheel as required to steer the car where we want it to go. If we don't turn the steering wheel the correct amount, we see our error and adjust the steering wheel accordingly. Then, when the next bend arrives, we repeat the process.

This process requires fast action; it involves our eyes and brain as well as our hands. Were the nervous system to respond too slowly, we'd be in trouble. In fact, our central nervous system is quite capable of meeting this demand, for it is highly nonlinear and extremely fast and efficient. It accomplishes this speedy response because our nerves, which conduct electrical impulses, are able to conduct those impulses much more rapidly than if the nerves were designed as wires. Instead of merely traveling along the nerves, the impulses carrying the desired signals *leapfrog* along the nerves via the Nodes of Ranvier, speeding up nerve transmission and so meeting the requirement for a rapid response.

Non-linear designs are found not only in humans but throughout nature. The area that provided a breakthrough involved studies of heat flow and how convection affects weather (heat rising, similar to mixing cream into a cup of hot coffee; the same thing happens with air).

15.9 Edward Lorenz

The case that led to the development of modern Chaos Theory came about due to a fortuitous coffee break. Edward Lorenz was a mathematician, but in WWII he served in the Army Air Corps as a weather forecaster and, following the war, he continued to work in meteorology.[555] On one occasion, Lorenz was attempting to model weather with nonlinear equations using a primitive (and very slow) computer. His computer was printing its answers numerically, and he would then plot those answers. One day he decided to allow his model to run for an extended period of time. After several hours, he noted how far the model had gone, then wrote down the number it had reached in the middle of the run. Rather than repeat the entire run, he typed in the mid-run number, restarted the computer, then went for a coffee break.[556]

When Lorenz returned from his coffee break he expected the model to repeat the second half of his previous run before continuing on, for he had typed in exactly what had previously been printed. To his surprise, his equations now gave answers that slowly diverged from the previous run. What had happened? Lorenz had used purely deterministic equations, and the weather model should have unfolded exactly the same each time it was computed. At first he thought the computer had malfunctioned—perhaps a tube had burned out. Then it hit him. His computer carried six decimal places internally but printed out only three—and it was the printed number that he had typed in when he restarted the run. The result, even though the difference between the two numbers had been only one part in 10,000 (0.506127 vs. 0.506, which he had *assumed* would make no difference—because most weather instruments record at best one part in 1,000), and that miniscule difference had led eventually to wildly different answers and a new understanding of what came to be known as "Sensitive Dependence on Initial Conditions," also known as the Butterfly Effect (the concept that a butterfly's wings could affect a far distant weather system), for this seemingly insignificant input would be the equivalent of a small puff of wind in the midst of a large weather system.

As this phenomenon was studied, it became apparent that, especially in large systems such as weather, sensitive dependence on initial conditions was an inescapable consequence of the way small scales intertwine with large. As one author described it, "Lorenz and other scientists suddenly became aware that in deterministic (causal) dynamical systems, the potential for generating chaos (unpredictability) crouches in every detail."[557]

Lorenz had found unpredictability, but as he delved further he also found pattern—if his system were perturbed, wiggled, interfered with, then when everything settled down, the system would return to the same peculiar patterns of irregularity as before. Others who followed also found structure within seemingly random behavior. This discovery of patterns within chaos, and of chaotic behavior from apparently orderly systems, was to prove revolutionary. What had been discovered was *deterministic disorder*. It appeared that a system's simple orders and its chaos are both features of one indivisible process.[558]

It was discovered, for example, that Jupiter's Red Spot—which remains stable even though the Jovian atmosphere is in constant motion, and has puzzled scientists for centuries—could be modeled by studying the planet's chaotic fluid flow. As one writer described it, "The spot is a self-organizing system, created and regulated by the same nonlinear twists that create the unpredictable turmoil around it. It is stable chaos."

One of the ways of examining equations that has proven useful is to plot the solutions in a phase space, composed of as many dimensions or variables as the scientist needs to describe a system's movement, and to plot the interactions of different variables against each other as time progresses. As the system changes, the motion of the point represents the continuously changing variables. When Lorenz made such a plot, he obtained a now famous diagram, that of a strange attractor that became known as the Lorenz Attractor. This owl's mask, or butterfly's wings, reveals a pattern that never exactly repeats itself, looping around and around forever. It is a strange attractor.

What are attractors? Think of an attractor as a region of phase space (e.g., plotting x versus dx/dt) that exerts a "magnetic" appeal for a system, seemingly pulling the system toward it. Attractors describe what the system does after a long period of time, and they come in three varieties: (1) a singular solution (e.g., the resting location of a pendulum damped by air resistance and not rewound), (2) a limit cycle (the final cyclic behavior of a periodic system, as in a clock whose pendulum is energized to overcome the air resistance), or (3) a strange attractor, such as the Lorenz attractor (found in chaotic systems). The last can really be understood only by graphic solutions, preferably plotted by a computer. Their phase space portraits demonstrate their behavior.

Lorenz's findings sparked a revolution, a paradigm shift. No longer would deterministic equations, even nonlinear ones, be sacrosanct, and this disturbed many. One physics professor, recognizing the impact of this shift, started quoting Tolstoy, "I know that most men, including those at ease with problems of greatest complexity, can seldom accept even the simplest and most obvious truth if it be such as would oblige them to admit the falsity of conclusions which they have delighted in explaining to colleagues, which they have proudly taught to others, and which they have woven, thread by thread, into the fabric of their lives." Such are the difficulties of new ideas, whether in science or in religion.

New insight into the interaction between orderliness and chaos came from a study of fish populations. Population growth can be modeled (with appropriate assumptions) by the simple equation $x_{next} = rx(1-x)$ where r is the population's rate of growth. However, r is highly nonlinear, and as it increases, its impact on the population's size is dramatic, exhibiting stable, periodic (with period-doubling appearing as r increases), or chaotic behavior, depending on the magnitude of r. The message became clear: Chaos is ubiquitous; it is stable; and it is structured. *Chaos and order exist intertwined in nature.*

The interrelationship between order and chaos has been found in biological processes as divergent as New York measles epidemics and Canadian lynx populations. Physiologists have begun looking at organs not as static but as complexes of oscillations, some regular and some irregular.

15.10 Benoit Mandlebrot

We are fortunate that Benoit Mandlebrot's father was far-sighted. A Lithuanian Jew living in Warsaw, he was wise enough to recognize the danger posed by Hitler in the 1930s, so he moved his family to Paris, where his brother was a mathematician. After Hitler invaded France, he moved his family to rural France, where Benoit spent his adolescent years. After the war, Mandlebrot studied at the École Polytechnique in Paris. (He had been admitted to the elite École Normale but left due to Bourbaki—a group of mathematicians at the École Normale devoted to mathematical rigor and distrustful of geometric solutions.) He later came to the US, where he found a home at IBM's Thomas Watson Research Center. He was a mathematician, but his insights into, and his understanding of, the behavior of equations was geometrical rather than analytical. He took advantage of the Center's computers to enable him to study the behavior of equations and of nature.

Mandlebrot studied a wide variety of disciplines, from linguistics to game theory to economics (and more). One of his studies was on the distribution of large and small incomes in an economy. A Harvard economics professor invited him to give a talk. When he arrived at the professor's office, he was startled to see his results already charted on the professor's blackboard. When he asked, "How could my findings have arrived ahead of my lecture?" the professor didn't know what he was talking about. The diagram on the blackboard had nothing to do with income distribution; it represented eight years of cotton prices. The cotton prices behaved in an odd way, however—they didn't follow the expected normal distribution, but contained too many large jumps.

To Mandelbrot, however, the cotton price picture looked familiar, so he obtained cotton price data back to the year 1900 and began a careful study of its behavior. He quickly found that, contrary to economists' belief that small, transient changes had nothing to do with large, long-term changes, (the latter believed to be caused by major forces such as wars or depressions), the data he was studying showed something quite different. He found that the key was not whether price changes were large or small, but that there was a symmetry of price change patterns whether the changes were on large scales or small. The sequence of changes was independent of scale: curves for daily price changes and monthly price changes were the same. Analyzed this way, the degree of variation in cotton prices had remained constant over a 60-year period that included two World Wars and the Great Depression. Within disorderly data he had found an unexpected order, and he had discovered that nature is often self-similar across scale; i.e., the patterns repeat at different scales.[559]

An illustration of this self-similarity was his (hypothetically) measuring the shoreline of England, from which he deduced that the length of the shoreline is infinite at the same time as the pattern is self-similar (a naturally occurring fractal, described below). He described the process of measurement with successively shorter measuring sticks, and he found self-similarity across scale—the degree of roughness is the same no matter what the scale. Each bay has its own smaller bays and headlands; and so on (this similarity extends even to indentations in a single rock). Mandelbrot liked to quote Jonathan Swift:

"So, Nat'ralists observe, a Flea
Hath smaller Fleas that on him prey,
And these have smaller Fleas to bite 'em,
And so proceed *ad infinitum.*" [560]

15.11 Fractal Geometry

Mandlebrot's use of computers and computer graphics to study the behavior of nonlinear equations led to the recognition of a new field of geometry—the geometric structure of irregular phenomena—which he named Fractal Geometry. These irregular systems exhibited self-similarity across scale, to a degree totally unexpected. *They can be described by their fractal dimension, a numeric indication of their degree of roughness, or irregularity.* There are mathematical ways of calculating the fractal dimension (the higher the fractal dimension, the greater the degree of irregularity). For example, an object has a degree of irregularity that is independent of its length, whether that length is finite (if a Euclidian shape) or infinite (as a coastline). *In general, fractals are characterized by infinite detail, infinite length, fractional dimension, self-similarity, and they can be generated by iteration.*

It turns out that the fractional dimension—the degree of irregularity—corresponds to the efficiency of an object in taking up space. And remember, fractal means not only irregular, but self-similar, symmetry across scale.[561]

Fractal dimension, a measure of the relative degree of complexity of an object, has proven highly useful in studying problems connected to the properties of surfaces in contact with each other, properties that may be quite independent of the materials involved but depend greatly on the bumpiness of the surfaces (e.g., contact between tire treads and concrete, or machine joints, or electrical contacts). For example, the fractal dimension of a metal surface often provides information corresponding to the metal's strength. The fractal dimension of the earth's surface can provide information valuable in understanding the earth's properties, including earthquakes.

In the human body, the circulatory system takes great advantage of its irregular, fractal structure, a structure that enables it to squeeze a huge surface area into a small volume. This structure is so efficient that no cell in the body is ever more than three or four cells away from a blood vessel, despite the fact that vessels and blood take up no more than about 5% of the body's volume.

The same complexity enables the digestive tract to have large area for food absorption and digestion, and the lungs to have a huge surface area (about the size of a tennis court) in a small volume. Similar fractal organization is found throughout the human body: in kidneys and liver, in cardiac innervations, and also in the frequency of heartbeat timing. The fractal dimension of the human brain is around 2.76, providing again the ability to have a large surface area in a relatively small volume. The same thing occurs in trees, where fractal branches and fractal leaves enable the tree to capture sun and resist wind. Clouds are fractal. Satellite images have shown clouds to have a constant fractal dimension over seven orders of magnitude. Astronomers are discovering that distant galaxies are clumped together in fractal distributions. Fractal design is ubiquitous in nature; chaos is all important to life.

Perhaps most important to scientists, *strange attractors are fractals*, tying together the studies of the behavior of nonlinear systems with fractal geometry. The same complexity that lets fractals model the irregular geometry of the natural world is what leads to random behavior in deterministic systems.

The most famous of these results illustrating fractals' self-similarity have been the graphics resulting from the iteration (using one answer as the starting point for the next computation) of what has become known as Mandlebrot's Equation, a nonlinear equation that describes the population growth of, e.g., insects ($z \rightarrow z^2 + c$, iterated for all possible (complex) values of z and c [i.e., take the answer of $z^2 + c$ as the new z and repeat the process]). Mandelbrot's Set is the set of all answers for z. Note the "gingerbread man" imbedded in the Mandelbrot Set.

$$z = z^2 + c$$

The Fork in the Road

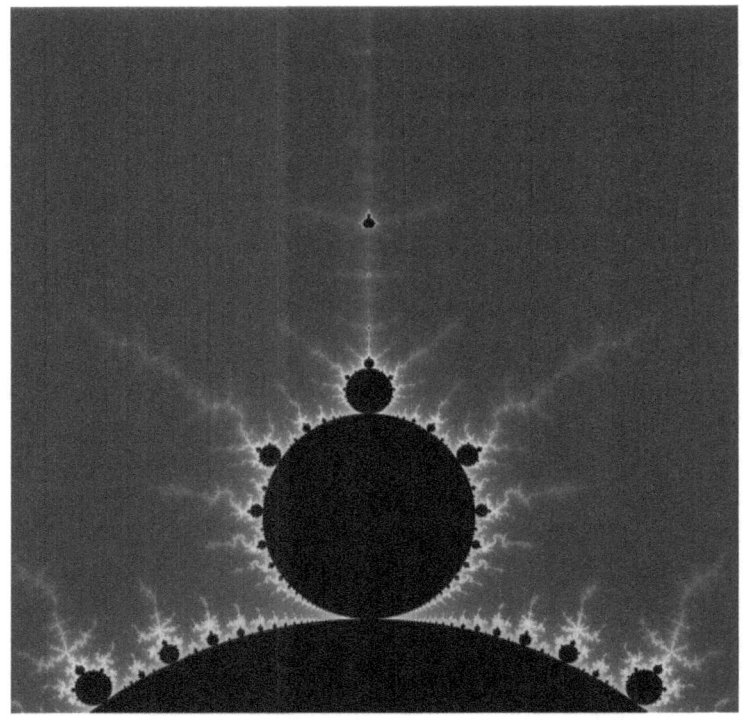

(Image credit: Creative Commons license.)

Note before leaving Chaos Theory: Thanks to modern developments in computers and astronomy, we can now answer King Oscar's question, "Is the solar system stable?" We can now solve the dynamical equations for the Solar System over billions of years. There is in fact a possibility that, in time, the orbit of Mars will drift close to the orbit of Earth and the possibility exists of a collision or near collision. The good news is that this won't happen for about 5 billion years!

15.12 Order in Chaos and Chaos in Order

Perhaps the most startling discovery that has come out of the study of chaotic systems is that, in the midst of chaotic systems is embedded orderly behavior, and that seemingly orderly systems go chaotic. The study of fractals has revealed features not hitherto suspected. Fractals have opened new windows into nature and provided new directions for mathematical modeling. Recall always, however, that mathematical models—as useful as they are in increasing our understanding of nature—are just that, models; they are maps, not territories. Nevertheless, it seems clear that in nature as well as mathematical equations, order and chaos exist side by side. Thus, Chaos Theory has led to a new recognition among scientists that many assumptions about orderliness must be reexamined. A new science is unfolding.

It is useful to summarize what we've learned about Chaos Theory:
1. Newton's Laws of Motion are only the beginning. Nature is *not* linear!—It is far more complex than Newton had envisioned, and in nature's complexity we find chaos as well as order.
2. Even deterministic models are incredibly sensitive to initial conditions—the Butterfly Effect.
3. Seemingly simple models can exhibit stable, periodic, or chaotic behavior under different conditions, and the same is true of nature.

4. Chaos is imbedded in order, and order is imbedded in chaos.
5. Attractors in phase space show the long term behavior of a system.
6. Strange attractors are fractals, and fractals exhibit self-similarity across scales.
7. Fractal geometry is the geometry of irregularity.
8. Fractal design enables a large surface area to be contained in a small volume.
9. Nature is chaotic—There has been a paradigm shift (in scientific recognition of this fact).

Footnote: The distinction between determinancy and randomness is determined by what takes place on short timescales. On a short timescale, a deterministic system will behave deterministically even though on a longer timescale it will exhibit chaotic behavior. And, even though the system may be governed by a deterministic rule, the behavior produced by that rule may appear random (for the system's behavior is determined by initial conditions as well as the rule). The growth rate of a small error with time (Butterfly Effect) provides a quantitative measure of chaos (Liapunov growth rate).

15.13 Implications of Chaos Theory, Fractals, Holograms

Reference has previously been made to the use of reductionism by science as a means of studying the behavior of matter. Looking at this issue further, it must be noted that reductionism only works with classical physics, describing a version of physics working independently of the surrounding environment (e.g., the "frictionless pendulum" studied by physics students). Newtonian physics is "linear," meeting restrictive mathematical requirements. Unfortunately, classical linear physics describes only a small fraction of the real world, and reductionism works *only* in a linear universe.

In the real, nonlinear, chaotic world, nature is heavily influenced by its environment, and the new science of Chaos Theory (developments in Chaos Theory have been possible due to computer technology and therefore due to quantum physics) has both given us an extraordinarily powerful way of viewing nature and, except for those frictionless pendulums, has rendered reductionism scientifically obsolete. We can study in great detail the bricks of a cathedral, but understanding the properties of those bricks does not give us an understanding of the cathedral itself.

Chaos theory, the study of non-linear systems, provides an understanding of the relationship between order and chaos. Edward Lorenz's study of meteorological records has led to the recognition of the Butterfly Effect. Benoit Mandelbrot's work on Chaos Theory has led to an understanding of fractals, the geometry of self-similar structures across scale. This has given us a way of describing, calculating and thinking about shapes that are irregular and fragmented, jagged and broken-up, from snowflakes to galaxies, from biology to economics. "A fractal curve implies an organizing structure that lies hidden among the hideous complication of such shapes."[562] There is regularity within seeming chaos, and chaos within seeming regularity. Chaos geometry (fractals) is to Euclidian geometry as quantum mechanics is to Newtonian mechanics. Fractals have given new understanding to complex systems in many areas of science, from meteorology and geophysics to physiology and economics.

Just as bricks do not define a cathedral, a detailed study of the biology of a cell, or how a drug interacts with that cell, gives us no assurance that we know how that drug will affect our bodies, with all their chemical, emotional, and electromagnetic complexities, non-linearities and interactions. It is for this reason that drugs developed under controlled laboratory conditions may react very differently when used in the real world of patients, and further, why their effect on one patient may be very different from that on another.

The same logic applies to the use of herbs. No two patients are alike; thus the imperative nature of iteration of the medical treatment loop to verify that the treatment plan is appropriate for *that particular patient*.

Chaos theory has given us a new understanding of complex systems, including how nature apparently violates the second law of thermodynamics, which says that entropy *must* increase and that the universe is "running down," and so creates complex interactions. The geometry of fractals gives us new insights into system similarities (macro to micro—reflecting the ancient concept, "As above, so below"), and the discovery of holograms has added understanding of phenomena previously unfathomable.[563] The key property of holograms, which are derived from the wave properties of light, is, from our perspective, that the whole is contained in each of the parts. The construction of a hologram is illustrated in Bentov's *Stalking the Wild Pendulum*.[564] A holographic image, wherein each piece of the film, when viewed with appropriate imaging techniques, captures the entire image (though with less resolution than if the entire film were present), provides a major tool for understanding many natural phenomena. Note that a hologram can be considered a snapshot of interference patterns, (e.g., of waves spreading across a pond after pebbles have been thrown into the pond, and it appears probable that nature makes good use of this tool).

Thus, apparently unexpected physiological phenomena, such as the representation of the entire body in a small portion of the body (the ear, the foot, the hand, a drop of blood, the face) begin to make sense when viewed from the perspective of a hologram. Similarly, some of the most compelling models of memory suggest that at least portions of our memory are represented in the brain (and, it appears probable, elsewhere as well) in a holographic fashion.

15.14 The Brain and a Holographic Universe

The question of memory is one with profound implications. Neuroscientist Karl Lashley had found that his attempts to find a location of memory in the brain demonstrated instead that there was no single location for a given memory. He would train animals in a task, then destroy different regions of the brain. Some functional deficit would result, but the memory always remained. Stanford neurosurgeon and scientist Karl Pribram built upon Lashley's work, and noted the similarity between the properties of a hologram and those of the brain and memory, eventually concluding that there are slow waves in the brain that perform mathematical operations on the sensory data our sense organs provide. The result is that we store memories as a hologram stores light information, and that memory is distributed throughout the brain (and perhaps elsewhere).

Then Pribram asked the question, "Who is interpreting the holograms?" Pondering this one evening, he suddenly thought, "What if the *world* is a hologram?" If the nature of reality is *itself* holographic, and the brain operates holographically, then the concreteness of the world is an illusion, the *maya* of Eastern religions. It was at this point that Pribram discovered the work of Einstein protégé, physicist David Bohm, and realized that *Bohm was describing a holographic universe.*[565] Without going into the details of Bohm's fascinating work, we can summarize the result of the Pribram-Bohm studies as saying that *our brains mathematically construct "hard" reality by interpreting frequencies from a dimension transcending time and space*, for waves have the properties of frequencies and amplitude, not time and space. Thus, *the brain provides a hologram, interpreting a holographic universe.*[566]

The concept of a holographic universe brings us back to the issue of a universal system of information storage. There is now good evidence for the existence of a universal energy field, storing information in holographic wave patterns. This field, variously called a Zero Point Field (the field existing in space at a temperature of absolute zero) or a Quantum Hologram by physicists, appears to be the same storage vehicle called the Collective Unconscious by Carl Jung, the Akashic Record by Edgar Cayce, the Mind of God by some, or simply the universal Field of information and energy. It is presumably this energy field of information that is tapped into by shamans, mystics, intuitives, and dowsers. We have had indirect evidence of such information storage in the past. Now we have an identified vehicle that contributes greatly to the solution of much seemingly contradictory information from fields as variable as cosmology, physics, biology and consciousness.[567]

A final observation before moving on: Note that Pribram's work on memory and Bohm's on reality, each concept long recognized by shamans and mystics, are the absolute antithesis of reductionism and so materialism.[568]

The concept of a holographic universe opens the door wide—just as do new models of nature developed from chaos theory—to a far greater understanding of reality than was previously the case. They also remind us again to consider *all* the elements that influence the health of individuals and the nature of illness.

15.15 Limitations of Mathematical Models: The Map Is Not the Territory!

A map provides only a very limited representation of a territory. As one increases the magnification, or scale of the map, the detail represented by the map increases until a closer and closer approximation of the territory results. The problem of the yardstick: the accuracy of the measurement is a function of the length of the measuring device. This problem was illustrated by attempting to measure Britain's coastline. As the measuring tool grew shorter, the length of the coastline apparently grew longer. It was finally concluded that the coastline must have infinite length—Chaos Theory comes to the fore here.

Mathematical models are maps. Flow charts are maps. To a first approximation they may represent the territory, but beyond that first approximation they fail to encompass the details of the system under study. This is quite aside from the issue that mathematics is a game based on postulates, on axioms that may or may not be applicable to the system under study. This pitfall has been illustrated by the use of statistical analyses based on the assumption of time invariance in experiments studying biological systems—an assumption particularly dangerous when applied to biological experiments on anesthetized animals!—such studies are not scientifically valid, yet too often such analyses are performed, albeit they have unknowable validity.

Further, almost all mathematical models are based on the assumption of linearity. We have already noted that very few physical or biological processes are in fact linear, so the model will inevitably fail once the narrow bound of approximately linear behavior is passed. As you may recall, a spring may obey Hooke's Law ($F = kL$) within a certain range and under certain conditions, but outside that range, or under different conditions, the equation fails to represent the spring's behavior.

Biological systems are far more complex than springs! We must turn to Chaos Theory, fractals and non-linear mathematics if we want to use mathematics to assist us in understanding biological systems.[569]

Notes

541 Kuhn, Thomas S., *The Structure of Scientific Revolutions*, 2nd Ed., Univ. of Chicago Press, 1970.
542 Gribbon, John, *In Search of Schrödinger's Cat: Quantum Physics and Reality*, New York, Bantam Books, 1984.
543 Wolf, Fred Alan, *Parallel Universes: The Search for Other Worlds*, New York, Simon & Schuster, 1988.
544 Bohm, David *Wholeness and the Implicate Order*, London, Routledge Kegan Paul, Ltd., 1980.
545 Prigogine, Ilya and Isabelle Stengers, *Order Out of Chaos: Man's New Dialogue with Nature*, Bantam Books, 1984.
546 Goswami, Amit et al., *The Self-Aware Universe: How Consciousness Creates the Material World*, New York, Tarcher/Putnam, 1993.
547 Bentov, Itzhak, *Stalking the Wild Pendulum: On the Mechanics of Consciousness*, New York, E. P. Dutton, 1977.
548 Laskow, Leonard, *Healing With Love: A Breakthrough Mind/Body Medical Program for Healing Yourself and Others*, San Francisco, Harper Collins, 1992.
549 Gleick, James, *Chaos: Making a New Science*. Science writer, accessible, recommended.
550 Velikovsky, Immanuel, *Worlds in Collision*, Dell, 1967.
551 *Nature*, 24 September 1981, p. 245 reviewing: Sheldrake, Rupert, *A New Science of Life: The Hypothesis of Formative Causation*, Tarcher, 1981. Related: Sheldrake, Rupert, *Morphic Resonance: The Nature of Formative Causation*, Rochester, VT, Park Street Press, 2009.
552 Briggs, John & David Peat, *Turbulent Mirror: An Illustrated Guide to Chaos Theory and the Science of Wholeness*. Psychologist and physicist, accessible.
553 Gleick, James, *Chaos: Making a New Science*, Viking Adult, 1987.
554 Ibid.
555 Ibid.
556 Ibid.
557 Abraham, Ralph, *Chaos, Gaia, Eros: A Chaos Pioneer Uncovers the Three Great Streams of History*, Epigraph Publishing, 2011.
558 Stewart, Ian, *Does God Play Dice? The New Mathematics of Chaos*, Wiley-Blackwell, 2002.
559 Herbert, Nick, *Quantum Reality: Beyond the New Physics*, New York, Anchor Books, 1985.
560 Swift, Jonathan, *Miscellanies in Prose and Verse*, Vol. 5, London, 1735.
561 Gleick, James, Chaos: Making a New Science, Viking Adult, 1987.
562 Ibid.
563 Wilber, Ken (ed), *The Holographic Paradigm and other paradoxes: Exploring the Leading Edge of Science*, Boulder, CO. Shambala Publications, 1982.

Also, lbot, Michael, *The Holographic Universe*, New York, HarperCollins Publishers, 1991.
564 Bentov, Itzhak, *Stalking the Wild Pendulum: On the Mechanics of Consciousness*, New York, E. P. Dutton, 1977, p16.
565 Bohm, David, *Wholeness and the Implicate Order*, London, Routledge Kegan Paul, Ltd., 1980.
566 Talbot, Michael, *The Holographic Universe*, New York, HarperCollins Publishers, 1991.
567 McTaggart, Lynne, *The Field: The Quest for the Secret Force of the Universe*, 2002.
568 Wallace, B. Alan, *Choosing Reality: A Buddhist View of Physics and the Mind*, Ithaca, NY, Snow Lion Publications, 2003.
569 Gordon, James S., *Manifesto for A New Medicine*, Addison-Wesley Publ. Co., 1996.
Also, Krieger, Dolores, *The Therapeutic Touch*, Gloria Press, 1995.
and Moyers, Bill, *Healing and The Mind*, Doubleday, 1995.

Conclusion
What We Have Learned About the Nature of Healing

16.1 On the Nature of Healing

Ancient sources reveal a sophisticated medicine that was far in advance of modern Western scientific medicine. Recent discoveries reveal that we are not at an intellectual peak, and that we have much to learn from the shamans and mystics, and from the mystery schools of the past. These reveal much about healing.

What is Healing? Plato wrote: "The part can never be well unless the whole is well." To heal is to make whole—body, mind, and spirit. Plato's insight is today reflected in psychiatrist Carlos Warter, M.D., Ph.D., when he noted that, for healing to occur, "a partnership with mind, body and spirit is essential." [570]

Warter further speaks of the importance of engaging the body *essence* (inner spirituality) in healing:

Everyone has a heart. Everyone wants love. Our true vocation is love. The core frequency that unites us all is love, and it flows through the heart. Wellness—spiritual, emotional, and physical—is related to our ability to open our hearts to God, which happens when we live from essence.

Overall health is a function of the balance between head and heart. The head transmits information. The heart activates wisdom. In this age of information, it is easy to forget about the function of the heart. The brain reaches our awareness with feelings, sensations, and imagery. The heart's communication is much more subtle. We hear the heart through the inner voice of silence—that quiet, still place from which creativity, inspiration, and deep kinds of knowing originate. [571]

We must examine not just physical symptoms, but the events in the patient's life that led to those symptoms. If the cause is an emotional injury, forgiveness is often needed, as well as care and compassion.

The mind and soul act to protect a person. The development of disease symptoms is a benevolent act, our mind and emotion's way of calling attention to a problem. As problems that are the *cause* of illness persist, symptoms will become more serious, often with cancer or heart disease as the ultimate warning signs. If *cause* is not dealt with, the symptoms may become life threatening.

Phineas Quimby, nineteenth century healer and founder of the New Thought movement, wrote? "Every disease is the invention of man, and has no identity in Wisdom, but to those that believe, it is a truth. It may seem strange to those in health that our beliefs affect us... There is one thing that man is ignorant of. It is this: that he is a sufferer from his own belief, not knowingly, but by his own consent."[572]

Healer Doreen Virtue comments, in *Awakening Your Spiritual Power to Know and Heal*, "Quimby emphasized mind treatment that focused upon the patient's thoughts." [573]

An emotional cause can be involved in acute as well as chronic illness—an immune system depressed by an emotional shock can be susceptible to a bacterium or virus that it would otherwise shrug off.

How is cause detected? There are many methods, with *careful history taking* being foremost. Dr. Lissa Rankin, in observing patients that ate a healthy diet, who exercised regularly, lived a presumably healthy lifestyle, and yet were chronically sick, expanded her patient intake form to include questions that would point to cause:? "Is anything keeping you from being the most authentic, vital *you*? If so, what is holding you back? What's missing from your life? What do you appreciate about your life? Are you in a romantic relationship? If so, are you happy? If not, do you wish you were? Are you fulfilled at work? Do you feel like you're in touch with your life purpose?" And most important of all, "*What do you think might lie at the root of your illness?* And, "*What does your body need in order to heal?*" Dr. Rankin, in her book, *Mind Over Medicine*, goes on to provide Marla's case history, a classic case of a change in lifestyle leading to the patient's healing of her chronic illnesses.[574]

Dr. Rankin's insights have been further validated by thousands of years of experience by indigenous shamans throughout the globe and by healers ancient and modern. Her book is highly recommended as a source of scientific data on the mind's importance in all healing, including self-healing.

The energy bodies that surround the physical body often reflect cause, and can be detected by many methods. *Vision* both normal and subtle is valuable, often used by indigenous shamans. Hawaiian *kahunas* have found *dreams* valuable in diagnosis, and even in specifying treatment, as did ancient Greek medicine. *Pulses* are studied in a meditative state by Chinese, Ayurvedic, Tibetan, ancient Greek healers, and by many others.

How is cause healed? If symptoms are life threatening, they must be managed, and Western scientific medicine (WSM) may be valuable. WSM is not the only approach—herbal practitioners are also capable of addressing acute symptoms, as are the spiritual and herbal treatments of shamans.

If symptoms are *not* life threatening, the practitioner must assist the body's innate self-healing ability. This may require balancing energies with acupuncture or herbs, counseling regarding lifestyle, exercise, and diet, possibly bodywork. The aim is to detoxify the body, to improve immune function, to improve circulation, and to enhance energy. All are often required in chronic disease.

Addressing emotional issues may be required if that is the cause of the patient's problem, or emotional issues may emerge from a careful and thorough intake interview. *Counseling regarding emotional cause* may be important, and referral to a psychiatrist, psychologist, or shaman, medicine man or woman may be appropriate. If an energy imbalance exists, or an organ system needs support, the practitioner must provide that support with diet, energy work, acupuncture, herbs, or bodywork.

Psychiatrist Carlos Warter, M.D., PhD., found the following perspective useful in developing a heart-to-heart connection between healer and patient:

1. First, one must remember that one is really one's essence, higher self or soul.

2. Second, one is aware of the patient as a whole human being, and envisions and discerns the essential self or soul within the patient. One must look beyond the labels—diagnosis, gender, situation—to accomplish this step.

3. Third, one examines the soul of the patient and acknowledges that the disease or discomfort can be an evolutionary step, that it can have purpose. The condition must be thought of as a transforming experience so that thoughts of victimization can be avoided.

4. Fourth, one suspends all judgments.[575]

Cause is frequently a function of thoughts or emotions, so we need to ascertain the cause, respect and deal with it. Then the body can heal. Traditional Tibetan medicine recognizes three mental poisons as the root causes of most disease:

  i. Acquisitiveness, greed → To heal, go to → Generosity, Gratitude

  ii. Anger, hate; → To heal, go to → Forgiveness, Compassion

  iii. Self-delusion → To heal, go to → Wisdom

Psychologist Jeanne Achterberg comments, in *Imagery In Healing*, "Healing is embracing what is most feared: healing is opening what has been closed, softening what has hardened into obstruction, healing is learning to trust life." [576]

Psychiatrist Martin Weiss has found that in his experience, the relaxation produced under hypnosis often leads to healing, perhaps enabling the subconscious mind to identify the underlying cause of an illness and to heal that cause.

Dr. Weiss has also found cases where a present illness is a holdover and has been caused by a past life incident. Tibetan medicine occasionally finds illnesses that are the result of a past life occurrence. Dr. Weiss's approach is outlined in his books, *Many Lives, Many Masters* and *Messages From The Masters*. [577]

If cause is truly external, then symptoms represent the way the body fights back. Examples are fever and local immune responses to a physical wound.

It must also be recognized that symptoms play an important role in communicating the body's needs (e.g., the hemorrhoids described by Dr. Upledger and referred to in Chapter One). There is real risk in the elimination of symptoms, and so disguising the underlying problem.

Effective therapy—whatever its form—initiates, facilitates, and supports the patient's self-healing efforts, whereas symptom management provides a more temporary and perhaps only palliative effect. It may remove the symptoms of a disease, but it usually leaves the underlying cause of the symptoms untouched, and new or recurring symptoms are likely to appear.

Traditional medicines do not separate the mental and spiritual from the physical. Dr. Lewis Mehl-Madrona comments, "Most indigenous cultures, including Native American, believe that *all* physical and emotional healing is first spiritual healing."[9] Traditional medicines' concept of healing is to bring about the restoration of balance and harmony, so the body can heal itself. The role of family and community is important in supporting the patient's self-healing and in serving as the unit for healing, in contrast to the often isolated individual.

Meditation and relaxation encourage self-healing. As Tibetan Lama Thortang Tulku Rinpoche taught, "Many diseases are the result of blockages in our physical bodies caused by our emotions. In Tibet there are very few cases of cancer, because the environment is tranquil and life is less stressful."

Dr. Lissa Rankin lists nine areas essential for robust health:
(1) *Healthy relationships*, including a strong network of family, friends, loved ones, and colleagues.
(2) *A healthy, meaningful way to spend your days*, whether you work outside the home or in it.
(3) *A healthy, fully expressed creative life* that allows your soul to sing its song.
(4) *A healthy spiritual life*, including a sense of connection to the sacred in life.

(5) *A healthy sexual life* that allows you the freedom to express your erotic self and explore fantasies.
(6) *A healthy financial life*, free of undue financial stress, which ensures that the essential needs of your body are met.
(7) *A healthy environment*, free of toxins, natural-disaster hazards, radiation, and other unhealthy factors that threaten the health of the body.
(8) *A healthy mental and emotional life*, characterized by optimism and happiness and free of fear, anxiety, depression, and other mental-health ailments.
(9) *A healthy lifestyle* that supports the physical health of the body, such as good nutrition, regular exercise, adequate sleep, and avoidance of unhealthy addictions.[578]

To respond to emotional stresses, Louise Hay and Mona Lisa Schulz, M.D., Ph.D., have this to recommend in their book, *All Is Well*:
(1) Becoming conscious of our emotions and those of other people in our life, making note of the warnings that come with fear, anger, and sadness
(2) Figuring out what thoughts accompany these feelings that keep swirling around our heads
(3) Identifying symptoms of distress and locating them in our bodies
(4) Decoding the intuitive/emotional thought-pattern information underlying the symptoms and understanding that every illness is also in part due to diet, environment, genetics, and injury."[579]

Note: Louise Hay is a pioneer in identifying emotional cause, and her book with Mona Lisa Schulz is highly recommended as a guide to identifying cause.

If a patient feels love, compassion, peace and joy, healing will follow.

Dr, Mehl-Madrona, adds, "Fundamentally, I believe that *all healing is spiritual healing*. Whatever else we do—including herbs, diet, radiation, surgery, or bodywork—we need to humbly ask for help from the spiritual realm. Spirit is the spark in the chain that creates healing and miracles."[580]

The Shoshone/Cherokee medicine man Rolling Thunder echoes Dr. Mehl-Madrona in the need for spiritual healing, including ceremony, herbs collected in a sacred manner, even water energized with prayer.

Healing a major illness may require a profound life change—a transformation of one's relationships to all aspects of life.

Always remember that *all healing is ultimately self-healing.* The task of the healer is to help the patient heal her/himself. A recurrent theme in traditional medicines is that key elements in healing are often *forgiveness, compassion,* and *gratitude.*

A Summary of Key Points in *The Fork in the Road*

16.2 The Invisible Reality

From ancient records—a sophisticated science, including medical science, existed in past ages.

From shamans—reality is only half visible. Half is matter, and half is invisible. By entering an altered state, one can contact the invisible. Mystics, shamans, and others have confirmed this.

From Amit Goswami, John von Neuman, John Wheeler, et al—consciousness underlies all reality, both matter *and* energy.

From Plato's Cave, Crazy Horse's dream, physicist David Bohm's insights—there is an invisible and implicit reality underlying our explicit (physical) reality.

From Ervin Laszlo—the Akashic Field contains a record of all events and thoughts since the Big Bang.

From Harold Puthoff (Zero Point Field)—there is an invisible field of (holographic) information, memory and energy.

From Bell's Theorem—We are all interconnected at superluminal speeds and have been since the Big Bang.

From Marco Bischof—Quantum physics tells us there is a fundamental interconnectedness *within* the organism as well as *between* organisms, and that of the organism *with the environment.*

From Amit Goswami—Consciousness is universal.

From indigenous cultures—We are interconnected with each other and with all of Nature.

From dowsers—We can tap into the Zero Point Field, to find out information at a distance. We can also tap into its energy (as can shamans and healers) to heal, to move underground streams, to heat rocks and move objects, etc.

From healers—We can use this energy to stimulate the self-healing ability of patients, and we can stimulate that healing at a distance.

From Albert Schweitzer—We can enlist the doctor within and the patient will heal him/herself.

From Rupert Sheldrake—Invisible Morphogenetic fields play a key role in physical and biological processes.

From Valerie Hunt (UCLA)—auric fields are at least in part electromagnetic.

From Hippocrates, Homeopaths, Scientific Research, Shamans & Clairvoyants—There is a vital force, *physis,* that enables the body to heal itself. There is a subtle energy field (the etheric template) within the body's aura. It reflects and guides the physical body, and that energy body has electromagnetic components.

16.3 An Important Invisible Aspect of Reality Is Emotion

From HeartMath—emotions affect the immune system, even DNA configuration.

From HeartMath—the heart's electromagnetic field is many times stronger than the brain's.

From Adam—emotions interact with and affect each others' energy fields.

From random event generators and satellite data—emotions affect the earth's geomagnetic field, which in turn affects weather, geological stress, human behavior, etc.

From Candace Pert—neurotransmitters are released in response to emotions from the heart, the immune system, and the gut, as well as the brain. Emotions affect cells and organ functions. This has led to the science of psychoneuroimmunology, also to an understanding of the placebo effect (see also Norman Cousins in Chapter Three).

From Emoto—water (70% of the body) is affected by emotions.

From Bruce Lipton—Cells have a consciousness located in the cell membrane. Epigenetics plays an important role in heredity as well as in the development of a child.

From Robert Jahns (Princeton Engineering Anomalies Research laboratory)—Mind can control matter, even time-displaced (until it is viewed by a consciousness). Distant viewing can also be time-displaced.

From Carlos Warter—A key question is often, "*Why* is this happening?"

From many sources—There are invisible dimensions that exist outside of time and space.

From Shamans, Mystics, ancient sources, and psychiatrist Dr. Martin Weiss—We are immortal, spirits who have taken physical bodies in order to learn and to grow.[581]

16.4 Healing

From Pythagoras—*health, as wholeness, means that body and soul must be examined together... human will ensures and completes the harmony between body, mind and soul.*

From Plato—The part can never be well unless the whole is well.

From Plato—man possesses within himself the power to heal the diseases of the body. In the end every man is his own priest and his own physician.

From Socrates—One cannot heal the body without healing the soul.

Hippocrates—Was a healer-priest who healed the whole person with diet, lifestyle changes, exercise and herbs, and who represented the culmination in the West of traditional medicine.

From Hippocrates and Avicenna—Food is the best medicine.

From Dr. Rankin—History and lifestyle are often the cause of disease.

From Dr. Mehl-Madrona and medicine man Rolling Thunder—*all healing is spiritual healing*.

From shaman Credo Mutwa—Do *not* name or give energy to what you *don't* want—focus on what you *do* want, giving energy to the desired outcome.

From Jeanne Achterberg—Your biography is your biology.

16.5 Chaos Theory and Fractal Geometry

From Mandelbrot and Lorenz—most physical, mathematical, and biological systems are self-similar across scale. They are non-linear and are critically dependent on initial conditions. Chaos Theory and fractal geometry provide an understanding of irregular objects. There is order within chaos, and there is chaos within order.

From Bells Theorem—We are all instantaneously interconnected.

From David Bohm—The universe is a hologram, and there is an underlying implicit reality behind the explicit reality we observe and measure.

16.6 The Healer

Dr. Lissa Rankin, in *Mind Over Medicine*, suggests fifteen steps healers can take that echo the theme of this book. The fifteen steps are:
(1) Listen
(2) Open your heart
(3) Make eye contact.
(4) Take your hand off the doorknob and sit down.
(5) Be present.
(6) Offer healing touch [energy medicine].
(7) Invite your patient to be your partner.
(8) Avoid judgment.
(9) Educate, but don't dictate.
(10) Choose your words with care and remain optimistic.
(11) Trust your patient's intuition.
(12) Be respectful of other practitioners who are treating your patient.
(13) Reassure your patients they are not alone.
(14) Encourage stress relief and let your presence relieve stress.
(15) Offer hope, because no matter how grim the prognosis, spontaneous remission is always possible.[582]

If all healers followed Dr. Rankin's recommendations, beginning with *listening to the patient with compassion* and ending with *always* giving *hope*, many of their patients would heal themselves. The answer to "*Why* is this happening?" may be the key to self-healing.

Notes

570 Warter, Carlos, M.D., Ph.D, *Recovery of the Sacred: Lessons In Soul Awareness*, Deerfield Beach, FL, 1994.
571 Warter. Carlos, M.D., Ph.D., *Who Do You Think You Are?: The Healing Power Of Your Sacred Self*, New York, Bantam Books, 1998.
572 Quimby, Phineas, *The Quimby Manuscripts*, Forgotten Books, 2008.
573 Virtue, Doreen, *The Lightworker's Way: Awakening Your Spiritual Power To Know And Heal*, Hay House, 1997.
574 Rankin, Lissa, *Mind Over Medicine: Scientific Proof That You Can Heal Yourself*, Hay House, 2013.
575 Warter, Carlos, M.D., Ph.D., *Recovery of the Sacred: Lessons In Soul Awareness*; Warter, *Messages From The Masters*. Deerfield Beach, FL, 1994.
576 Achterberg, Jeanne, *Imagery In Healing: Shamanism and Modern Medicine*, Boston, Shambhala, 1985.
577 Weiss, Martin, MD, *Many Lives, Many Masters*, New York, Simon & Schuster, 1988.
578 Rankin, Lissa, *Mind Over Medicine: Scientific Proof That You Can Heal Yourself*, Hay House, 2013.
579 Hay, Louise L. and Mona Lisa Schulz, *All Is Well: Heal Your Body with Medicine, Affirmations, and Intuition*, Carlsbad, CA, Hay House, 2013.
580 Mehl-Madrona, Lewis, M.D., *Coyote Healing: Miracles in Native Medicine*, Bear & Company, 2003.
581 Weiss, Martin, MD, Many Lives, Many Masters, New York, Simon & Schuster, 1988,
582 Rankin, Lissa, *Mind Over Medicine: Scientific Proof That You Can Heal Yourself*, Hay House, 2013.

APPENDIX A:
Prehistory Timeline

65,000,000 BCE	Presumed extinction of dinosaurs.
130,000 BCE	Founding of Atlantis, Lemuria, Sumer?
100,000 BCE	Paleolithic Age: Estimated date of earliest shamans.
80,000 BCE	Pleistocene Ice Age: Cro-Magnon in Asia, navigation and land bridge to Australia.
77,000 BCE	Shamanic inscriptions engraved on stone
60,000 BCE	Submergence of Lemuria, per Waitaha descendants
50,000 BCE	Culture established in Brazil.
35,000 BCE	Cro-Magnon man in Europe; settlements in Egypt.
32,000 BCE	Agriculture in Brazil; carvings in Germany; settlements in Pacific islands.
30,000 BCE	Cave art in Brazil, France; marine culture in Chile.
24,000 BCE	Cave art in Africa.
15,600 BCE	Navigator gods in Mexico, Sumer; Bön Buddhism established in Tibet.
15,000 BCE	Peak of Nazca culture (Peru).
11,000 BCE	Cataclysm/Deluge: Per Mayan records, 11,202 BCE; per Sumerian records, 11,000 BCE.
10,000 BCE	End of Ice Age Sumer developed; Malta built; Peruvian navigation; Piri Reis map; Thoth arrived in Egypt; agriculture in Belize, Mexico; mummies in Chile; Sphinx built in Egypt; megaliths; Tiahuanaco (Bolivia) built. Rising sea level inundated much of Lemuria, Atlantis.
8,000 BCE	Neolithic man in Europe; mummies in Brazil; Caucasians in Northwest America; major Mayan site in Belize; sudden warming in Gulf of Mexico between 8,000 – 9,000 BCE per geologic records; land bridge

	between Asia and Australia subsides; urban farming culture in Egypt.
6,500 BCE	Bronze Age in Mesopotamia, Egypt City of 7,000 in Turkey (Catal Hüyük).
4,000 BCE	Mesopotamian Flood Cities, hospitals, royal graves in Sumer Olmec trade between Mexico and Africa.
3,114 BCE	Mayan calendar begins Comet Enke's first brush with earth; major impact on Lemuria (lands submerged); Atlantis. Malta destroyed by tidal wave; first pharaonic dynasty in Egypt; Karnak; writing in Egypt; Egyptian mummies; pyramids; Sumer flourishing; beginning of Mayan cycle.
2,193 BCE	Comet Enke returns: Worldwide catastrophe.
2,023 BCE	Destruction of Sumer per Sumerian texts, due to an "Evil Wind," possibly nuclear fallout
1,960 BCE	Sacking of Ur of Chaldees and emigration of Abraham's family from Sumer.
1,628 BCE	Comet Enke returns Final destruction of Lemuria; barrage of meteoric material causes gigantic tsunamis; most remaining Lemurian lands submerged or destroyed.
1,334 BCE	Moses leads exodus from Egypt.
1,198 BCE	Comet Enke returns Final Destruction of Atlantis; great cataclysm.
1,000 BCE	Iron Age Navigation between Middle East and America came to an end.
586 BCE	Babylonian captivity of Hebrews; first books of Old Testament written using Babylonian and Sumerian records.

146 BCE	Carthage and its library destroyed by Romans.
0-800 CE	Moche pottery (Peru) depicting dinosaurs with humans.
642 CE	Library of Alexandria destroyed Final destruction of Library was by Muslims; following previous major destruction by Christians
1500s CE	Destruction of Mayan, Toltec, Inca libraries by Christian priests.

APPENDIX B: Assumptions of Western (Materialistic) Science

a) It is possible to understand nature by observation. In truth, all observations are influenced by the theory espoused by the observer. Einstein: "The answer you get is determined by the question you ask."
b) The experimenter understands all the influences that may affect the experimental outcome.
c) The experimental outcome is independent of the experimenter.
d) The phenomenon under study can be represented by a mathematical model.
e) The experimental testing and/or analytic procedures used are relevant to the real state of the phenomenon under study.
f) Accepted scientific laws are appropriate for the interpretation of the experimental data.

About the Author

Dr. Robert Elphin Smith spent the bulk of his professional career teaching in the Department of Human Physiology in the School of Medicine at the University of California, Davis. During this allopathic-centered period, he became aware of the extent of patients' influence over their own health outcomes. Attitudes, beliefs, and practices all had an effect. From there he became the President of the Traditional Chinese Medical College of Hawaii and consulted the University of Hawaii on shamanistic and non-allopathic healing techniques. During the same period, he pursued his own shamanistic training under the tutelage of Papa Awae. He died unexpectedly shortly after completing the draft manuscript of *The Fork in the Road*.

His wife, Maryse Bader Smith—well-versed in spiritual approaches to healing herself—took on the task of bringing the book to fruition. She mourned his loss heavily and, perhaps as a final proof of the power of attitudes, she also died just as the final chapters went to the editor.

Out of respect for the tremendous effort that they both poured into producing this book, it has now been ushered through its final stages and is available to everyone interested in learning about the split and rejoining of Western and traditional medicine.

Dean Elphin Smith
August 2019

www.ingramcontent.com/pod-product-compliance
Lightning Source LLC
Chambersburg PA
CBHW030607220526
45463CB00004B/1197